baby care
book

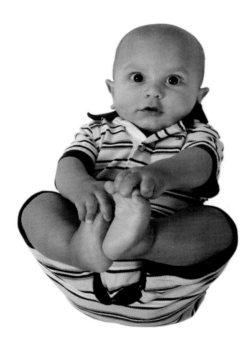

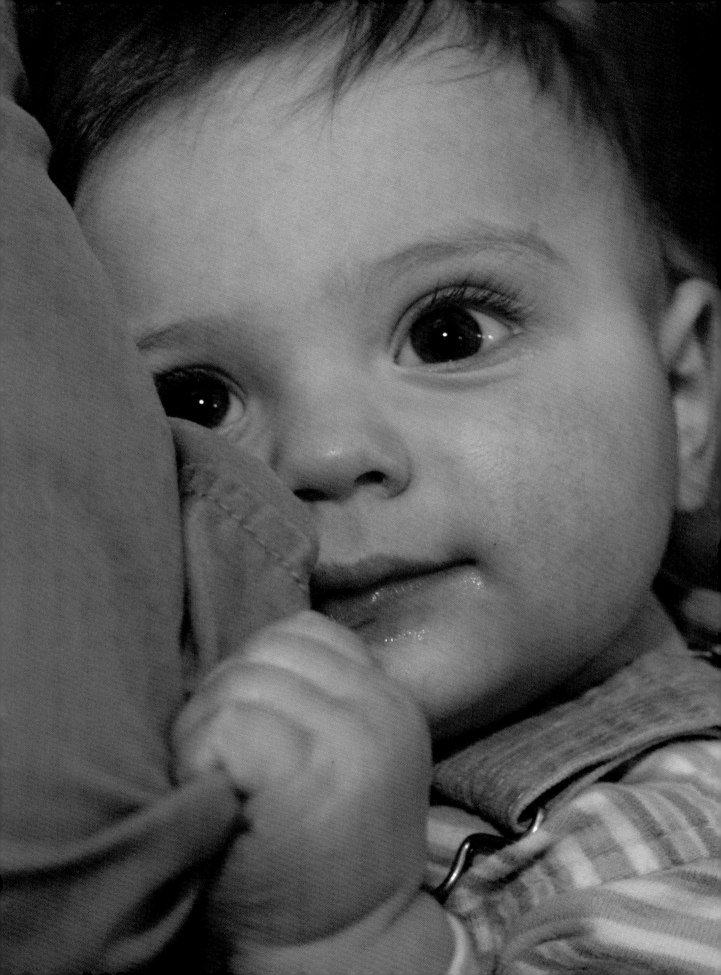

baby care book

A Complete Guide from Birth to 12 Months Old

Dr. Jeremy Friedman, MB.ChB, FRCP(C), FAAP
Dr. Norman Saunders, MD, FRCP(C)

The Hospital for Sick Children

Robert ROSE

For a complete list of photo credits, see page 440.
For complete cataloguing information, see page 441.

Editor: Bob Hilderley, Senior Editor, Health
Copy editor: Sue Sumeraj
Proofreader: Sheila Wawanash
Indexer: Gillian Watts
Design & production: PageWave Graphics Inc.
Illustrations: Kveta/Three in a Box
Sam's Diary teddy bear illustration: iStockphoto.com/Helle Bro Clemmensen
Front cover image: Jim Craigmyle/Veer
Back cover image: Diogenes Baena/The Hospital for Sick Children

The publisher acknowledges the financial support of the government of Canada through the Book Publishing Industry Development Program.

Published by Robert Rose Inc.
120 Eglinton Ave. E. Suite 800, Toronto, Ontario, Canada M4P 1E2
Tel: (416) 322-6552   Fax: (416) 322-6396

Printed in Canada

4 5 6 7 8 9 TCP 15 14 13 12 11 10 09

To two of the finest mothers I have ever known:
my wife, Lynn, and my late mother, Fanny Saunders.
And to my friend and colleague Jeremy Friedman, who serves
as a wonderful role model for physicians everywhere. — NS

To my wife, Shelley, for being the best mother and wife
anyone could wish for, and for allowing us to use part
of Sam's diary to help illustrate some of the ups and downs of
the first year. To Norman, my mentor and friend, whose
wisdom and courage continues to astound me — I will always
remember and cherish our collaboration and friendship.
And to my own babies, Sam and Dani. — JF

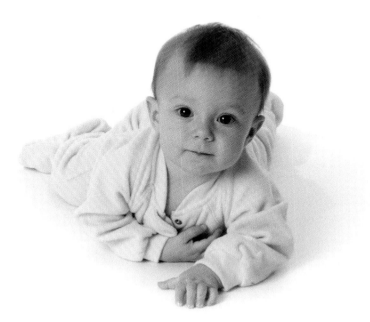

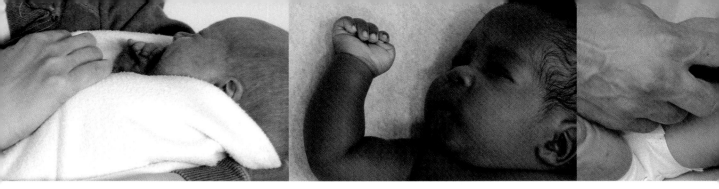

Contents

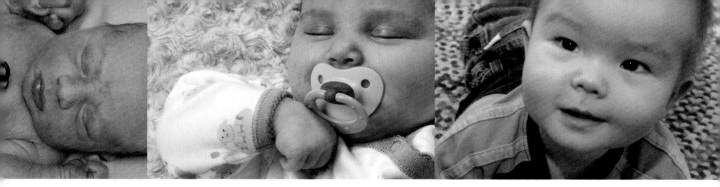

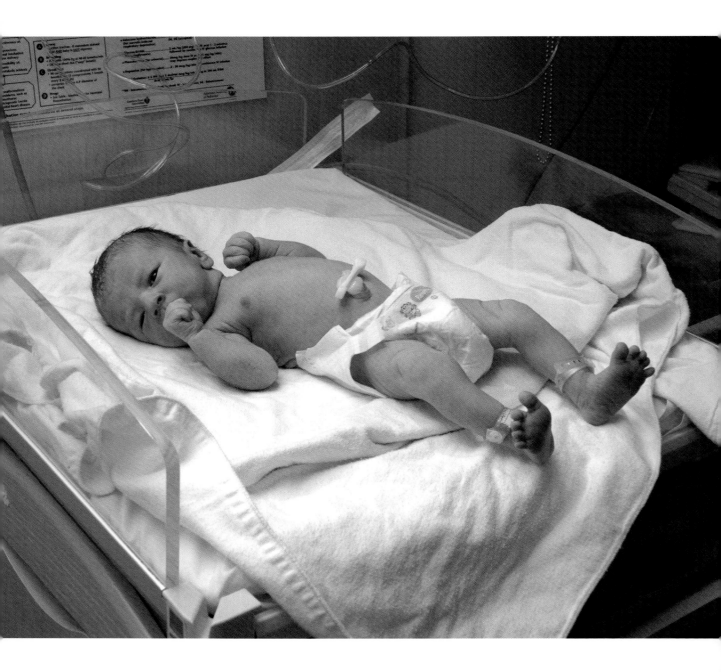

Contributing Authors

Sherri Adams, RN, MSN, CPNP
Division of Paediatric Medicine
The Hospital for Sick Children
Faculty of Nursing
University of Toronto

Carolyn Beck, MSc, MD, FRCP
Division of Paediatric Medicine
Department of Paediatrics
The Hospital for Sick Children
Assistant Professor
Faculty of Medicine
University of Toronto

Catherine Birken, MSc, MD, FRCP
Division of Paediatric Medicine
Department of Paediatrics
The Hospital for Sick Children
Assistant Professor
Faculty of Medicine
University of Toronto

Jeremy Friedman, MB, ChB, FRCP, FAAP
Division of Paediatric Medicine
Department of Paediatrics
The Hospital for Sick Children
Associate Professor
Faculty of Medicine
University of Toronto

Sheila Jacobson, MB, ChB, FRCP
Division of Paediatric Medicine
Department of Paediatrics
The Hospital for Sick Children
Assistant Professor
Faculty of Medicine
University of Toronto

Norman Saunders, MD, FRCP
Division of Paediatric Medicine
Department of Paediatrics
The Hospital for Sick Children
Associate Professor
Faculty of Medicine
University of Toronto

Michelle Shouldice, MD, FRCP
Division of Paediatric Medicine
Department of Paediatrics
The Hospital for Sick Children
Assistant Professor
Faculty of Medicine
University of Toronto

Michael Weinstein MD, FRCP
Division of Paediatric Medicine
Department of Paediatrics
The Hospital for Sick Children
Assistant Professor
Faculty of Medicine
University of Toronto

Introduction

Does the world really need another parenting book? The chances are pretty good that this book came off a shelf containing a handful of similar baby care books, all claiming to be unique, authoritative, and invaluable. We make no such claims. This book may not be "essential" for caring for your baby. A lot of great parenting goes on without reference to a book. You could probably do a fine job of raising your children without advice from us. But if you're looking to do the best job you can as a parent, and do it with confidence in your parenting skills, you might find this book very useful indeed. Here's why.

The Hospital for Sick Children is the largest pediatric health science center in Canada, and one of the most respected in the world. Founded in 1875, Sick Kids (as it is widely known) has evolved into an international institution. Its stated mission is "to deliver exemplary patient care, train the next generation of child health leaders and develop new interventions and treatments." This goal is achieved through the efforts of more than 3,200 hospital staff members, 600 medical professionals, and 1,100 dedicated individuals at the Hospital for Sick Children Research Institute. Trainees come from all over the world to learn the best and most up-to-date practices in child health care.

From this talented group, we have carefully selected eight contributors to produce this work. Seven are pediatricians, while one is a nurse practitioner. Three are

men and five are women. All are parents; in fact, three have given birth in the last year. Some are community pediatricians with almost 30 years experience in primary care, while others are hospital-based. We also called on some of our highly skilled allied health professionals, including a dietitian, a lactation consultant, and a sleep expert, to review and augment relevant sections. In short, we wanted our authors to bring diverse perspectives to this book. The chief common denominator among this team of writers is pediatric expertise and a dedication to serving children.

Recruiting a capable group of experts was certainly a good start to the project, but it doesn't explain why this parenting book is so different. The complete answer requires a confession. When we were asked to write this book, we realized we had no particular ax to grind, cause to champion, or egos to stroke. Producing a book is hard work. Most books are written by people with a strong point of view. They feel the need to express their opinions, an innate personal bias often amplified by the fact that a book is more likely to sell if it is dramatically opinionated.

Our goal was not to present a strongly held dogmatic opinion, but rather to provide a clear, objective, and, above all, practical guide to help parents better raise a young infant. We want parents to use this book day in and day out. That's why you will find more "How to" and "Guide to" features in our book than in other baby care

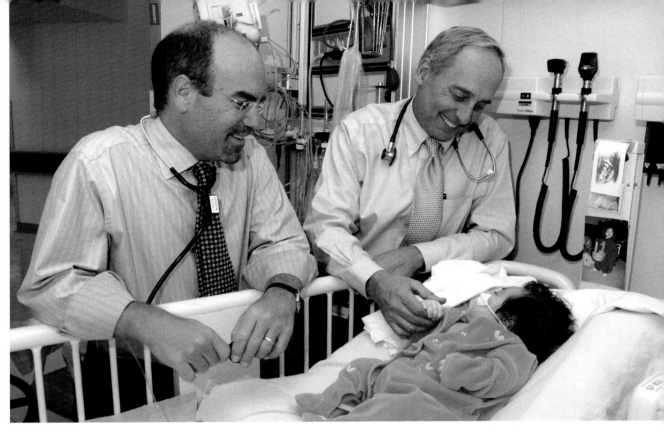

book. You can use this book to learn how to change a diaper, treat a cold, and breast-feed; how to select a stroller and safety proof your home; and how to follow the curve of your baby's growth and development. We've even included a diary of one mother's experience with her infant son, from pregnancy to his first birthday, so you can compare the challenges and joys of parenting your baby. This book will help you build and hone your parenting skills, whether or not you have previous experience.

When it comes to questions about baby care, the advice offered by "authoritative" sources is often contradictory. It's a fact of life that, as soon as a couple announce they are expecting a baby, they are bombarded with unsolicited instructions that are usually confusing. This can be quite unsettling, undermining an expectant couple's confidence. What's a new parent to do? That's where this book comes in. It does not insist on a particular formula

for parenting or extol only one rigid "best way" of doing things. Rather, it empowers parents with knowledge. It explains, informs, and demonstrates. We aimed to be comprehensive in presenting information and advice. Where possible, we incorporated the latest scientific "cutting edge" research findings. If there is no particular evidence to support a parenting practice, we present what is known so that parents can make informed choices that will work best for their particular circumstances.

We trust that the *Baby Care Book* will help replace uncertainty with knowledge, insecurity with confidence. We don't want you to do things our way; rather, we want you to feel comfortable raising your child in your own unique style. If this book helps you through the wonderful first year of your baby's life, we will be amply rewarded. Enjoy!

Dr. Jeremy Friedman
Dr. Norman Saunders

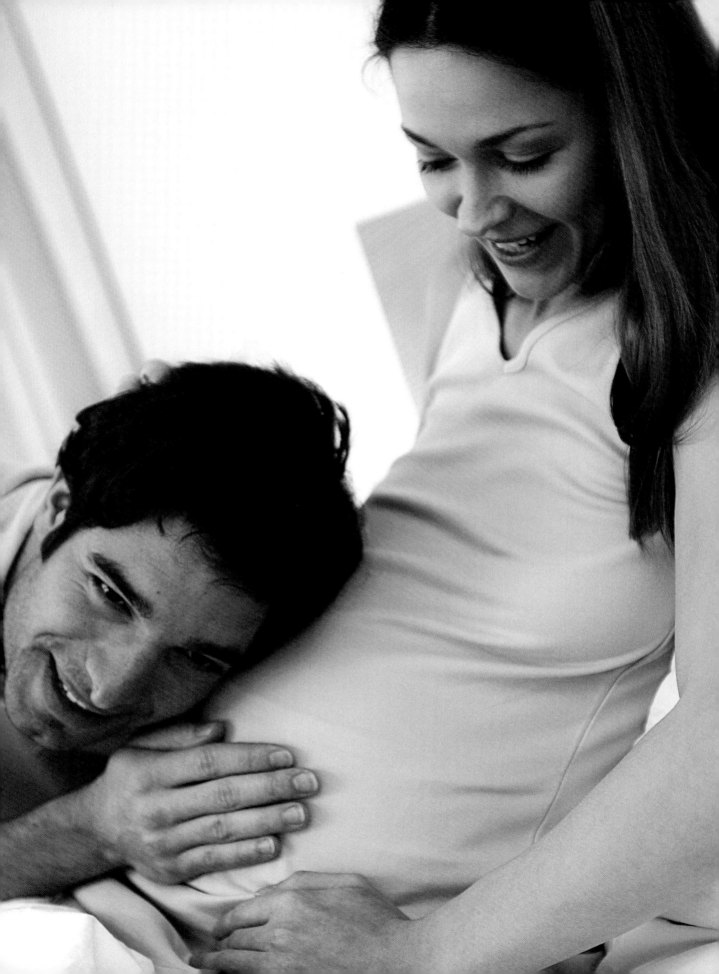

PART 1

Getting Ready to Have Your Baby

So you are planning for a new baby

Congratulations! You are about to embark on a wonderful journey that will enrich your life forever — probably even more than you can imagine. Most expectant parents wonder just how their lives will change with the arrival of their new baby. This time tends to be a mixture of anticipation, excitement, and some trepidation. There is no question that the addition of a new member to your family will require planning and adjustments to established routines.

Changes at home

Simply accept the fact that you will need to adjust. Certainly your sleep patterns will be altered! However, the various changes that you, specifically, will experience with the arrival of a new baby will depend on many factors that are particular to you, your family, and your baby.

A baby's routines will change frequently throughout her first months. At first, it often seems that a newborn's only consistency is inconsistency! Flexibility and patience will be needed. While most new parents talk about their lives becoming busier with feeding, diapering, bathing, and washing their baby's clothes, some families find the initial days unexpectedly quiet, due to the considerable sleep requirements of a newborn.

New parents find that an activity or outing that used to be simple now requires planning and much more time than it did before. There is a baby to feed and then a diaper to change, a supply bag to pack and naps to consider. It is not unusual for any outing, such as a trip to the doctor for a checkup, to take half a day or more.

If you have other children, you will be juggling several schedules. Planning becomes essential. Setting your priorities, focusing on those things you and your baby really need, and leaving less important tasks undone will help. Vacuuming can probably wait for another day … or even week.

Everyone's got advice

When you begin telling family, friends, and acquaintances that you are expecting a baby, you will probably find advice, invited and unsolicited, coming at you from all sides! Although some advice can be helpful, many expectant parents find too much information stressful, overwhelming, or confusing. Remember, this experience is different for everyone. There is often no one right way of doing things. Don't be afraid to change the subject or tune out if you have had enough.

If you like to gain information through reading, pick one reliable source of information and stick with it. You will also want to develop a good relationship with your health-care provider, who will see you through your pregnancy and your baby's birth.

HOW TO
Prepare siblings for a new baby

Based on alterations in your behavior or routines, as well as discussions they may overhear, children, even young ones, tend to know when any significant change is occurring in their lives. You need to prepare them for the arrival of a new member of the family. Besides, they should be included in the excitement and anticipation you are experiencing!

Siblings adjust better to an approaching birth if they have an understanding of what is happening. How you tell your children about the impending new arrival will depend on their age and level of understanding:

For young siblings, talking about "the baby in mommy's tummy" is appropriate. Allowing them to feel the baby move or kick will make the anticipated arrival more real.

For older children, make them feel part of the experience by involving them in planning. Discussing ways they can help once the baby arrives will make them feel included.

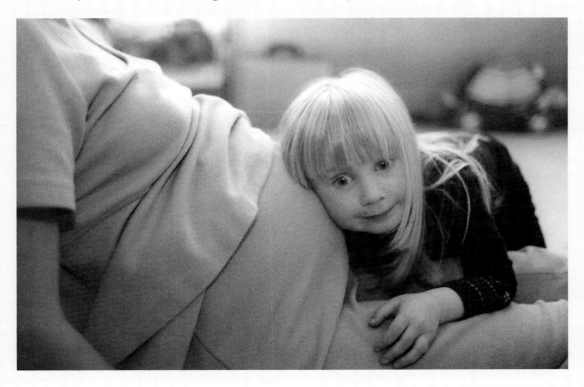

Decisions, decisions

Yes, you need to prepare for many changes, but you will also need to make many decisions for the welfare of your baby during your pregnancy. No one said parenting would be easy, but it will certainly be easier if you properly prepare for it. Getting ready for your new baby should be fun and exciting. Enjoy yourself!

Health-care options

One of the first decisions you need to make involves choosing the health-care professional who will monitor your pregnancy and assist with your baby's birth. There are several options, including a family doctor, a midwife, or an obstetrician. Your choice is an individual decision, based on your family's preferences and health histories. Whichever option you choose, it is important for expectant mothers to be examined regularly to ensure that any problems are addressed promptly. You should make this decision as early as possible and set up an appointment with your health-care provider to discuss the next steps.

Family doctor

Many expectant parents elect to have their family doctor follow them throughout the pregnancy. If this is your choice, ask your doctor if she provides prenatal care and does deliveries. Some family doctors will also attend the delivery of patients in their practices or work with a group of doctors who will be on call for deliveries.

Midwife

Other families choose to be followed by a midwife, who is a person trained to provide advice about events before, during, and after childbirth.

Obstetrician

Some couples prefer an obstetrician. Obstetricians are doctors who have special training in the care of pregnancies in which there are health problems in the mother or baby and have expertise in the management of complex births, difficult deliveries, and Caesarian sections.

Tests and more tests

A number of screening tests are typically done during a pregnancy to monitor the fetus and assess the expectant mother for conditions that might affect the baby's health at birth and beyond. Early detection and treatment of health conditions in the mother have been shown to prevent significant health problems in the baby.

Pre-eclampsia test

You will be asked to provide a urine sample to assess the protein in your urine; an excess may indicate a common problem associated with pregnancy called pre-eclampsia. Also known as toxemia, this condition can occur during the second half of pregnancy, and manifests with high blood pressure, protein in the urine, and swelling that doesn't go away.

Diabetes test

Blood tests to evaluate blood sugar levels for diabetes are routine during pregnancy.

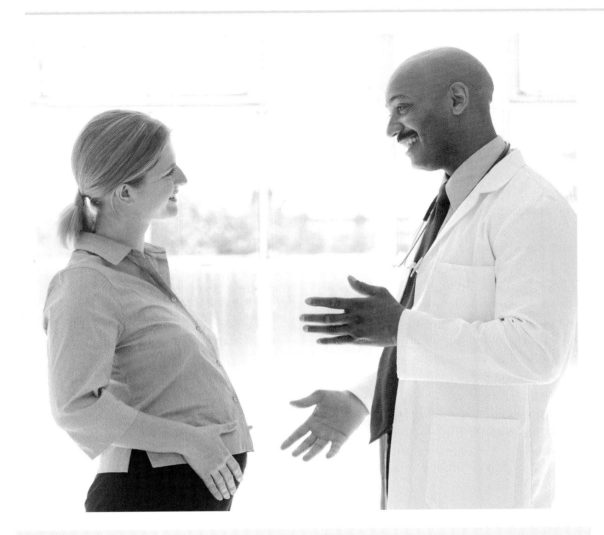

Did You Know?

First visit

At your first visit with your health-care provider, the expected date of delivery will be determined based on the first day of your last menstruation. Of course, this date is not set in stone and may be off by 2 weeks in either direction. In fact, very few women actually deliver on their "due" date.

You will also likely discuss where the birth will take place — at home, in a birthing center, or in a hospital. Don't forget to ask when and where health assessments will occur and what tests are recommended during the pregnancy.

As the pregnancy progresses, information will be provided about prenatal classes, which are offered to expectant mothers and fathers. In these classes, you will learn more about the course of your pregnancy, consider birth options, and learn how to care for your new baby.

Your urine will also be checked for sugar. If detected, diabetes can be treated by dietary changes, although medications, such as insulin, are sometimes required.

Rubella test

Blood tests to detect immunity against rubella (German measles) are also routine. Rubella, if contracted by women during pregnancy, is associated with a number of birth defects. Fortunately, most women have been immunized against rubella. While women who are currently pregnant cannot be immunized against rubella even if they are not immune, women who have not been immunized or who no longer have antibodies against this infection should be immunized before their next pregnancy.

Hepatitis B test

Routine blood tests include a test for hepatitis B, a liver infection that requires immunization of the baby immediately after birth if the mother has an active infection.

Blood type test

The expectant mother's blood type will also be determined. Certain differences between a mother's and her baby's blood types may result in health problems that require urgent treatment in the newborn infant.

HIV test

Pregnant mothers are offered a test for HIV infection. Treatment of HIV infection during pregnancy has been shown to reduce transmission of the virus to the baby by 80%.

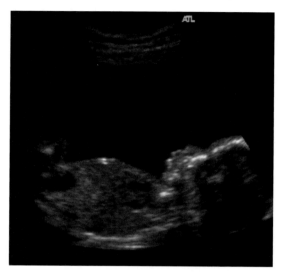

■ An ultrasound at 18 weeks, with the fetus lying on her back, with the head on the right side.

Ultrasound tests

At least once during the pregnancy, an ultrasound of the growing baby is recommended, typically around 18 weeks of pregnancy. Ultrasounds are safe during pregnancy. They allow for assessment of the size and growth of the fetus, enable visualization of the placenta's placement in the uterus, and provide a picture of the baby's body structures.

If you would like to know the baby's gender, this is the time to find out! However, ultrasound technicians may not tell you the final results of the ultrasound — they require confirmation by a radiologist, who will send a report to your health-care provider.

Fetal disorder tests

Other tests may be done during the pregnancy to assess the potential for congenital malformations or birth defects due to inherited or genetic disorders in the fetus. Much can be learned from your family's health history. Ultrasound testing of the developing neck area can be used to screen for genetic problems such as Down syndrome, as can blood tests. Blood tests are also used to screen for spinal cord problems, such as spina bifida.

Other screening tests for rare diseases, such as Tay-Sachs disease or cystic fibrosis, may be suggested, particularly if your ethnic background suggests a greater risk for such conditions. Amniocentesis, which tests the amniotic fluid surrounding the baby, or chorionic sampling from the growing placenta, may be recommended, depending on your family's health history and risk factors.

Some families wish to have all of these tests, and others do not. Consider whether knowing the results will help you prepare better for your baby's birth or will make a difference in your decision to continue the pregnancy.

Did You Know?

Ongoing monitoring

Once your pregnancy has been confirmed with a blood or urine test, some basic monitoring will be completed periodically during your pregnancy. At each visit to your health-care provider, your weight will be measured and the size of your uterus assessed to ensure that the baby is growing appropriately. The baby's heartbeat will be measured using a small ultrasound probe placed on your abdomen or, later in your pregnancy, using a stethoscope. Your blood pressure will also be checked.

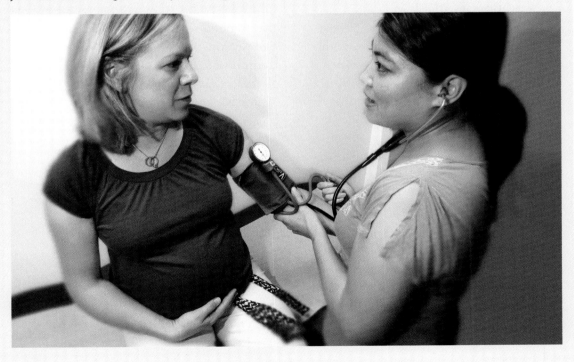

Feeding your baby

In planning for your baby's birth, you should also learn about breast-feeding. Breast-feeding is recommended by all authorities for your baby's growth and development, but infant formula can be used if you choose not to breast-feed or because you have certain medical conditions. How you feed your baby is ultimately up to you, so do some research to make an informed decision.

Breast-feeding

Breast-feeding is recommended by health-care professionals because of its benefits for the baby. For example, breast-feeding offers increased protection against certain infections and may help to prevent some health conditions, such as obesity, diabetes, allergies, and sudden infant death syndrome (SIDS). In addition, many parents find this to be the easiest method of feeding. Breast milk is readily available and requires no preparation. Once breast-feeding is established with your baby, breast milk can be expressed and fed by bottle if feeding by other caregivers is necessary or desired.

Breast-feeding may be slightly difficult initially, so you may need help. Prenatal breast-feeding classes are often available through community agencies, such as La Leche League, and most hospital postnatal units have a breast-feeding class for new mothers or a consultant available to provide hands-on guidance. Make use of these resources before you leave the hospital. Be sure to have contact information for a breast-feeding consultant or clinic in case you require additional support when you get home with your baby.

Formula-feeding

Some parents choose to formula-feed from the outset because of an inability to breast-feed, difficulty in breast-feeding, lifestyle requirements, or personal choice. If you choose to formula-feed your new baby, you will need to purchase infant formula and bottle-feeding equipment.

Select an iron-fortified formula. When purchasing formula in anticipation of your

Did You Know?

Formulas and bottles

There is a wide variety of infant formula brands, several different formulations (powder, liquid concentrate, ready-to-serve), and an endless number of bottle and nipple designs on the market. For healthy infants, there is no clear-cut advantage to any one of these formulations or designs. The choice is yours.

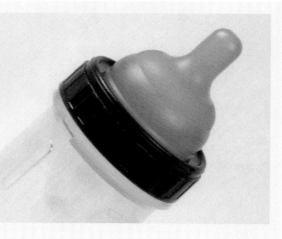

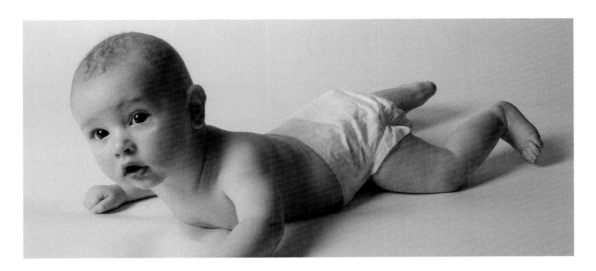

baby's arrival, check the best-before date on the label.

Do not plan to feed your newborn cow's milk or goat's milk; it will not meet your baby's nutritional needs and can result in health problems.

Circumcision

If your new baby is a boy, you will need to decide whether he will be circumcised. While circumcised men have a lower incidence of urinary tract infections and less risk of developing penile cancer and some sexually transmitted diseases, such as HIV, there is no overriding advantage to circumcision, so the decision is an individual one based on your religious or personal preference.

Circumcision involves the surgical removal of the foreskin covering the head of the penis. This procedure is relatively simple, with few complications, although it can be painful, and there is a small risk of bleeding, infection, and poor healing. To reduce the pain associated with this procedure, an anesthetic cream can be applied to the foreskin or freezing injected around the nerve supplying the penis; the latter works in a similar way to the technique used by dentists to "freeze" teeth. Many health-care professionals now feel that pain reduction should be a regular part of the circumcision procedure.

Not all doctors will perform circumcisions, and there might be an additional cost for the procedure.

Diapers

Disposable or washable? That is the question. Disposable diapers are convenient, particularly for use out of the home. And rashes are less likely when using disposable diapers than when using cloth diapers.

However, disposable diapers are expensive and environmentally unfriendly, creating a significant amount of garbage. Cloth diapers are reusable but must be changed promptly to avoid diaper rashes. You may choose to wash them yourself or use a diaper service, which picks up soiled diapers and replaces them with new ones.

The choice is yours!

Eating for two

Although it does not justify overeating or overindulging food cravings, there is some truth in the old expression that you are now "eating for two." As your pregnancy progresses, your nutrient requirements do increase. Balanced consumption of the three macronutrients — carbohydrate, protein, and fat — will provide you with the energy you need to feed the two of you, while supplementation of the key micronutrients — calcium, vitamin D, folic acid, iron, and zinc — will promote the general health of mother and child during pregnancy and after delivery. Before making any changes to your diet, be sure to consult your health-care provider or a dietitian registered with the American Dietitians Association or the Dietitians of Canada.

Energy needs

During the first trimester, your energy needs will increase by 100 calories a day, and during the second and third trimester, by 300 calories a day, to an optimum 2,300 to 2,700 calories, spread across three meals and one or two snacks.

Special requirements

Several specific minerals and vitamins are needed to ensure a healthy pregnancy. These nutrients can be obtained from food sources, but you may need to take a supplement.

Adequate calcium is essential for the growth of the fetus, while adequate vitamin D leads to an increased chance of giving birth to a healthy child. Folic acid, taken as a supplement before you become pregnant and until the end of the first trimester, can reduce the risk of neural tube defects, such as spina bifida. Iron is crucial, because an iron deficiency can lower immunity, increasing the risk of infection and illness. Extra zinc is required by both the fetus and the mother.

Food guides

One of the best ways to ensure a healthy diet before, during, and after pregnancy is to follow the nutritional advice in the United States Department of Agriculture's MyPyramid guidelines or in Canada's Food Guide to Healthy Eating.

Daily recommended intake of macronutrients and micronutrients during pregnancy

Carbohydrate	Protein	Fat	Calcium	Vitamin D	Folic acid	Iron	Zinc
175 g	71 g	20–35% of total energy intake	1,000 mg	200 IU	600 µg	27 mg	11 mg

Adapted by permission from Daina Kalnins and Joanne Saab, *Better Food for Pregnancy* (Toronto: Robert Rose, 2006).

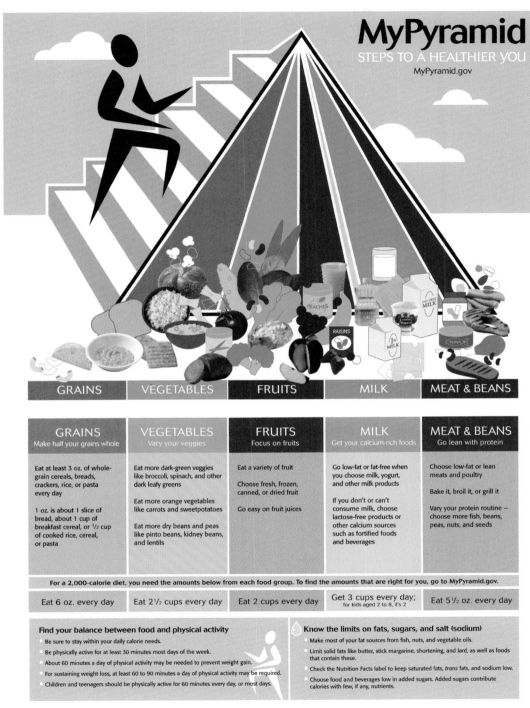

MyPyramid
STEPS TO A HEALTHIER YOU
MyPyramid.gov

GRAINS	VEGETABLES	FRUITS	MILK	MEAT & BEANS

GRAINS Make half your grains whole	VEGETABLES Vary your veggies	FRUITS Focus on fruits	MILK Get your calcium-rich foods	MEAT & BEANS Go lean with protein
Eat at least 3 oz. of whole-grain cereals, breads, crackers, rice, or pasta every day 1 oz. is about 1 slice of bread, about 1 cup of breakfast cereal, or ½ cup of cooked rice, cereal, or pasta	Eat more dark-green veggies like broccoli, spinach, and other dark leafy greens Eat more orange vegetables like carrots and sweetpotatoes Eat more dry beans and peas like pinto beans, kidney beans, and lentils	Eat a variety of fruit Choose fresh, frozen, canned, or dried fruit Go easy on fruit juices	Go low-fat or fat-free when you choose milk, yogurt, and other milk products If you don't or can't consume milk, choose lactose-free products or other calcium sources such as fortified foods and beverages	Choose low-fat or lean meats and poultry Bake it, broil it, or grill it Vary your protein routine — choose more fish, beans, peas, nuts, and seeds

For a 2,000-calorie diet, you need the amounts below from each food group. To find the amounts that are right for you, go to MyPyramid.gov.

Eat 6 oz. every day	Eat 2½ cups every day	Eat 2 cups every day	Get 3 cups every day; for kids aged 2 to 8, it's 2	Eat 5½ oz. every day

Find your balance between food and physical activity
- Be sure to stay within your daily calorie needs.
- Be physically active for at least 30 minutes most days of the week.
- About 60 minutes a day of physical activity may be needed to prevent weight gain.
- For sustaining weight loss, at least 60 to 90 minutes a day of physical activity may be required.
- Children and teenagers should be physically active for 60 minutes every day, or most days.

Know the limits on fats, sugars, and salt (sodium)
- Make most of your fat sources from fish, nuts, and vegetable oils.
- Limit solid fats like butter, stick margarine, shortening, and lard, as well as foods that contain these.
- Check the Nutrition Facts label to keep saturated fats, *trans* fats, and sodium low.
- Choose food and beverages low in added sugars. Added sugars contribute calories with few, if any, nutrients.

MyPyramid.gov
STEPS TO A HEALTHIER YOU

U.S. Department of Agriculture
Center for Nutrition Policy and Promotion
April 2005
CNPP-15

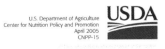

Recommended Number of *Food Guide Servings* per Day

	Children			Teens		Adults			
Age in Years	2-3	4-8	9-13	14-18		19-50		51+	
Sex	Girls and Boys			Females	Males	Females	Males	Females	Males
Vegetables and Fruit	4	5	6	7	8	7-8	8-10	7	7
Grain Products	3	4	6	6	7	6-7	8	6	7
Milk and Alternatives	2	2	3-4	3-4	3-4	2	2	3	3
Meat and Alternatives	1	1	1-2	2	3	2	3	2	3

The chart above shows how many Food Guide Servings you need from each of the four food groups every day.

Having the amount and type of food recommended and following the tips in *Canada's Food Guide* will help:

- Meet your needs for vitamins, minerals and other nutrients.
- Reduce your risk of obesity, type 2 diabetes, heart disease, certain types of cancer and osteoporosis.
- Contribute to your overall health and vitality.

What is One Food Guide Serving?
Look at the examples below.

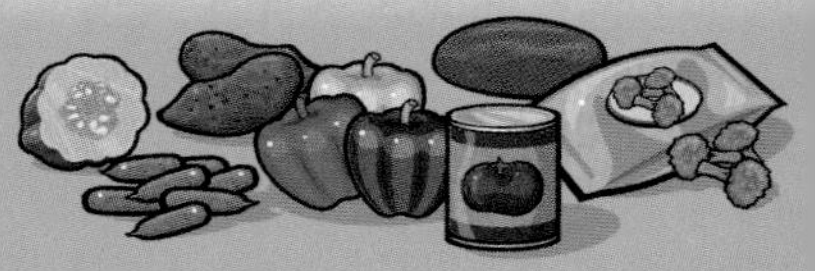

Fresh, frozen or canned vegetables
125 mL (½ cup)

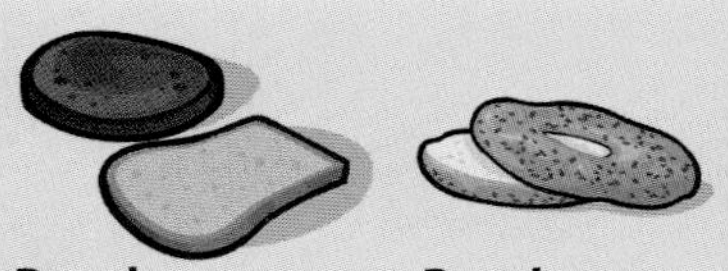

Bread
1 slice (35 g)

Bagel
½ bagel (45 g)

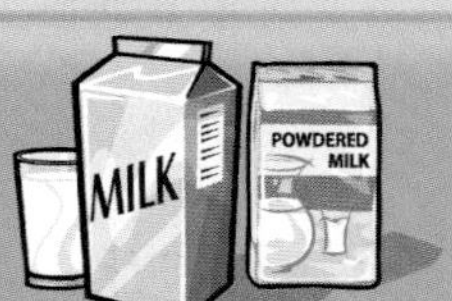

Milk or powdered milk (reconstituted)
250 mL (1 cup)

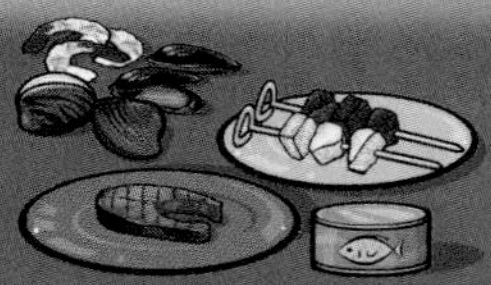

Cooked fish, shellfish, poultry, lean meat
75 g (2 ½ oz.)/125 mL (½ cup)

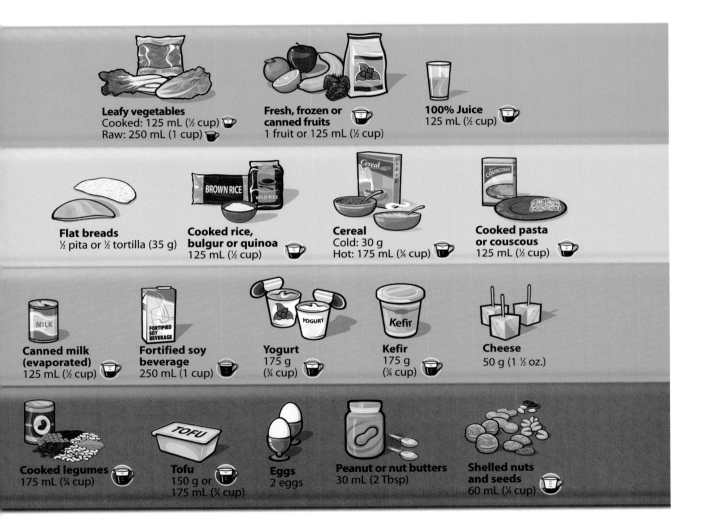

Leafy vegetables
Cooked: 125 mL (½ cup)
Raw: 250 mL (1 cup)

Fresh, frozen or canned fruits
1 fruit or 125 mL (½ cup)

100% Juice
125 mL (½ cup)

Flat breads
½ pita or ½ tortilla (35 g)

Cooked rice, bulgur or quinoa
125 mL (½ cup)

Cereal
Cold: 30 g
Hot: 175 mL (¾ cup)

Cooked pasta or couscous
125 mL (½ cup)

Canned milk (evaporated)
125 mL (½ cup)

Fortified soy beverage
250 mL (1 cup)

Yogurt
175 g
(¾ cup)

Kefir
175 g
(¾ cup)

Cheese
50 g (1 ½ oz.)

Cooked legumes
175 mL (¾ cup)

Tofu
150 g or
175 mL (¾ cup)

Eggs
2 eggs

Peanut or nut butters
30 mL (2 Tbsp)

Shelled nuts and seeds
60 mL (¼ cup)

Planning a safe and healthy pregnancy

Planning is a big part of a successful pregnancy. You will want to think about everything from your emotional readiness for raising a child to more immediate concerns about finding the right caregiver after your baby is born. But even before you become pregnant, you will also want to decrease your risk of exposure to known teratogens — medications, chemicals, and infections that can cause birth defects.

Ten Steps

If your pregnancy is not planned, don't worry. Nearly half of all pregnancies are unplanned, and the vast majority of children born in North America are normal and healthy. Still, you'll want to get the facts from the experts on the "do's and don'ts" of exposure to drugs and other substances.

In the meantime, here are 10 steps to a safe and healthy pregnancy:

1. Take folic acid to prevent neural tube defects.
Why is folic acid so important before pregnancy? It's simple. With sufficient amounts of folic acid in your diet, you dramatically decrease the risk of spina bifida and other forms of neural tube defects. Neural tube defects are major congenital anomalies of the brain or spinal cord that occur when the brain or spine fails to close properly. This crucial event occurs very early in pregnancy — so early, in fact, that many women run the risk of a neural tube defect before they even know they have conceived. Planning your pregnancy and taking folic acid supplements before conception will ensure that your unborn child is protected in those very early days of development.

Folic acid is one of the B vitamins, found naturally in green, leafy vegetables, nuts, and oranges. In North America, flour is fortified with folic acid, so it is present in breads and pastas.

With a minimum intake of 400 micrograms of folic acid every day, the risk of neural tube defects decreases by 75%. But most people do not get that much through their daily diet. That's why women planning a pregnancy should take a daily supplement tablet containing folic acid. The best way to do this is to start taking a prenatal multiple vitamin pill *before* you become pregnant or, even better, if you have unprotected sex.

All prenatal multivitamin tablets contain around 1,000 micrograms (1 mg) of folic acid, so you are well covered if you take one a day.

2. Stop drinking alcohol to prevent fetal alcohol spectrum disorder.
Fetal alcohol spectrum disorder (FASD) is the leading cause of preventable brain

damage. The great beauty of planning your pregnancy is that you can take steps to avoid exposure to alcohol in plenty of time to ensure that your baby is safeguarded against its harmful effects.

Unfortunately, not all women (and their babies) are so lucky. Nearly 50% of all pregnancies are unplanned. What's more, nearly 50% of women of childbearing age consume alcohol in varying amounts. This means that nearly 25% of all babies will be exposed to some level of alcohol before they are born. Their growth and development will depend in large part on the amount of the prenatal exposure.

If a lot of alcohol causes the worst harm, and less alcohol will produce different effects, what, you may ask, is a safe amount to drink during pregnancy? The answer is, we just don't know. That's why the most prudent choice when planning your pregnancy is to avoid alcohol entirely. If avoiding alcohol is a challenge for you, ask your health-care provider for help.

3. Stop smoking cigarettes to help prevent stillbirth, prematurity, and SIDS.
When planning a pregnancy, you should stop smoking. Smoking in pregnancy may decrease the baby's birth weight and increase the risk of stillbirth (fetal death after 20 weeks of gestation) and prematurity (baby born before 37 weeks of pregnancy). It also increases your risk for miscarriage. Smoking in pregnancy is also associated with sudden infant death syndrome (SIDS) or "crib death," where infants die during their sleep for no apparent reason. If you're having trouble kicking the habit, think about getting help. Talk to your doctor.

Nicotine replacement therapy (nicotine patch, gum, or spray) or Zyban (bupropion) tablets may be right for you. Both methods have been shown in controlled randomized trials to be effective in smoking cessation.

4. Treat drug or chemical dependencies.
If you are chemically dependent on or addicted to a recreational drug, such as cocaine or marijuana, you should seek addiction counseling and treatment before pregnancy. Drug abuse may affect your baby directly by entering the baby's body, or indirectly by affecting your health and/or your ability to care for your baby when it is born. Remember, too, that drug dependency is not limited to the use of "street drugs," but may also involve common medications, such as pain relievers. If "kicking the habit" is a challenge for you, ask your health-care provider for help.

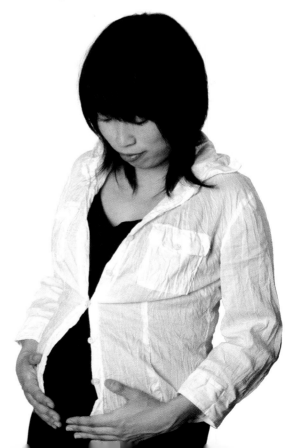

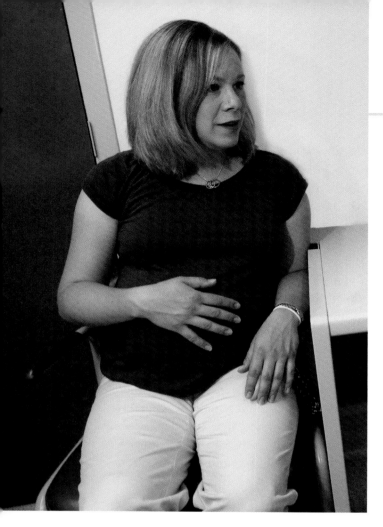

teacher or caretaker), it is even more important to be vaccinated.

The other virus that can adversely affect the fetus and for which there is a vaccine is chicken pox (varicella). When contracted by pregnant women who have not previously had chicken pox, the varicella virus can cause fetal varicella syndrome — which affects the brain, the eyes, and limb formation — in a small percentage of unborn babies (1% to 2%). You can get the vaccine from your doctor after a blood test shows that you are not immune.

6. Seek proper treatment of medical conditions.

If you have a medical condition, this is the time to ensure that you are treated with medications that are safe for the fetus. Discuss with your health-care provider whether pregnancy will affect your medical condition, and whether your medical condition will affect the pregnancy.

Don't stop medications "cold turkey." Many medications do not pose a risk to the fetus. What's more, if you have relied on certain prescription medications to control conditions such as hypertension or depression, you may do more harm than good by suddenly going off your medication. You can often continue your medication during pregnancy, but your doctor may want to prescribe another, safer medication. Remember that many untreated conditions themselves pose a risk to the fetus. If you have a chronic medical condition and are planning a pregnancy, it is advisable to get your condition under control with the help of a medical specialist who is experienced in the management of pregnancy.

5. Immunize against dangerous infectious diseases.

When planning your pregnancy, you should ensure that you are immunized against viruses that are dangerous for the unborn baby. The most important one is rubella (German measles). If you have not had rubella, or have not been immunized against it, your unborn baby will not be protected. If the rubella virus attacks the fetus, the result may be congenital rubella, characterized by deafness, mental retardation, and other adverse effects, such as heart anomalies. Vaccination against rubella is crucial because you may contract it from young children (your other children, neighbors, friends, family members) who have been exposed to it in daycare or at school. If you work with children (as a

7. Do not self-prescribe.

You may be used to treating your coughs, colds, aches, and pains with one or more of the thousand of products for sale at your local drugstore, but once you are pregnant (or planning a pregnancy), over-the-counter self-help must end. What is safe for you may not be safe for your unborn baby.

Also be cautious with the use of herbal medicines. Be guided by evidence-based information about the risk or safety of the medicines and products you use during pregnancy. In general, we have more information on the safety of older medications than we do on those that are newer. When it comes to herbal medicines, there is little human data on their safety or risk in pregnancy.

8. Avoid exposure to dangerous chemicals in the workplace.

If your occupation involves or may involve exposure to chemicals, find out what chemicals are involved and seek advice on their fetal safety. Exposure to chemical solvents and heavy metals can pose a risk to your baby. The ones you have probably heard the most about are carbon monoxide, formaldehyde, lead, mercury, and organic solvents, but there are others.

9. Seek pre-conception genetic counseling.

If you or your partner has a family history of children born with congenital malformations or developmental delays (your own children or those of your siblings), your health-care provider can refer you for genetic counseling, which usually involves a detailed assessment of your medical, obstetric, and family history.

10. Be confident.

There is plenty of excellent, evidence-based information to guide you through your pregnancy and while you breast-feed your child. Your health-care providers are there to guide you. Ask questions, be positive, and learn the facts. The list of known teratogens (medications, chemicals, and infections that have been proven unsafe to an unborn baby) is relatively short. The list of substances that are not compatible with breast-feeding is even shorter. Stay informed, and your odds of having a safe pregnancy and a healthy baby are excellent.

Teratogen Information Services

There are a number of teratogen information services in North America.

The Organization of Teratogen Information Services (OTIS)

For local teratogen information services in most states and provinces in North America, contact OTIS at: (866) 626-OTIS or (866) 626-6847. Information about OTIS is also available online at www.otispregnancy.org/index.htm.

Motherisk

The Motherisk Program at the Hospital for Sick Children in Toronto is one of the largest teratogen research, counseling, and education centers in the world. Contact Motherisk at (416) 813-6780, or online at www.motherisk.org.

Guide to

Selected drugs and chemicals that are unsafe in pregnancy

A number of common drugs and chemicals have been proven to cause malformations in the fetus when the mother has been exposed to them. If you believe you have been exposed to these teratogens before or during pregnancy, contact your health-care provider immediately.

Guide to unsafe drugs and chemicals

Drug or chemical	Teratogenic effect
Alcohol	Fetal alcohol spectrum disorder (FASD)
Alkylating agents Anticancer drugs such as busulfan, chlorambucil, cyclophosphamide, mechlorethamine	Growth retardation; cleft palate; heart defects; other malformations and anomalies
Antimetabolic agents Anticancer drugs such as azauridine, cytarabine, 5-FU, 6-MP, methotrexate	Hydrocephalus and other developmental anomalies; skull, ear, eye, palate, and limb malformations
Carbamazepine	Increased risk for neural tube defects
Carbon monoxide	Cerebral atrophy; mental retardation; microcephaly; convulsions; spastic disorders; intrauterine or postnatal death
Corticosteroids	Oral cleft; reduction in birth weight and head circumference
Danazol and other androgenic drugs	Masculinization of female fetuses
Hypoglycemic drugs	Hypoglycemia in the newborn
Lead	Lower scores in developmental tests

Drug or chemical	Teratogenic effect
Lithium	Ebstein's anomaly of the heart
Methyl mercury, *Mercuric sulfide*	Microcephaly; eye malformations; cerebral palsy; mental retardation; malocclusion of teeth
Misprostol	Moebius syndrome (paralysis of cranial nerves)
Nonsteroidal anti-inflammatory drugs *(NSAIDs)* Such as ibuprofen, naproxen	Possible gastroschisis; when used in third trimester, may prematurely close the fetal ductus arteriosus
PCBs (polychlorinated biphenyls)	Stillbirth; children who survive do not meet milestones and show signs of central nervous system damage
Penicillamine	Skin hyperelastosis
Phenytoin	Growth retardation; central nervous system damage
Systemic retinoids Such as isotretinoin (Accutane) and etretinate.	Central nervous system damage; skull, face, heart, and other defects
Tetracycline	Anomalies of teeth and bone
Thalidomide	Limb-shortening defects; internal organ defects
Valproic acid	Neural tube defects
Warfarin	Skeletal and central nervous system defects; Dandy-Walker syndrome

Adapted by permission from Gideon Koren, *The Complete Guide to Everyday Risks in Pregnancy & Breastfeeding* (Toronto: Robert Rose, 2004).

HOW TO
Choose your baby's doctor

Before your baby is born, you should choose a health-care provider to follow your baby's growth and development after birth. You may choose to have your own family doctor, a pediatrician, a nurse, or a health clinic care for your baby. Some pediatricians, who are specialists in child health, do "well baby" visits, while others only follow children with health problems. Here are some points to consider when you are making your decision.

1. Convenience: During the first months, frequent visits are required to monitor your baby's growth and development, so convenience is important. It will make your early days and months with your baby easier if you select a health-care provider who works in a location close to your home.

2. Comfort: Pick someone you trust and with whom you feel comfortable asking questions. Set up a prenatal appointment to discuss important logistical issues. Does the health-care provider have "privileges" at the hospital to see your baby before you are discharged? If you have a concern about your baby's health at night or on a weekend, how do you get help? How is the practice set up — is it a solo practice or a partnership of practitioners who share on-call duty?

3. Consideration: Take your time in making this important choice. Ask family members and friends for their advice. Your own doctor may also have good recommendations.

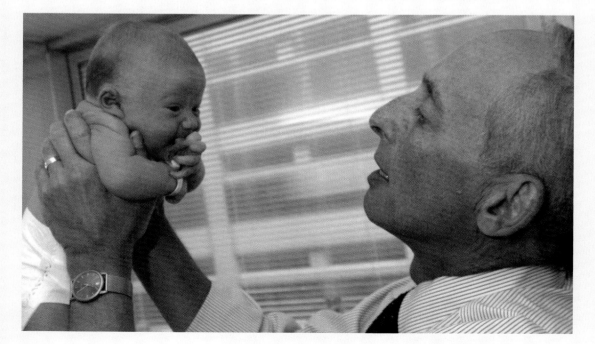

What will your baby need?

There is an overwhelming quantity of baby products awaiting you. Despite changes in fashion and technical advances, the paramount concern remains the safety of any product.

Initially, your baby's needs are simple: a place to eat, a place to sleep, a place to have her diapers changed, and a place to be bathed. If you want to be mobile, you'll also need a safe means of transportation. Here is a guide to meeting these basic needs.

A place to eat

Whichever feeding method you choose, you will spend considerable time feeding your baby. You might as well make yourself comfortable. Create a peaceful place where both you and your baby can feel relaxed. Of course, if you have other children, this is easier said than done.

Many parents choose a simple rocking chair or a glider rocker (a particular favorite due to its smooth rocking motion), but any comfortable chair with a cushioned seat, footrest, and armrests will do. Place a table beside your chair to keep a glass of water, a damp cloth, reading material, and the telephone close by.

A place to sleep

You will need to decide where your baby will spend her first days in your home. Some parents choose to have the newborn sleep in their room, while others prefer to have a dedicated baby's room. Some parents prefer to use a bassinet, some a crib. Others prefer to co-sleep with their newborn.

Bassinets

Some families choose to use a bassinet initially. However, your baby will very quickly outgrow a bassinet and require a larger sleeping space. Be aware of safety issues — some bassinets have handles, allowing transport of a sleeping baby from room to room, but the bassinet can easily be dropped by a tired parent. Others attach to the side of an adult bed, but care must be taken to ensure that there is no gap or possibility of entrapment between beds. If you are a mobile family that travels frequently, you may choose a playpen with a removable bassinet. Be sure the playpen is used only when your baby is the recommended age.

Safe bedding

The mattress you use should be approved for newborns by health agencies. It should be firm, not too soft. Use only a thin or porous blanket and do not give your baby a pillow. Never place your baby to sleep on a couch or waterbed — there is a risk of suffocation. The current recommendation is that infants sleep on their backs. Sleep positioners (wedges used to prop a baby on her side) are not recommended, and some may pose a suffocation risk.

Co-sleeping

Some families plan to co-sleep with their newborn for ease of nursing. Be cautious if you do so. Co-sleeping with adults who are obese, overtired, or under the influence of alcohol or drugs may be associated with a higher risk of sudden infant death syndrome (SIDS).

■ To reduce the risk of sudden infant death syndrome (SIDS), parents are advised to place their baby on her back while she is sleeping.

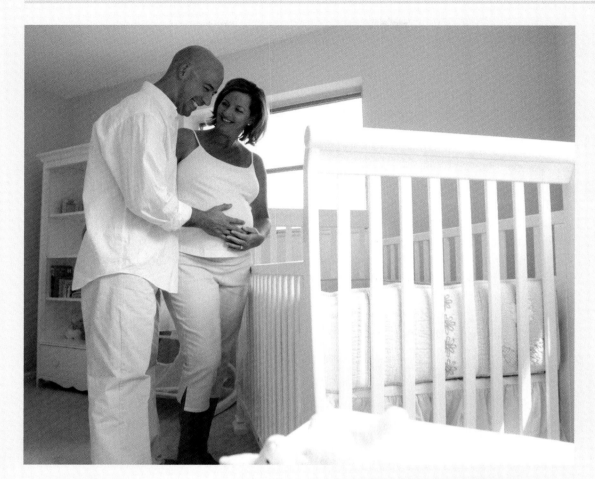

HOW TO
Choose a crib

Many parents choose to have their baby sleep in a crib, but there's some planning to do beforehand.

1. If you are buying a new crib, check the label to ensure that it meets current safety standards. Look for a product certification from a reputable testing agency.

2. If you are planning to use a second-hand or older crib, make sure it meets current safety standards. For example, are the slats or spindles set apart at the recommended distance? The National Safety Council and the Consumer Product Safety Commission provide guides to these safety features.

3. Ensure that the railing on one side can be lowered so you can easily place your baby in the crib.

4. Check that the railing's raising and lowering mechanism is relatively quiet and smooth.

A place to have diapers changed

If there is one thing your baby will require frequently, it is diaper changes! You will need a stable, clean surface for this job. Some parents use a blanket or change pad on the floor. A portable change pad to take with you for diaper changes outside your home is especially handy.

Many parents opt to purchase or borrow a change table. The advantage of change tables is their comfortable height, which allows an adult to change a diaper without getting a backache. The disadvantage is that babies can wiggle or roll off change tables if you're not watching. Be sure to keep a hand on your baby at all times.

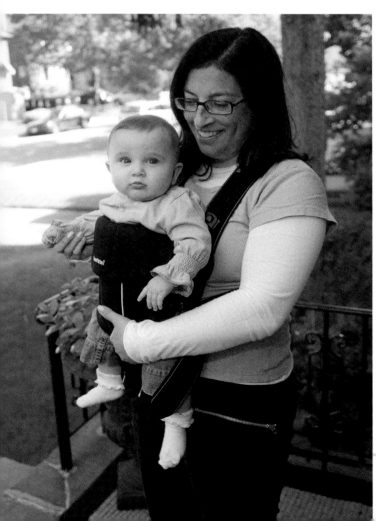

Place the necessities for diaper changing (diapers, cream, and wipes) within reach.

A place to be bathed

Many new parents choose to purchase a baby bathtub rather than use the adult tub or the sink for bathing their baby. Keeping several small facecloths around is helpful for wiping small hands and face while bathing and after eating. Mild baby soap can be used to wash your baby's skin and hair. Some cloths to place over your shoulder as you burp or hold your baby will help protect your clothing and cut down on your laundry.

On the move

Baby bags

Of course, you won't always be at home to feed and change your baby, especially as you get past the first month or two. As you become more mobile, it will be helpful to have a diaper bag ready to go with supplies for the road. Select a bag that can hold a few diapers, wipes, a small change pad, a change of baby clothes, and a blanket or burp cloth. It's a good idea to have a small insulated bottle bag, which can hold bottles of expressed breast milk or formula. Later, you can use this to carry baby food and a "sippy" cup.

Snugglies

Some caregivers prefer to carry their young infants in an infant carrier or "snuggly." There are several brands on the market and many different styles. Try them out and pick the one that feels most comfortable and secure.

Guidelines for

Choosing a stroller

You will need a stroller to keep you mobile. Your choice of stroller should be based on where you intend to use it (outside versus inside); the weather conditions in your area; whether you intend to take it in the car or on a plane; and, of course, price restrictions. You will likely use your stroller for a few years, so durability is another important factor.

The many strollers on the market differ in size and weight, the number of wheels, the suspension, the folding mechanism, the available storage area, and the number of seats. Several models allow you to clamp your car seat onto the frame of the stroller so you don't have to move your sleeping baby. If you choose this option, ensure that the car seat and the stroller are compatible. The car seat must be securely clamped in place when attached to the stroller. The combination of car seat and stroller may be more susceptible to tipping over.

If you have more than one child, there are various double strollers available. Tandem strollers (one child seated in front of the other) are easier to maneuver in public places, but are large and heavy. Side-by-side strollers are another option. They look pretty wide, but they do fit through most doorways.

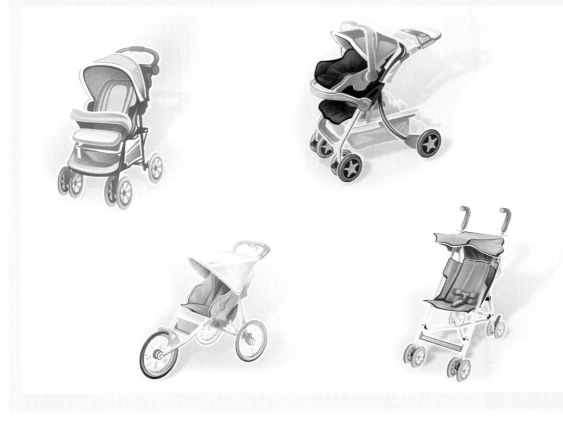

Car seats

There is considerable evidence that infants and children are safest in cars when they are secured in special child car seats. Car seats should be placed in the back seat; the front seat of newer cars is not safe for children until they are at least 12 years old or taller than 5 feet because of the presence of air bags, which may cause significant injuries to a child when activated. Car seats that are used until the child is 4 years old or 40 pounds (18 kg) have an internal seat belt that fastens the child to the seat. They are secured to the vehicle's seat using the vehicle seat belt or a "LATCH" Universal Anchorage System (metal clips secured to the car frame).

Your child's car seat must be placed properly in your car and held tightly in place as recommended by the seat and car manufacturers. The internal seat belt must be tightened properly, leaving a maximum of two finger widths between the chest clip and your child's body, with the chest clip at the level of your child's underarms. In many larger centers, professionals can check the seat installation for you — ask about this service when you purchase your car seat.

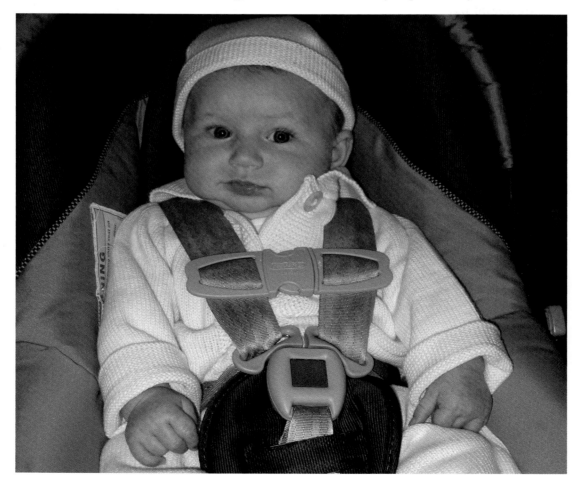

Did You Know?

Three car seat requirements

In general, there are three stages of car seat requirements for children: those for newborns and infants; those for toddlers; and those for school-age children. There are combination seats and convertible seats that may cover two to three of these stages, but they are generally more expensive. Choose the car seat that fits most securely into your vehicle.

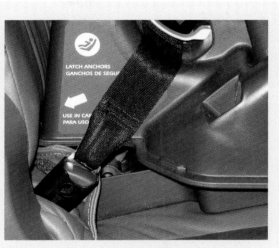

■ Car seats are necessary to ensure the safety of your baby ... but they must be properly secured according to the manufacturer's instructions.

1. NEWBORNS AND INFANTS

Because newborns and young infants have poor head control, they require a seat that is relatively reclined. This style of seat is used until your baby reaches 20 pounds (9 kg), around 1 year of age. The seat is placed in the vehicle with the infant facing the rear of the car, permitting maximal head support in the event of a crash. The seat can be secured directly to the car using the car seat belt or clipped into a base that remains in the car and is secured by the car's seat belt. This type has a handle that can be raised or lowered, and the baby can be carried outside the vehicle within the car seat. If your child reaches 20 pounds (9 kg) before 1 year of age, she can be moved up to a toddler car seat, but should remain facing the rear until she is 1 year old.

2. TODDLERS

Once your child reaches 20 pounds (9 kg) and 1 year of age, she should be seated in a toddler car seat facing the front of the car. From this point until she reaches 40 pounds (18 kg), at approximately 4 years of age, your child should remain in this seat. This type of seat is placed in an upright position and contains an internal seat belt. A strap from the car seat tethers it to a bolt secured to the vehicle frame or to metal clips between the seat cushions intended for this purpose. To protect your child from injury, the seat must be secured tightly to the car frame.

3. SCHOOL-AGE CHILDREN

Once she reaches 40 pounds (18 kg), and until she reaches 80 pounds (36 kg), at about 8 years of age, your child should remain in a "booster" seat to protect against lower spinal cord injuries. A booster seat has no internal seat belt, but simply raises the child slightly to allow the vehicle's seat belt to be used in the proper position over the hips. Shoulder strap positioners allow the shoulder strap portion of the seat belt to be positioned correctly. Booster seats do not require tethering to the car frame.

Getting ready for the delivery

The delivery date seems to approach all too quickly. Once you have decided where the birth will take place, it's a good idea to arrange a visit to familiarize yourself with it. Now you'll know where to go once those contractions become regular! You certainly don't want to get lost trying to find the parking lot when the baby has decided to make her appearance.

Check out visiting policies if you plan to deliver in a hospital or birthing center. Don't forget to include in your plans any family members or friends whom you want to be there at the time of your baby's birth.

Start packing

Start packing everything you will want to take with you to the hospital or birthing center — for your own needs and for your baby's needs.

You may want to prepare and freeze some meals ahead of time: you're unlikely to find much time to cook in your first week at home. From time to time, you may feel a bit overwhelmed with family and friends anxious to visit your new arrival. It's okay to let people know you all need some rest and ask them to come another day. If friends and family offer help, ask them to bring you a meal so you can focus on resting, feeding your baby, and getting settled into your new routine.

What to pack for your trip to the hospital or birthing center

For you:	For baby:
Underwear, nursing bra	Newborn-size diapers and petroleum jelly (Vaseline), if not provided
Comfortable, loose, dark clothing	
"Overnight" pads	Clothing appropriate for the weather, and a hat
Slippers or comfortable shoes	Blanket
Some favorite foods, snacks, and drinks	Car seat if you plan to drive home
Phone numbers of people you may wish to call before or after the baby is born	

And then there were two

For the first month or two, at least until skills are honed and routines successfully established, parenting can be exhausting for any young couple. When twins appear on the scene, the situation might well be described as "magnificent chaos." Yet the parents of twins almost invariably manage to cope beautifully with their double burden. Necessity is a great stimulus. After the initial adjustment, the experience of raising twins provides many extra rewards for their parents. Although nothing can fully prepare you for raising twins, getting ready in advance certainly helps.

Identical and fraternal twins

Twins are described as being either identical or fraternal. Identical twins are produced by the same fertilized egg that splits into two during the earliest phase of development. The genetic composition of the two fetuses is therefore identical. As a result, identical twins are always the same sex and very similar in their appearance. They often share a common temperament and, over time, seem to develop unusually close emotional bonds with each other.

Fraternal twins are somewhat more common than identical ones, occurring in about 1% of pregnancies. Fraternal twinning occurs when two different eggs are fertilized by different sperm cells at approximately the same time and then grow together in the womb. These twins will not have the same genetic makeup: they might be different sexes, and they will have unique appearances. They may have very different personalities and may even see each other as rivals. Because of their common experiences, fraternal twins may also be each other's best friend.

Early arrival

Twins often arrive early, so wise parents will want to prepare for this. You don't want to be rushing around at the last minute buying and borrowing all that you need.

Feeding options

You can make several decisions ahead of time. For example, will you breast-feed or formula-feed your twins, or even use some combination of the two? There is no reason not to try breast-feeding twins — most mothers produce sufficient milk for the task, though the technique for feeding two babies simultaneously requires some instruction. Breast milk provides the best nutrition for twins as well as for singletons. Still, be prepared to provide supplemental formula should the need arise. It's not so terrible: it can ease a mother's burden and allow fathers to participate more fully in raising their twins.

HOW TO
Raise twins

Most parents of twins learn what works well for them by experience, but there are some basic guidelines you can follow in caring for your babies based on the collective wisdom of parents with twins.

1. **Learn to do things in tandem:** With twins, efficiency is not an option; it is a necessity. Nurse your twins together, walk them together, and definitely try to get them on the same schedule. When you can't, double up, alternate, or, better yet, have someone work with you.

2. **When you are alone with your twins, attend to their needs one at a time:** Infant swings and toys can entertain one baby while the other is looked after.

3. **Know your limits:** If you need extra help or a short break, get it! Don't let yourself become totally sleep deprived. Parenting twins should be more than desperate survival — it should be fun.

4. **Treat each twin as an individual:** They will have their own traits and needs. Although it is natural to view twins as a pair, it's much better if they are encouraged to develop their own unique personalities.

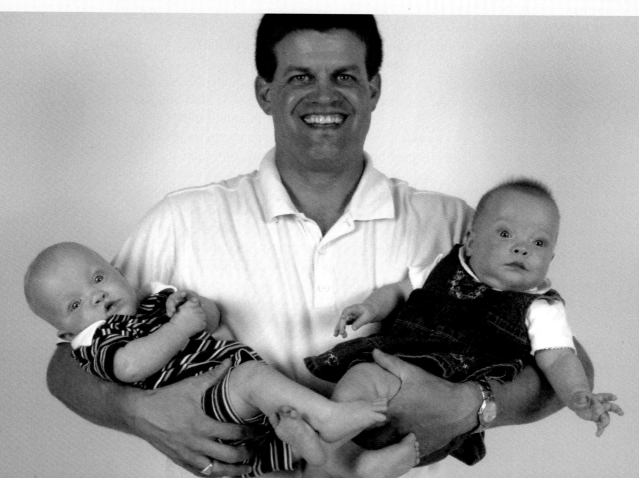

Duplication

You will need to obtain duplicates of most of the usual items needed for the care of infants. If you don't have to buy two of a given product, you will likely have to purchase an equivalent specialized item, such as a tandem stroller. As part of getting set up for twins, it's a good idea to contact parenting organizations specializing in multiple births. They can direct you to sources of the items you'll need and can provide other useful guidance.

Support

Obviously, preparing for twins requires more than just having your home set up. You will want help — lots of it — so arrange it in advance. The best support will be your spouse. Wonderful family bonds tend to be forged when you're parenting twins. Mothers, in-laws, siblings, and close friends are all potential assistants, and are usually overjoyed at the thought of helping out. Arranging this support will make parenting twins a lot easier.

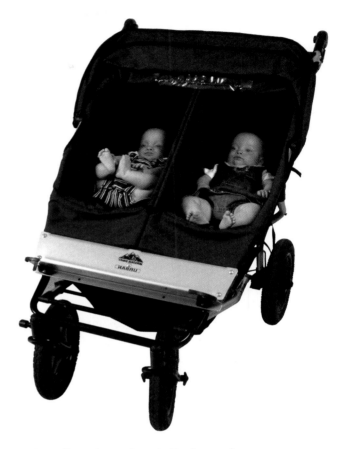

■ You will need a tandem stroller to care for your twins.

Did You Know?

Twin challenges

Things may not initially go as you imagined. Be ready for that and try to be flexible. Twins tend to arrive prematurely, sometimes early enough to need special care. They may need to be monitored in an intensive care nursery, need to be fed with a feeding tube, or require supplemental oxygen. They might become jaundiced and need phototherapy. They might not be ready to come home with you when you are discharged from the hospital. That will likely prove disappointing. When premature twins do come home, their schedules tend to be more erratic for a while. None of these hurdles are insurmountable, but they are challenges you may need to face.

Single parents

When young girls play house or otherwise fantasize about their future roles as parents, it's not likely they dream of becoming single parents struggling to make ends meet or to find enough time in their day to get their chores done. But childhood dreams don't always become reality. Many parents, either by circumstance or choice, are on their own. However rewarding that may be, it's never easy.

Single-parent variations

Single parents are quite a large, heterogeneous group. Many are teenagers who, upon becoming pregnant, elect to keep their baby; some are successful career women who choose single parenthood for personal reasons; others are the victims of family tragedy, such as an accident or disease or unanticipated marital breakdown.

Single parents often worry that, by not providing their baby with the idealized family model, they are somehow putting their child at a disadvantage in life. Nonsense. Single parenting itself is not a roadblock to future success. Just provide the love and guidance that all children need and remember to smile and enjoy life's better moments. The future will look after itself.

Single-parent challenges

There are some harsh realities to life as a single parent. Daily household responsibilities can be hard, if not impossible, to share. Fatigue is a constant companion. If a single parent is busy raising an infant, where does the money needed to pay the bills come from? When can a young teenage mother find time to educate herself — or just have time to be with friends? Who will support the single mother when the burdens lead to understandable tears? Certainly, it is easy to be overwhelmed by circumstances, but, with a little planning, it doesn't have to be that way.

Did You Know?

Single-parent facts

- Approximately one-third of all births in the United States are to unmarried women.
- There are 12 million single parents in the United States.
- Single parents account for 27% of households with children under 18 years of age.
- 84% of children who live with only one parent live with their mother.
- More than 2 million fathers are the primary caregiver to children under 18 years of age.

HOW TO
Succeed as a single parent

Identify your support systems: Who's there to help? Can your parents or siblings help look after the baby some of the time so you can get out? Can they provide financial assistance? How can your friends contribute? Do you have a social worker who can arrange supports to which you are entitled? Explore these sources of support before your baby arrives.

1. Decide how you want to live your life: You should feel in control, not like you are being helplessly swept downstream on the river of life. Set long-term goals and then make short-term plans that will help you fulfill those dreams. For example, if you think you would be happier spending some time at a paying job in the company of your peers, look into daycare options.

2. Clarify your legal rights and obligations: Lawyers aren't cheap, but you need to make sure you and your baby are protected. If applicable, child support payments should be set realistically and payments made promptly. Any custody issues should be clearly resolved before your baby is born.

3. Don't become your own slave driver: You can't work 24 hours a day, 7 days a week. Set aside at least 1 hour each day for yourself — work out, play a sport, go out for a coffee with a friend. Even go out on a date! Just make sure you are recharging your batteries. You will be happier and, therefore, a much better parent.

4. Do something nice for yourself at least once a week: It doesn't have to be something big, just self-indulgent. You deserve that hour-long bubble bath with scented candles and soft music.

5. Don't take your frustrations out on the baby: If the stresses in your life are starting to overwhelm you, get help … right away! Call your trusted loved ones, your doctor or social worker, or Parents Anonymous. Never let things build to the point where you feel like shaking or otherwise hurting your baby.

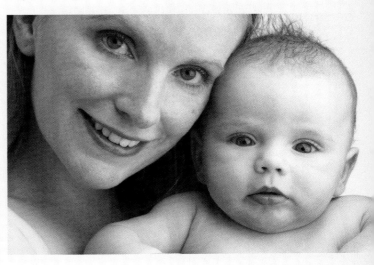

Same-sex parenting

There are many ways to create a family. While it is true that most children join their families after their parents procreate "naturally," modern reproductive technology has provided many other options to allow a couple to become parents, such as artificial insemination or in vitro fertilization.

Although families with parents of the same sex are still relatively rare, rough estimates suggest that between 1 and 9 million children in the United States have at least one parent who is gay. Gay couples considering parenthood face the same issues as heterosexual couples, including major adjustments to time and priorities, as well as the financial and general responsibilities of parenthood.

Gay parenting options

There are two likely scenarios for same-sex parenting. In the first, a biological parent formerly in a heterosexual relationship may "come out" and publicly acknowledge his or her homosexuality. That parent may subsequently become involved in a new relationship with a same-sex partner. This scenario, however, rarely occurs in a baby's first year.

In the second scenario, a gay couple may have a child via donor sperm fertilization or a surrogate, or may arrange an adoption, either domestically or internationally. This issue is still controversial. The various legislative jurisdictions in North America have reacted with a wide range of tolerance, from none to complete acceptance.

Did You Know?

Being raised by same-sex parents

What are the effects on a child of being raised by parents of the same sex? Objectively, not much, based on the available research. Adopted children follow common paths and have similar outcomes regardless of their parents' gender. There is no apparent difference between gay and heterosexual parents with regard to emotional health, parenting skills, and attitudes toward parenting. There do not seem to be any differences between the toy, game, activity, dress, or friendship preferences of boys or girls with same-sex parents and those with heterosexual parents. The same holds true for gender identity and sexual orientation in adulthood.

Clearly, additional issues must be faced by families with same-sex parents, but, for the most part, these families tend to cope with them.

As a result of these findings and to guarantee that children adopted by same-sex couples enjoy their full legal benefits concerning custody issues, health insurance, and death benefits, the American Academy of Pediatrics has issued a position statement on adoption that is favorable to same-sex couples.

Adoption options

Since ancient times, children have been adopted by parents who legally care for the child as their own. How a family comes into being is not as important as how well that family functions as a loving entity.

International adoption

Recently, there has been a sharp increase in the number of children being adopted from overseas, particularly from China and the countries of the former Soviet Union. In the past 10 years alone, nearly 20,000 newly adopted children have arrived in Canada and about a quarter of a million have come to the United States.

The experiences of these foreign-born youngsters are often quite different from those of domestic adoptees. They often come from orphanages or similar institutions where care is suboptimal: some degree of malnutrition and neglect is common. These children come to a better life in North America, and the fulfillment they usually provide to their new parents can bring tears to the driest eye. But, to be fair to all, adoption of a child from overseas must be a carefully thought-out decision. There are often special problems that must be faced; proper preparation is essential for success.

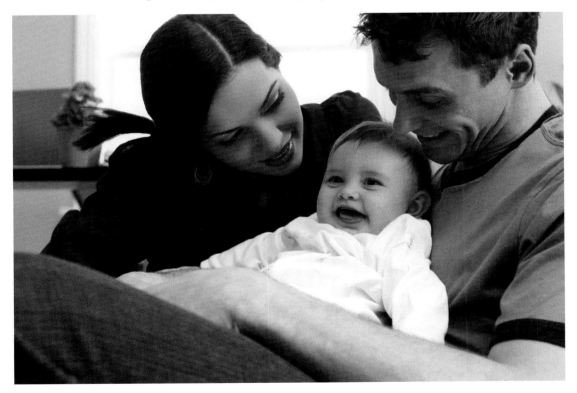

Guide to

Adopting internationally

To help parents who have adopted or are considering adopting internationally, the Canadian Paediatric Society has offered some useful suggestions. For additional information, consult the Amercian Academy of Pediatrics.

BEFORE YOU GO
- Consult an international adoption group specializing in adoptions in the country you are considering.
- Check with your doctor to ensure that both you and your household members are properly immunized.
- Find out if you will need anti-malaria medication while you are overseas.
- Arrange for expert medical care to be available for your new son or daughter when you return. About 50% of internationally adopted children will have a medical diagnosis that is not obvious from a physical examination. Developmental problems, fetal alcohol syndrome or effect, and nutritional problems, such as rickets, are all too common.
- Ask the adoption agency to obtain reliable hepatitis B and HIV testing.

WHILE YOU'RE THERE
- Get your child's medical and immunization records.
- Be skeptical about their accuracy.
- Get to know and enjoy your baby.

WHEN YOU BRING YOUR CHILD HOME
- In addition to the prerequisite immigration physical examination, have your baby carefully checked by your doctor.
- Bring all of the routine immunizations up to date, or at least have your baby tested for immunity.
- Other tests, such as for tuberculosis, may be needed.
- Give yourself and your child time to bond. Adjustment problems and difficulties with eating and sleep are understandable.

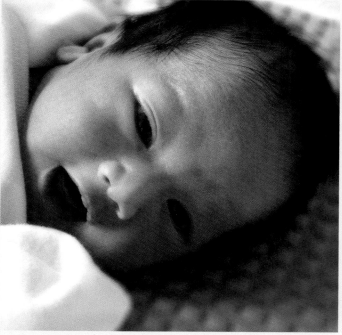

HOW TO
Care for an adopted child

Parenting, for all its rewards, is never easy. Adopting a child doesn't make it any simpler. How, then, should adoptive parents best prepare for parenting, and what special advice should they receive during their baby's first year? No single set of guidelines will deal with every scenario, but some common principles are worth following.

1. Do your homework: Make sure you have learned and understood your various options for dealing with infertility and parenting. Meet with your doctor or gynecologist. If, for whatever reasons, you decide to adopt, discuss the matter with the appropriate family services agencies in your community. If you are considering an international adoption, you may want to contact a social worker who specializes in this type of adoption and consult with parents who have chosen this route.

2. Before you adopt, feel comfortable with the idea of adoption: It's an emotional topic. At some level, you will likely feel disappointed about your infertility, and you will have to deal with these feelings. Often, you have to examine what creating a racially mixed family will entail, not just for the adopted child but also for your family and friends. What about the financial stress that goes with parenting, adoptive or otherwise? Remember, most problems are best resolved when they are handled honestly and openly.

3. Always protect your child's rights: Insist that friends, relatives, and society view your adopted infant as a full and equal family member. Furthermore, ensure that a trans-racially adopted child is respected as an individual and yet is encouraged to have pride in her ethnicity and heritage.

4. Accept that there are bound to be some uncomfortable moments: Some comments that were not made maliciously will still bother you. Somebody, somewhere, sometime is bound to say something like, "My, your baby must really look like her father!" You might want to prepare for these sorts of questions in advance.

5. Finally, never forget that the little baby you nurture and feed, whose diapers you change and whose fever you treat, is your baby: In every respect, you have earned the right to be called "Mommy" and "Daddy."

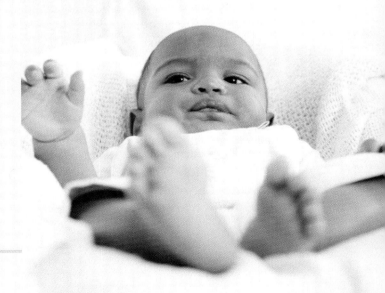

Frequently asked questions

As family doctors and pediatricians, we answer many questions from parents. Here are some of the most frequently asked questions. Be sure to ask your health-care providers any other questions that arise. If they don't have the answers, they will refer you to a colleague who does.

Q: Everybody thinks I'm going to have a boy. What is the best test to predict the sex of my baby?

A: There are a lot of popular myths, theories, and old wives' tales that claim the ability to predict a baby's sex. How you are "carrying" your baby, whether you have indigestion, and many other signs have been put forward as trustworthy indications of fetal sex. But the only reliable way to determine the sex of your child is to have a health-care provider examine the genitals on an ultrasound or the chromosomes in a sample of amniotic fluid taken by amniocentesis. Discuss with your partner whether you really want to know — it is a very personal decision. If your answer is yes, ask your health-care provider to check for you.

Q: I have heard about cord blood banking. Is this a good idea?

A: There is no simple answer to this question. Since the first cord blood banking service started in 1991, many programs have been created to collect blood from the umbilical cord at the time of delivery and store it for potential transplantation at a later stage. Some programs are funded by large not-for-profit organizations, such as the National Institutes of Health and the American Red Cross, while others are private for-profit businesses. In most not-for-profit programs, the cord blood collected is available to anyone who needs it and is a "match," while the for-profit businesses encourage parents to bank their infant's cord blood as a form of "biological insurance" for their own private use.

No accurate estimates exist of the probability that children will need their own stored cord blood cells in the future (estimates range from one in 1,000 to one in 200,000). While cord blood has been shown to be curative in patients with a number of serious genetic, blood, cancer, and immune disorders, there is no evidence yet of its safety or effectiveness for the treatment of a cancer in the child (donor) at a later stage.

The latest recommendation from the American Academy of Pediatrics is that cord blood donation should be discouraged if it is to be directed for later personal or family use (biological insurance) because most conditions that might be helped by cord blood stem cells already exist in the infant's cord blood. However, if a sibling in the family has a known condition that may potentially benefit from cord blood transplantation, directed cord blood banking should be encouraged. Cord blood donation should also be encouraged when the cord blood is stored in a bank for public use, but parents need to realize that this blood may not be accessible in the future for private use.

If you wish to have your baby's cord blood collected, you must give your consent in writing. The procedure is not painful for you or for your baby. The blood is taken from the umbilical cord, which would otherwise normally be discarded.

Q: Getting ready for our new baby seems to require making a lot of purchases. With my wife starting maternity leave, how will we be able to afford all these necessary items?
A: Truthfully, parenting is never cheap, nor does it come without sacrifice. Kids have expensive needs at all ages: first, tons of diapers; then, hundreds of outfits; next, sports equipment and music lessons; and later, college tuition. Fortunately, we can convince ourselves that it is all worthwhile. Like all projects, preparing for a new baby requires budgeting. If you are joggers, you might choose to splurge on a special stroller, but that might mean the rocking chair in the nursery comes from a garage sale. As long as your purchases meet the safety code, used or less expensive items are just fine. Friends and relatives are always trying to find the perfect baby gift. A tactful suggestion or a creative partnership can transform an unwanted teddy bear into the change table you really need. Finally, it's important to remind yourselves that the happiest children aren't always the ones with the most expensive stuff: as the song suggests, love is all you really need.

Q: My husband is adamant that our baby boy be circumcised. My reading suggests that it is better to leave the foreskin alone. This is one of our first decisions as parents, and I want to get it right … without a fight. What should I do?
A: Parents often disagree about what is best for their child. Now is as good a time as any to establish some general guidelines on how you, as a couple, will handle these disagreements. For starters, it's best to review the facts involved in this or any issue. A little extra information can sometimes be quite persuasive. Then, see if there is some strong emotional reason behind the adamant viewpoint. A non-practicing Jew, for example, may still want to retain some cultural bonds with his past. For him, circumcision takes on extra importance.

Do your best to understand your spouse's position. You would be surprised at the number of men who want their son to look just like them, ignoring the obvious fact that their infant son will lack pubic hair. A little extra skin should be no big deal. Try to retain your sense of humor. If the issue is still unresolved after forthright discussion, meet with your health-care provider, who can mediate the dispute.

Sam's Diary

June 30 (birth minus 34 weeks)

What an amazing day — we found out we were pregnant using a home pregnancy test, and today we saw Dr. Murphy, who is going to be your doctor — she is really nice, you'll really like her! She confirmed that you are expected to arrive on February 23rd — we are excited and can't wait to see you. We told your grandparents, but asked them to keep it a secret until you are 12 weeks old. Now we need to find an obstetrician.

July 29 (birth minus 30 weeks)

We saw Dr. Barrett, the obstetrician, for the first time today — he is going to take great care of you and Mom when you arrive. You are now 10 weeks old, and we had our first ultrasound a few weeks ago.

September 28 (birth minus 21 weeks)

In the beginning, we had to see Dr. Barrett every 4 weeks. Daddy came

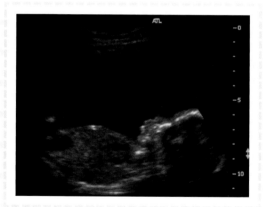

with us to our last visit, on August 24th. Today, you are 19 weeks old, and we got to see you really nicely on the ultrasound. You were moving around so much that the technician had a difficult time seeing all of you in detail. Then you must have been really tired, because you seemed to be asleep and so still. We saw your spine, your legs and arms and fingers.

October 21 (birth minus 18 weeks)

We felt you for the first time a few weeks ago. You were making gentle little movements, kind of like a bubble popping. After a while, you started to kick very gently, and Dad could feel that too. Last night, while we were lying in bed, we felt you moving about and kicking like we have never felt before — you went on for quite a while, and we loved it. Dad loves to put his hand on Mom's tummy and feel you.

October 27 (birth minus 17 weeks)

We heard your heartbeat quite a while ago through a special machine called a Doppler. Last night Dad tried listening to your heartbeat by putting his ear on Mommy's tummy — and he thought he could hear you quite clearly. You even gave him a gentle kick in the ear while he was trying to listen.

November 17 (birth minus 13 weeks)

You are now 6 months old, and you've really grown in the last 2 weeks. There is no mistaking that Mom is pregnant now. Your Mom is attending aquafit classes — a special exercise program for moms-to-be. It is interesting to be with and talk to other expectant mothers. You just received your first present: a pair of knitted booties from your Auntie Rae. We went out to buy you a car seat and a crib for your room. It was exciting and fun to be shopping for you, although there were so many choices to pick from.

February 8 (birth minus 2 weeks ... or maybe not)

Mom and Dad saw Dr. Barrett this morning after an ultrasound to make sure you were safe and sound in Mom's tummy. What a surprise! On examination, Dr. Barrett found that Mom was already 3 cm dilated and that it was time for us to meet you. He decided to induce you 2 weeks early, as Mom's placenta was a little calcified. Luckily, Mom had packed her bag yesterday, because we had to go straight over to the hospital. We were given a really nice big birthing suite, and the nurses broke Mom's water and administered a drug called pitocin, which gets labor started. Dad went home to get Mom's bag and called all her clients to tell them that you were on your way and that their appointments would have to be canceled.

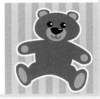

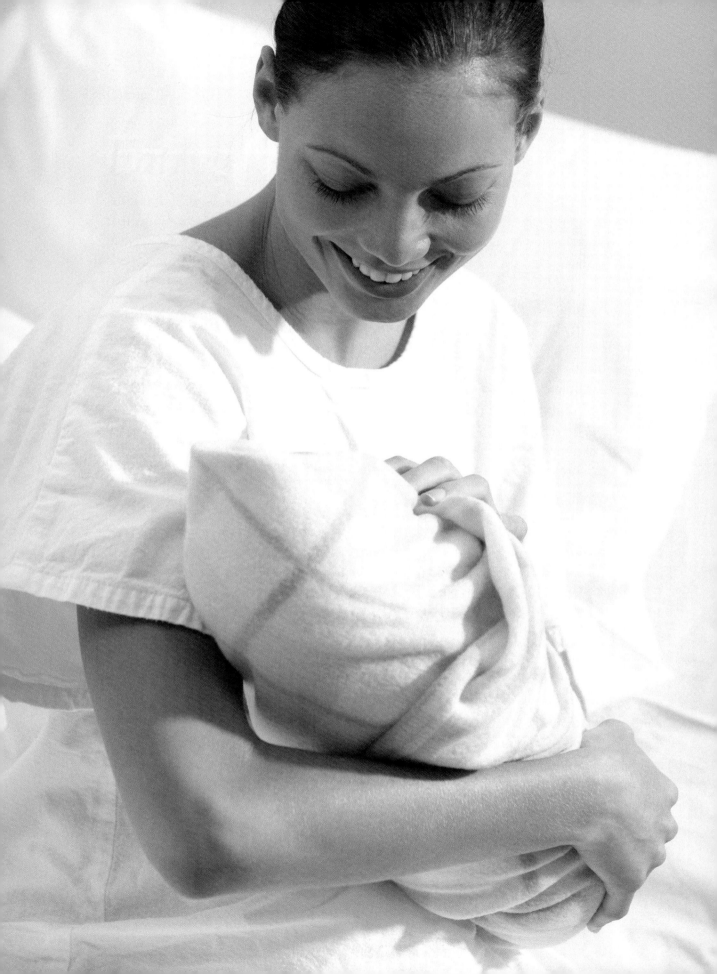

Your Baby's
First Few Days

In the beginning

You've probably spent months anticipating your baby's arrival, daydreaming about life with your baby and making plans for your family's future. The nursery is painted, the receiving blankets are folded, and the car seat is installed.

But if this is your first child, you may not have considered what exactly will happen during the first few moments of your baby's life. Who will be present in the delivery room to help out with this amazing transition? How will your baby react as he moves from the comfort and warmth of his mother's womb to the strange air-breathing world? If anything goes wrong, what can be done?

Who will be present?

This is a short, exciting, and crucial time. What exactly takes place will differ depending on the setting in which you've chosen to deliver and the ease with which your labor has progressed. While we will attempt to answer most of your questions, as always, speak to your health-care provider beforehand about what to expect.

By now, you have probably decided on the people you would like with you in the delivery room, whether it be just you and your partner or another support person who will provide assistance and encouragement. Besides your personal choices, the faces in the delivery room will largely depend on the setting in which you have chosen to give birth.

Remember that it is your right to know the role of everyone in the delivery room, so if they do not introduce themselves, be sure to ask. Regardless of how your birthing center is run, you should be confident that team members are specialists and know their own skills and limitations. It is better to discuss any questions or concerns you might have, rather then let them fester and grow.

Midwife

If a midwife will be attending your delivery, she will likely be at your side throughout the active stages of labor, working with you to deliver your baby and attending afterwards to the needs of the newborn and the mother.

Family doctor "on call"

Alternatively, you might choose your family doctor to serve a similar role. Increasingly, family physicians work as part of a larger group who rotate being "on call" for deliveries. In this scenario, one of your doctor's trusted colleagues may deliver your baby. Your prenatal records will be available, of course, to the physician on call. Be sure to speak with your doctor beforehand so that you know the specific arrangements of this practice.

Obstetrician

Another option is to have an obstetrician — a surgeon who specializes in delivering babies — attend you. If yours is a complicated situation, the obstetrician may be consulted by your midwife or family physician to provide expertise and help you with the delivery.

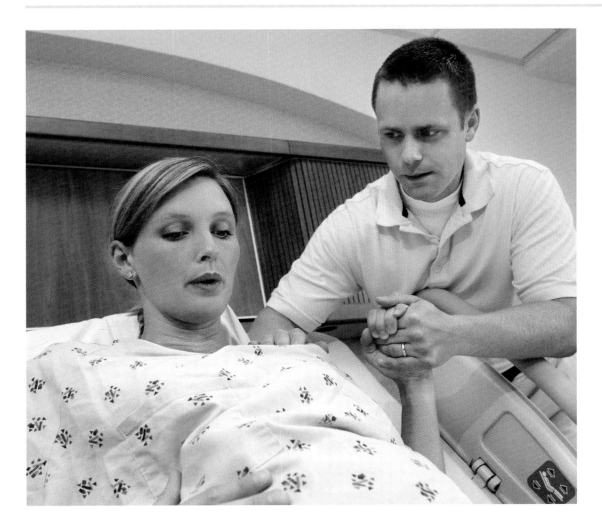

Nurses

Labor and delivery nurses are also an integral part of the birthing process. One specific nurse will usually be assigned to you and will follow your progress in the labor and delivery room. This nurse is often the key to good communication, as she will liaise between you and the other health-care professionals. If you have specific requests or wishes about your labor and delivery experience, make sure to inform your nurse. If your labor has progressed without complication, do not be surprised if the physician on call is not present until the last minute, to aid in the baby's delivery.

Respiratory therapist

Respiratory therapists are often part of the health-care team, particularly at larger centers. They are expert in the baby's airway and breathing. At some hospitals, they attend each birth; at others, they are called when needed, to ensure that your baby's lungs are adapting appropriately to the air-breathing world.

Anesthesiologist

Last but not least, an anesthesiologist, a physician with expertise in pain control, will follow your case. The anesthesiologist can help reduce the discomfort of a vaginal birth or provide anesthesia in the event a Caesarian section is required. Pain control is usually achieved with an epidural or, more rarely, with a general anesthetic.

Baby's first moments

Presentation

Most babies have a vertex presentation, meaning the head is the first part to be delivered. After this happens, there may be a brief pause as the baby's mouth and nose are suctioned with a small catheter or suction bulb to clear the airway, preparing your baby for his first breath. Then it's time for the rest of the body to emerge. The moment you've been waiting for has finally arrived!

Umbilical cord

The umbilical cord, which connects the baby to the placenta, will then be cut using a pair of surgical scissors. This is painless. Cutting the umbilical cord can sometimes be a ceremonial act done by the mother's partner.

Warming your baby

After ensuring a clear airway, drying and warming your baby are the first items on the agenda. Cold air is a shock to a newborn, who has spent 9 months surrounded by warm amniotic fluid. Warm blankets are used to wrap your baby, and delivery rooms are equipped with a radiant warmer

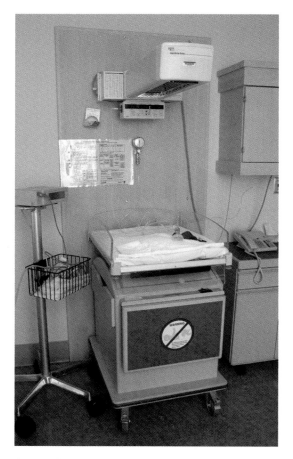

(a small table with overhead heaters) to help regulate your baby's temperature.

If there are no other concerns, your baby can be placed immediately on your abdomen to be warmed with his skin against yours. Once your baby is warm, dry, and breathing comfortably, he will be weighed, swaddled in a receiving blanket, and given to you or one of your support people to hold.

First breast-feeding

If you have decided to breast-feed your baby, it's time to start right then and there. After all, a mother's job doesn't end with the delivery — it's just beginning!

Did You Know?

Apgar score

More than 90% of newborns make the transition from fetal to extrauterine life smoothly and do not require any more intervention. To aid the health-care team in assessing the baby's ease of adaptation, an Apgar score is assigned at the baby's first and fifth minutes of life. The Apgar score, developed in 1952 by Dr. Virginia Apgar, is a numerical score between 0 and 10. It is based on the baby's heart rate, respirations, muscle tone, response to stimulus, and color.

Keep in mind that the score is *not* a predictor of long-term health. A low score alerts the health-care team that the newborn may need continued medical intervention or simply further observation. A difficult labor and delivery or prematurity are the more common reasons for lower

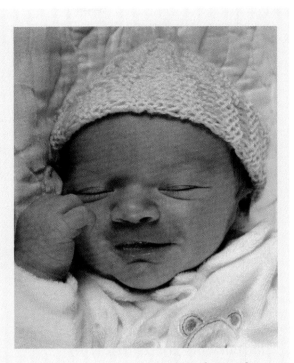

Apgar scores. It is important to know that even a perfectly healthy baby usually does not score 10 out of 10.

Apgar score card

(bpm = beats per minute)

Sign	Score			Total
	0	1	2	
Heart rate	absent	slow (<100 bpm)	>100 bpm	
Respirations	absent	slow, irregular	good, crying	
Muscle tone	limp	some flexion	active motion	
Reflex irritability (catheter in nares, tactile stimulation)	no response	grimace	cough, sneeze, cry	
Color	blue or pale	pink body, blue extremities	completely pink	
				/10

Assisted delivery

No matter how well you try to prepare yourself for your labor and delivery, it will remain somewhat unpredictable. Like so much in your baby's first year of life, there will be some things out of your control. You will need to be flexible in your approach. Rest assured that the team you have assembled to help you with your labor and delivery will have the expertise to guide you on a safe journey into parenthood.

Induction of labor

Some women may not go into labor spontaneously, or, when they do, the labor may progress very slowly. Health-care providers may need to induce or augment labor to protect the health of the baby and the mother.

Indications for induction

- Post dates. The pregnancy has gone past 42 weeks, and there is concern about the placenta's ability to provide adequate oxygen and nutrition to the baby.
- High blood pressure or diabetes that could harm the baby.
- Uterine infection.
- The waters have broken, but contractions haven't begun, which raises the risk of infection reaching the baby.

Common ways to induce labor

- Ripening the cervix. This is done by inserting a small tablet in the vagina, against the cervix, which softens and thins the cervix and helps start the process of labor.
- Medications to start uterine contractions. Oxytocin (Pitocin) is given intravenously to start or strengthen uterine contractions.

- "Breaking the waters." This involves breaking the membrane that encircles the baby and amniotic fluid (waters), which can be felt through the opening of the cervix. It is done with a small, sharp instrument. The procedure is not painful and is usually followed by a sudden gush of warm fluid.

Fetal monitoring in labor

During your labor, your baby's condition will be closely monitored, which generally involves monitoring the fetal heart rate. The fetal heart rate usually varies between 120 and 160 beats a minute. It often drops during a contraction, but should recover shortly thereafter.

External monitors

Externally, a contraction stress test is used to monitor the fetus. Very sensitive ultrasound monitors are placed on your abdomen, held by a belt, with a jelly-like substance (which usually feels cold) applied to the skin to help conduction. These monitors sense both the baby's heart rate and your uterine contractions. They tell your caregivers how well the placenta is providing oxygen to the baby while under the stress of your contractions.

Internal monitors

If external monitoring is not working well, or if your health-care provider is concerned that the baby might be distressed, she may decide to proceed to internal fetal monitoring, which is more accurate. A thin wire electrode connected to a monitor is placed in a plastic guide that is moved through the cervix (after the membrane has been ruptured) and placed on the baby's scalp. The plastic guide is removed, and the electrode remains in place.

Caesarian section

A Caesarian section (C-section) refers to the delivery of the baby through a surgical incision made in the mother's lower abdominal wall and uterus. This is generally done by a specialist (obstetrician or gynecologist). In North America, the incidence of C-sections has almost doubled in the last 10 years. Rates vary among different jurisdictions, but in the United States, 30% of deliveries are now by C-section.

In some cases, your health-care provider may recommend that an elective, or planned, C-section be performed before you have a chance to go into labor on your own. If, during your labor, there are concerns that the fetus is becoming distressed and could suffer some damage, an emergency C-section may be required.

Indications for a Caesarian section

- The baby's position in the uterus (feet, buttocks, or shoulder first) makes it unlikely that you will be able to deliver vaginally.
- There is an anatomical problem. For example, if the placenta (afterbirth) is implanted very low in the uterus, the baby's descent could cause massive bleeding.
- There is a high risk that the uterus will rupture, because the mother has undergone previous uterine surgeries, such as C-sections. (Some women are able to deliver vaginally after a C-section; it depends on the indication for the C-section and the type of incision that was used.)
- The mother has an underlying medical condition, such as heart disease, high blood pressure, genital herpes, or diabetes.
- There is more than one baby. Twins or triplets may sometimes be delivered more safely by C-section.

Procedure

Caesarian sections are often done while the mother is awake, but with an epidural or spinal anesthetic administered. This means that you will feel no pain in the area of the surgery while it is being performed. If the baby becomes unexpectedly distressed, there may not be enough time to perform an epidural. In that case, the mother may be put to sleep with a general anesthetic for the duration of the surgery.

The average hospital stay after a C-section varies from 3 to 5 days, although mothers are encouraged to get out of bed as early as possible. Full recovery can take 4 to 6 weeks. Mothers who deliver vaginally usually require only a 1- to 2-day hospital stay, and they make a full recovery more quickly.

Risks associated with C-section

Caesarian sections are a common and generally safe method of delivering a baby, and most mothers and babies will do very well, but you should discuss the indications, risks, and benefits in your case with your health-care provider. The risks involved include:

MOTHER
- Bleeding
- Infection
- Injury to the bladder or bowel
- Blood clots in the legs and lungs

BABY
- Possible increased risk of some breathing problems, as the fluid on the lungs hasn't been "squeezed" out by the trip down the birth canal
- Anesthetic used in the mother can cross the placenta and make the baby a little more sleepy and sluggish

Episiotomy

This procedure involves cutting the skin and subcutaneous tissues between the vagina and anus to enlarge the vaginal opening, providing extra space for the baby to emerge through at the time of birth. An episiotomy may also prevent these tissues from tearing. The area will be numbed with a local anesthetic.

Estimates of the incidence of this procedure vary from 65% to 95% of vaginal deliveries in the United States. However, episiotomies are not considered routine and are not always necessary. Episiotomies do not always prevent the skin from tearing at the time of the birth, although the tear is likely to be smaller and to heal more easily. Episiotomies do not necessarily speed up a normal birth, and there is no indication that they help to prevent the bladder control problems that some women get after having a baby. Speak to your health-care provider about her approach to episiotomies, and discuss the pros and cons ahead of time.

Forceps and vacuum extraction

There are certain circumstances in which other forms of assistance are required to help the mother deliver her baby.

Forceps

Forceps, which are shaped like big steel spoons, are placed into the vagina, around the baby's head. When they are correctly in place, the forceps click together. When the uterus contracts and the mother pushes down, the forceps are used to pull the baby's head through the vagina. They are then removed, and the rest of the baby is delivered normally. You may see some temporary bruising over the baby's cheeks or ears, but this tends to disappear within a few days.

Vacuum extractor

The vacuum extractor includes a pump mechanism to create a vacuum, and a big suction cup that fits on top of the baby's head. With each contraction, as the mother pushes down, the doctor pulls on the suction cup, helping to guide the baby's head out of the vagina. The pump is then switched off, and the rest of the baby is delivered normally. You will likely see some swelling of the scalp tissue, below where the suction cup was placed, but this disappears over a few days.

Indications for forceps or vacuum extraction

- The mother is exhausted, and the baby's head is just ready to be delivered.
- The mother has had an epidural and doesn't feel the urge to push.
- The baby's head is in a posterior position.
- The baby is in a breech position (feet or buttocks first).

Did You Know?

Breech babies

Although many babies are "heads-up" early in the pregnancy, most of them will rotate into a head-down position in the mother's uterus prior to delivery — which is why the head emerges first. If the baby has his head up and either his buttocks or feet pointing down close to the time of delivery, this is called the breech position.

Situations that make a breech position more likely include:

- Multiple pregnancies
- Too much or too little amniotic fluid
- An abnormally shaped uterus
- Premature delivery

If your health-care provider suspects that the baby is in a breech position, this can be confirmed by ultrasound. Most doctors prefer to deliver breech babies by C-section because they consider it safer for the baby. Some doctors may try to turn the baby in the mother's uterus, using a procedure called external cephalic version, but this is not appropriate for all mothers.

Birthing features

Most babies are not picture perfect, at least not immediately, so don't be surprised! Features to be prepared for include the vernix caseosa, which is a white waxy coating covering the baby's skin. Some blood may be on the baby from the delivery process. There may be bruises, and possibly marks from instruments (forceps or vacuum extractor) used during the birth. Your baby's face may be puffy and slightly misshapen, and the head may be molded as a result of having been delivered through the vaginal canal. Many babies with significant molding have an accompanying caput, a diffuse swelling of the scalp, which heals on its own in just a few days. Some babies have one or two well-demarcated bumps called cephalohematomas, which are large bruises under the scalp. While they are usually benign, cephalohematomas usually take a few weeks or even months to heal. Acrocyanosis (bluish hands and feet) is both common and normal at this early stage and produces a point deduction in the Apgar score.

Regardless of these slight physical imperfections, your baby will be beautiful, and your memories of your baby's birth will undoubtedly be indelible. Still, be sure to pack a camera so that your memories of these precious moments may be preserved.

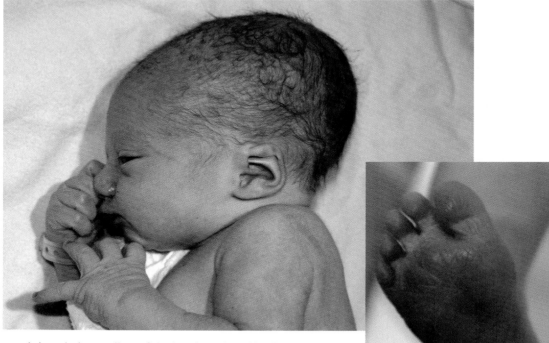

■ (Above) The swelling of the head produced by the tight squeeze through the birth canal in labor is called caput. This swelling disappears in a few days. (Right) The reddish blue color of the foot is called acrocyanosis. It is quite normal.

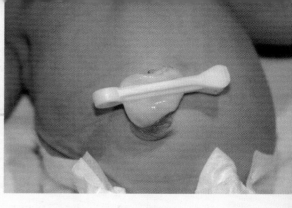

HOW TO
Care for the umbilical cord

The umbilical cord is the vital connection between a baby and the mother's placenta. In the womb, the umbilical cord is the lifeline delivering all the nutrients and oxygen the fetus requires. Despite its vital role in pregnancy, this cord is not needed after birth.

Immediately following your baby's delivery, a plastic clamp will be placed on the cord, close to the baby, and the cord will then be cut. What remains is the stump of the umbilical cord. This residual stump is initially white and fleshy. You may even be able to see the ends of the three vessels through which blood has flowed over the past 9 months. The plastic clamp will probably be removed before you leave the hospital, and, gradually, the stump will shrivel, dry, and fall off, resulting in the baby's "belly button." The time that the umbilical stump takes to fall off or separate can vary, but it usually occurs within the first 2 weeks after birth. Until that happens, most new parents naturally wonder how they should best care for the cord.

Infection risk

Because the umbilical stump is an "open" connection between the baby and the outside world, it is at risk of infection. You may have heard or read a lot of differing advice about what to use to clean the cord and how to care for it properly. Studies show that measures such as cleaning the cord with antiseptics or protecting it with gauze dressings offer no advantage over simply keeping the cord clean and dry. In fact, using rubbing alcohol to clean the cord may prolong the time before it falls off, thus increasing the time it is at risk of infection. Sponge baths have historically been recommended until the cord separates, but again, there is no evidence that this is a better practice than giving your baby a total body wash and patting the stump dry afterwards.

How do I care for my baby's belly button?

So, what should you do? As with most parts of a healthy baby's body, you don't need to do very much!

1. Wash the cord with baby soap and water as part of your newborn's bath and keep it dry between baths.

2. To prevent irritation, try folding down the top of the diaper so that it's not rubbing against the cord.

3. Be mindful of signs of infection: warmth, redness, or swelling in the skin immediately surrounding the stump, or the presence of pus or other foul-smelling discharge. If any of these arise, contact your baby's doctor.

4. Don't worry if there is a drop or two of blood on the diaper in the first day or two after the cord falls off: that's normal. You should only be concerned about a steady or persistent oozing of blood.

5. Finally, do not try to hasten the umbilical stump's separation. This will happen naturally.

Before you know it, your baby will have a cute little belly button as a reminder of his attachment to you!

HOW TO
Swaddle your baby

Many babies find comfort in being tightly bundled, perhaps feeling closer to their 9 months spent warm and snug in the womb. You can learn how to swaddle your baby from the nurse or midwife caring for you and your baby after the delivery, but the basic approach is as follows:

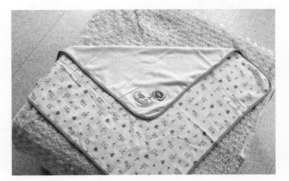

1. Use a large, square receiving blanket, if possible.

2. Lay it in front of you like a diamond and fold the top corner down to the blanket's center.

3. Lay your baby on his back with his head just above the folded corner.

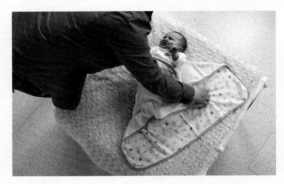

4. Holding his right arm down alongside his body, bring the right side of the blanket over his shoulder and down across his body, tucking it snugly under the left side of his body.

5. Bring the top of the left side of the blanket down just a little, to cover the left shoulder, and wrap the remaining blanket across your baby's body, tucking it under him on the right.

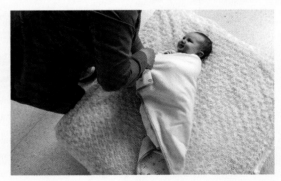

6. Straighten his left arm along his side while you bring the bottom corner up, tucking the blanket under his left shoulder and around his side.

7. Make the wrap fairly snug — loose blankets are unsafe for little babies.

8. If your baby enjoys being swaddled but prefers his hands free, or if you rely on his hand and mouth cues for hunger, you can still follow the technique above, but simply bend your baby's arms at the elbows, leaving his hands free.

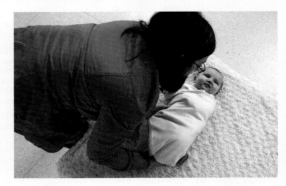

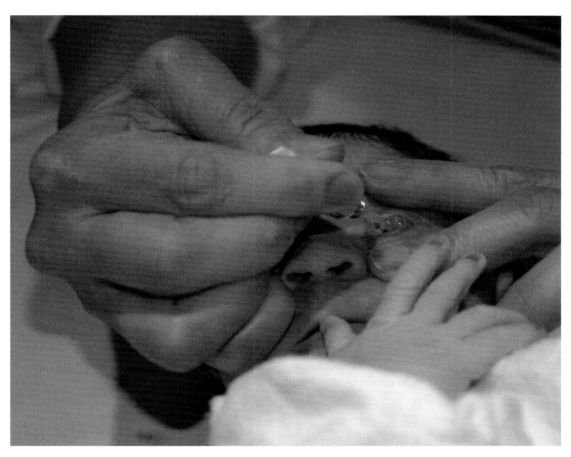

Eye ointment

From the moment your child is born, the health-care team will be concerned with preventing serious newborn diseases. Antibiotic eye ointment is given to all babies soon after birth to prevent serious eye infections that might occur in the first month.

While most eye infections and discharge are minor, some may be caused by a bacterium (*Neisseria gonorrhea*) that can lead to permanent visual loss. Gonorrhea is a sexually transmitted infection that often causes no symptoms in affected women, but may be contracted by the baby during delivery. You should not feel judged by your health-care team when they provide the eye ointment for your baby: the American Academy of Pediatrics and the Canadian Paediatric Society, for example, recommend that *all* women be screened for this infection during their pregnancy and that every infant be treated the same way with an eye ointment.

This ointment is an antibiotic, generally erythromycin, which is squeezed from a small tube into each eye. Years ago, a silver nitrate solution, dropped into each eye, was commonly used for this purpose, but it often caused a chemical irritation, so it is used much less often now.

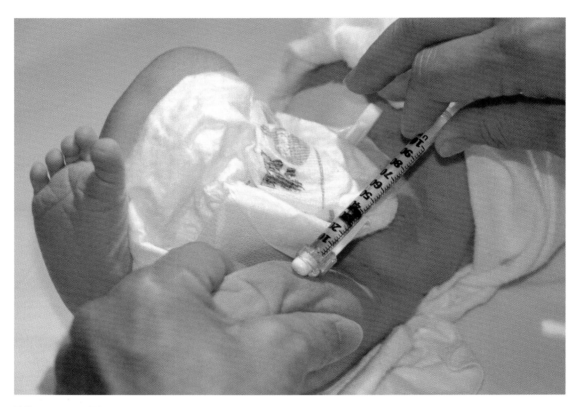

Vitamin K

Vitamin K is essential for normal blood clotting to occur. It is given to all newborns within the first 6 hours of birth to prevent serious bleeding, a condition called "hemorrhagic disease of the newborn." This bleeding can occur unexpectedly, as early as the first day of life and as late as 2 months of age.

The most effective way to give vitamin K to the newborn infant is via an injection into the muscle of the baby's upper thigh. This method of administration is the same as the one used later for your baby's early immunizations. Obviously, parents do not enjoy seeing their children being given a needle, especially so early after birth. But it's worth it. Many studies have shown that vitamin K given by mouth is considerably less effective than the injectable form, especially in preventing bleeding that may occur between 3 and 8 weeks of age. This form of bleeding is more likely to occur in the brain, clearly a serious event.

Given these risks and benefits, the Canadian Paediatric Society and the American Academy of Pediatrics both recommend the injectable form of vitamin K for all babies. If parents do refuse the needle for their baby, oral vitamin K is available, but the increased risk of serious bleeding is an important consequence to understand.

Most parents look back at their baby's first few hours and have no recollection that this medication was given. Parents should feel good that they helped get their baby off to the best possible start in life.

Nursing right away

If you have chosen to breast-feed your baby, there is no better time to start than right in the delivery room. Most infants are awake and ready to learn how to nurse in the first 2 hours of life. Provided that your baby has adapted to life outside the womb and is stable, he can be placed on your abdomen, skin to skin, within minutes of birth.

Many babies in this position, when given time, will find the breast on their own, latch on, and begin to feed. Even if the baby doesn't feed right away, the skin-to-skin contact itself has been shown to be good for the newborn: it keeps him warm and stabilizes vital parameters, such as heart rate and breathing.

Breast-feeding anxiety

While breast-feeding is natural, it is also a learned skill, one that you and your baby will become expert at over time. Remembering that both of you will learn with experience helps to alleviate the anxiety about breast-feeding that many mothers feel. The most important initial step is to ensure that your baby has a proper latch. This will help to avoid sore or cracked nipples and will optimize your baby's milk intake. With this in mind, don't hesitate to ask for help. Nurses, midwives, and lactation consultants are all valuable resources. Take advantage of classes offered by hospitals or as part of prenatal courses, which will help prepare you before your baby is even born.

Quality, not quantity

Nursing at this early stage is not about quantity. Healthy full-term babies do not need to be fed immediately. When they do begin to nurse, they will benefit from colostrum, the special breast milk that is produced before regular breast milk comes in, usually after 3 to 5 days. Colostrum is high in immunoglobulins — proteins that will strengthen your baby's immune system — and while it is not produced in large quantities, it is all your baby needs for the first few days.

Be flexible

Of course, there are sometimes circumstances in which the baby requires medical attention and is not able to nurse right away. It is important to be flexible — you may initially be disappointed to miss this bonding experience you had imagined having with your newborn. Rest assured that your baby's caregivers have his best interests at heart. The nursery staff will assist you with expressing milk and preparing you for the time when breast-feeding becomes possible. Remember that many babies who are not nursed "right away" are still successfully breast-fed.

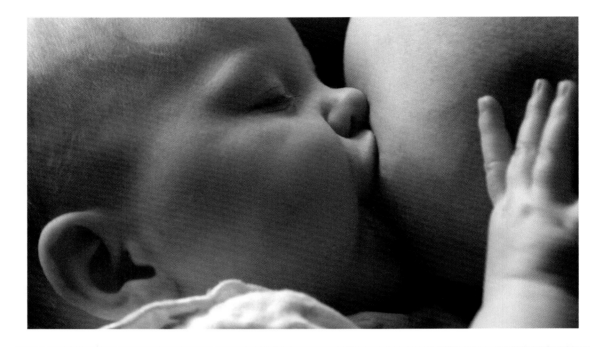

Did You Know?

Rooming in

Gone are the days of a central nursery where healthy babies were cared for primarily by the nurses and brought to their mothers only for periodic visits or feeding.

- In the current age of family-centered care, provided that you are both healthy, you and your baby will stay in the same room from birth until hospital discharge. A small bassinet for the baby is usually set up alongside your bed, and the two of you will be cared for by the same nurse.

- This is a time for you to begin to get comfortable handling your baby, swaddling him, feeding him, and hearing his cues. You will begin to understand and respond to your baby's needs. Of course, if yours has been an uncomplicated delivery, your stay in the hospital may be as brief as 24 to 48 hours. You're certainly not expected to learn all about your baby in that short a time, but it's an important start.

- Remember that your nurse is there to help, so don't hesitate to ask questions as they arise.

- You may not be able to room in with your baby if you are too unwell to care for him or if he requires closer observation or treatment in the nursery. In this situation, your caregivers will make it easy for the two of you to spend as much time together as you both can handle. In most cases, you will have an opportunity to spend at least one night rooming in together before you are discharged.

The first days and nights

Newborns' sleep patterns

Countless hours lie ahead when you will interact with your wakeful new baby: just don't expect this to start immediately. Nature seems to have told our little ones that mothers need rest following labor and delivery.

In the first day or two of life, babies are usually very quiet and sleepy. They have some recovering of their own to do! By the second night, newborns are often much more awake, and you will more than likely hear their frequent cry. Over the first few weeks, babies generally sleep for periods of 2 to 4 hours, wake with a cry, feed, and settle back to sleep. Babies often even doze off during a feed. A diaper change midway through, or between sides if you're nursing, will help to stimulate the baby and allow him to finish his meal. Though a newborn's alert periods are initially very brief, they will gradually lengthen, and by a month of age, babies are usually alert for a few hours a day.

Keep in mind that there is considerable individual variation in these patterns; as long as your baby is thriving, there is no "right" or "wrong" amount of time for him to be awake or asleep.

Sleep when your baby sleeps

Whatever your baby's pattern, you should try your best to sleep when the baby is sleeping. This is a period when mothers are recovering from the birthing process, learning how to breast-feed if they've

chosen to do so, and adjusting to their baby's round-the-clock feeding schedule. Few new parents are well rested, but making an effort to sleep when you can will help to keep your body healthy and your mind clear, allowing you to take better care of your newborn.

Evening routine

Some babies differentiate day from night faster than others, sleeping longer stretches at night. As long as your baby is growing well, there is usually no need to wake a thriving full-term newborn for feedings, though you should check your individual circumstances with your baby's doctor. To encourage your baby to recognize when it's nighttime, try to initiate an evening routine early on. This may include a warm bath, reading a story, and listening to or singing the same lullaby each night.

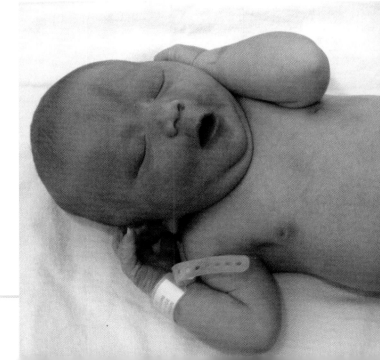

Rapid eye movement

During longer stretches of sleep, you may hear your baby murmuring or stirring; he is likely in the REM (rapid eye movement) stage of sleep, which is naturally accompanied by movement. By picking him up in response to every little sound, you may actually be disturbing the natural rhythm of sleep. If he seems comfortable but is simply stirring or making gentle sounds, let him be until he truly cries, indicating that his sleep cycle is over. That said, when your baby does cry, it's important to respond. The newborn stage is too early to follow the adage "let your baby cry." For at least the first 4 to 6 months, it is important to foster a sense of security. You can accomplish this in part by responding to your baby's cues, teaching him that you are there for him when he needs you.

Stool and urine patterns

After having a baby, you will probably discuss bowel movements and voiding patterns much more than you ever thought possible! Rest assured that it's not just because changing a baby's diaper may be new to you.

A newborn's stooling and voiding patterns are, in fact, very important because they indicate whether your baby is getting enough to eat. This is particularly true in breast-fed infants, because the quantity of their intake is difficult to assess.

Meconium

Your baby's first bowel movements, formed in the intestines before birth, will be black and sticky. This excretion is called meconium and should be naturally eliminated over the first 2 to 3 days of life. If it persists beyond the first few days, it may be a sign that your baby is dehydrated and at increased risk for jaundice, something you should check with your baby's doctor. Following the meconium, stools will gradually transition from brown to green to yellow. Breast-fed babies have very loose and seedy bowel movements, whereas the stools of bottle-fed babies tend to be more pasty yellow.

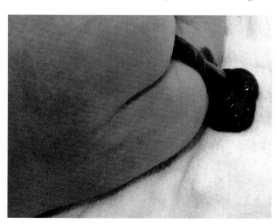
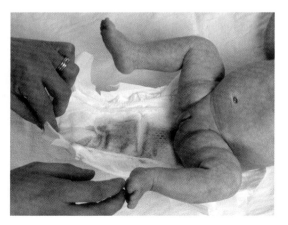

■ Your baby's first bowel movements will appear black and sticky. This stool is called meconium. Once your breast milk comes in, the stools will become a yellowish color with a soft and seedy consistency.

Newborn urine and stool patterns

If you're breast-feeding, don't expect your baby's diapers to be soaking wet until your milk comes in, usually after the first few days. Remember that, at first, your baby will be getting colostrum, the initial form of breast milk. Generally speaking, colostrum is about quality rather than quantity, so don't fret too much about the volume produced. It can often be difficult to estimate urine production. Absorbent disposable diapers make judging whether your baby has voided, and how much, particularly difficult. So can the mixing of urine with soft stools.

Other signs, such as your baby's meconium, weight, and a physical assessment of hydration by your health-care provider, can serve as indirect indicators that the baby is voiding well. If you have a boy, you may catch him urinating between diaper changes. If you have a girl, you can put cotton balls in her diaper to reassure yourself that she is passing urine.

Baby's age	Wet diapers each day	Stools each day
1 day old	At least 1 wet diaper (a wet diaper feels like at least 2 tablespoons/25 mL of water poured on a dry diaper)	At least 1 to 2 sticky dark green/black stools
2 days old	At least 2 wet diapers	At least 1 to 2 sticky dark green/black stools
3 days old	At least 3 heavy wet diapers (a heavy wet diaper feels like at least 4 to 5 tablespoons/50 to 75 mL of water poured on a dry diaper)	At least 2 to 3 brown/green/yellow stools
4 days old	At least 4 heavy wet diapers	At least 2 to 3 brown/green/yellow stools
5 days old	At least 5 heavy wet diapers	At least 2 to 3 stools, getting more yellow
6 days old and after	At least 6 heavy wet diapers At all ages, urine should be clear to pale yellow with almost no smell	At least 2 to 3 large yellow stools Stools can be soft like toothpaste or seedy and watery
After 1 month		After 1 month, some breast-fed babies may have 1 very large yellow stool every 1 to 7 days. This is normal as long as the stool is soft and the baby is healthy. It is also normal for some breast-fed babies to have many stools each day.

Adapted by permission from Toronto Public Health, *Breastfeeding Your Baby* (Toronto: Toronto Public Health, 2000; rev. 2002).

HOW TO
Change your baby's diapers

Of all the joys that accompany having a baby, endless diaper changes are probably not high on your list! However, they're a necessary part of parenthood and will become so much a part of your routine that you will (hopefully) come to think of diapering as no big deal. This is a skill you will learn very quickly, but here are a few pointers to get you started.

How often do I need to change my baby's diaper?

There are no rules. Clearly, when he has had a bowel movement or when he is uncomfortable, it's time for a diaper change. Otherwise, a good routine in the newborn period is to change the diaper either before, in the middle of, or after a feed. You might find that changing your baby at the start of a feed is a good tactic, not only to ensure a clean diaper, but to stimulate him so he is alert for his feeding. There is no need to wake a sleeping baby just to change his diaper.

What equipment do I need?

Newborn diapers

A supply of clean diapers is, of course, essential! Though you'll need to buy some diapers before your baby is born, don't stock up on too many in the newborn size. Even average-sized babies will quickly outgrow them, and it's better for diapers to fit slightly big than too small.

Count on using about 80 diapers per week for the first month of your baby's life. Once you're sure that he will be in one size for a while, check out discount stores or bulk sections, where disposable diapers will often be boxed in larger quantities at much lower prices.

Baby wipes

You will also need baby wipes to wipe the baby's diaper area after a bowel movement. For sensitive newborn skin, either use a hypoallergenic, fragrance-free commercial brand or buy a supply of cotton pads or towelettes, which can be wet with warm water. The latter are often available at medical or surgical supply stores, and a small spray bottle of water kept by the change table will make wetting them convenient, eliminating a last-minute dash to the closest sink.

Skin cream

A petroleum jelly, such as Vaseline, may be useful for minor irritations or keeping dry skin moist. A zinc-based barrier cream will cure many diaper rashes by providing a barrier between the baby's stool and his skin. If a rash is not responding to these simple solutions, have your doctor take a look. A mild steroid cream may be prescribed to reduce the inflammation. A simple yeast infection, which is easily treated, may be diagnosed. If your baby's diaper area is clear, clean, and dry, no ointment or cream is necessary.

Change of clothes

Despite proper diapering technique, babies often soil or wet not just their diaper, but their clothes too, so make sure to have a change of clothes or an extra sleeper available!

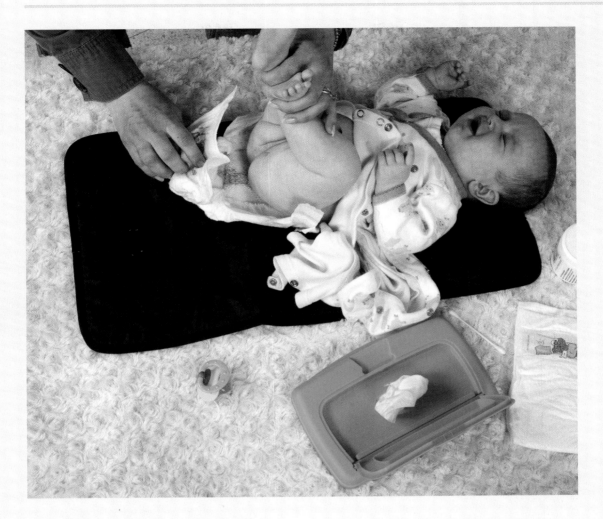

How do I change a diaper?

Your baby's first diaper changes will take place while you're still in the hospital or, if you've delivered at home, in the presence of a midwife. This provides an ideal opportunity to have the nurse or midwife demonstrate how to change a diaper.

1. With your clean diaper and wipes ready to go, place your baby on his back and undo his current diaper by undoing the tapes at either side.

2. If there's a bowel movement, you can use the dirty diaper to wipe away some of the stool as you pull the diaper out from under the baby. Roll the dirty diaper up and secure it with the tapes, creating a little bundle that can be set aside until you can properly dispose of it.

3. Lifting your baby's legs up by the ankles, wipe him clean with a baby wipe or wet cotton pad, being sure to get into the creases. For girls remember to wipe from front to back.

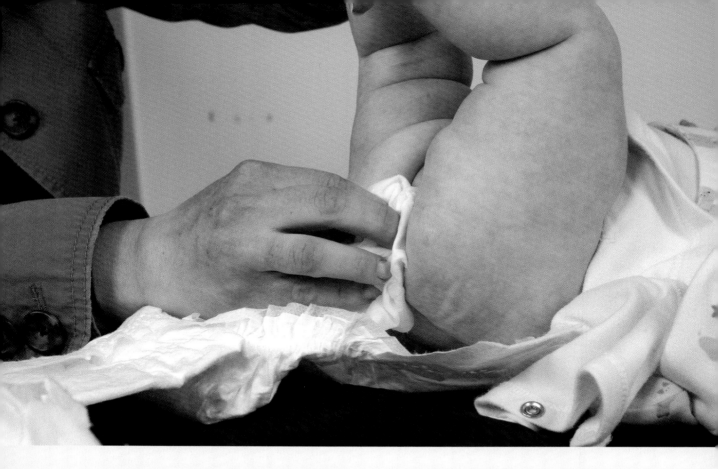

4. Next, slip a clean, open diaper under your baby, with the tapes at the back.

5. Bring the front of the diaper up between his legs, open the tapes, and fasten them snugly on either side. If you're using cloth diapers, there are often systems available with Velcro tabs, so that you don't need to use pins. If you do use pins, be sure to keep them well out of the baby's reach, and aim them away from him when fastening his diaper. Until the umbilical stump has fallen off, remember to fold the top edge of the diaper down below the cord.

6. For baby boys, ensure that the penis is aimed down when securing the clean diaper to minimize leakage out of the top of the diaper. Also, try to keep the penis covered with a clean diaper during the diaper change to protect everybody in the vicinity!

7. In the newborn period, bowel movements can also be fairly sudden and explosive, so try to make the changing process as quick as possible, and remember to keep a change of clothes or an extra sleeper handy.

8. When your baby's clean diaper is secure, dispose of the dirty one in either a diaper pail or a well-sealed garbage can. There are also several types of odor-free diaper disposal bins on the market. If you are using disposable diapers and your municipality has a composting program, check to see whether diapers are accepted. Given the number of diapers you will go through, you'll feel good about helping to save the environment!

9. Always wash your hands after a diaper change. If it is difficult to get to the sink with baby in tow, try keeping a bottle of alcohol-based hand sanitizer by the change table.

Where should I change my baby's diaper?

It's important to have a change table or dresser with a plastic change pad, preferably in your baby's room. Make sure that this table is the right height for you, so that you can comfortably keep a good grip on your baby without getting unnecessary backache. If you're on the go or changing your baby in a different room, any surface, including the floor, is fine, as long as you can keep a firm hand on him the entire time. Keep a cloth or plastic sheet handy to put under him to keep both the baby and the surface as clean as possible. Keep some colorful rattles or small toys close by: your baby will begin by gazing at them; as he gets older, he'll be able to play with them, which will help to distract him while you're changing his diaper. Of course, this is another good time to chat or sing to your baby, calming and entertaining him throughout the process.

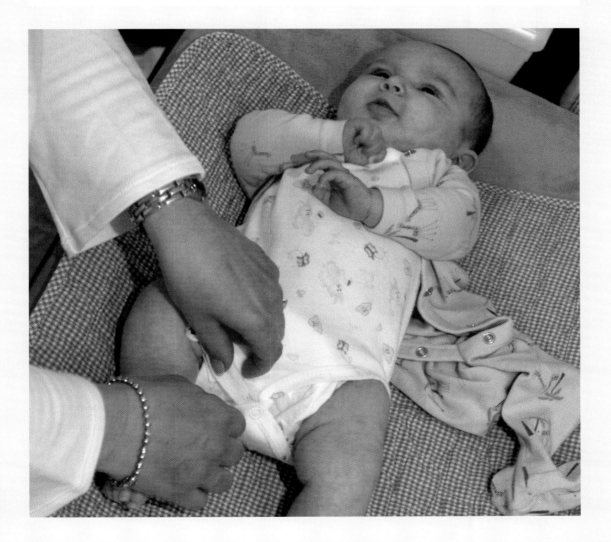

Spitting up

Once breast milk comes in and the volume a baby receives with each feed increases, it is normal for babies to spit up. Called gastroesophageal reflux, this is different from forceful vomiting; it's an effortless regurgitation of milk, due to an immature valve action between the baby's esophagus and stomach.

Reflux facts

Reflux usually does not bother the baby. If the milk made its way to the stomach before coming back up, it may have curdled and will smell sour, but otherwise the contents will be just like the milk your baby was fed. Like most things, there is much variation in how often each baby spits up. Some do so only occasionally, while others spit up many times each day.

The reality is that, if your baby is a "spitter," there is little you will be able to do to change this! Rest assured that it will come to an end. Spitting up usually lasts at least 6 months, but it may persist for up to a year. Many parents find that it settles down when their baby begins to sit upright or starts on solid foods.

Thriving

To parents, the quantity of regurgitated milk often makes it look as though the whole feed has come back up. The reality is much less alarming. Despite appearances, the majority of babies who spit up are keeping down all the milk they need, and the amount that is regurgitated is relatively insignificant. The ultimate test is whether or not your baby is gaining weight. If he is feeding well and thriving, his spitting up is an annoyance but not a concern, even if it looks like nothing is staying down.

Spitting-up strategies

Though there is no cure for simple spitting up, you may find these strategies helpful:

- Avoid overstimulating your baby following his feeds.
- Burp him in the middle of each feed, as well as at the end.
- If you're bottle-feeding, ensure that the bottle is tilted up to minimize the amount of air in the nipple.
- Stay as dry as possible by keeping a burping cloth over your shoulder (cloth diapers work well), carry a change of clothes for your baby when you go out, and stock up on laundry detergent!

Red flags

There are a few "red flags" that signal that your baby's spitting up might be worrisome. If you notice any of these features, consult with your baby's doctor:

- Your baby is not gaining weight.
- He is arching with feeds.
- He is refusing to feed.
- He is gagging or coughing persistently.
- There is green, brown, or blood in the spit-up.
- He is vomiting forcefully.

Gagging and choking

When your baby is born, he transitions from the fluid-filled womb to an air-breathing environment. It's not surprising that, despite having his mouth and nose suctioned at the time of delivery, your baby may sputter and spit up some remaining fluid and mucus within the first few hours of life. Once his lungs are clear, however, this should not be a regular occurrence.

What to do

Once an infant's feeding is established, it is normal for him to occasionally choke on breast milk or formula after taking a big gulp. This is particularly true if you are nursing and have a fast let-down reflex or if your baby spits up and sputters on the regurgitated milk. When this happens, lean your baby forward or over your shoulder, gently rub his back, and allow him to cough and catch his breath.

If your baby is choking and is unable to clear his own airway, call for an ambulance immediately. If necessary, and if you know how, you can initiate infant CPR. Every parent should be prepared with knowledge of infant CPR. Ask your local hospital or public health unit for available courses.

Household safety considerations

If you have a toddler running around, be careful that he doesn't inadvertently give the baby something he can choke on. This is of particular concern when your baby is a little older and begins to explore everything with his mouth — including his sibling's belongings. Keep small objects out of reach, ensure that toys don't have little pieces that can break off, and be sure to supervise your infant when he begins transitioning to solid foods. Keep in mind that Band-Aids are a choking hazard for babies. As an alternative, use gauze and tape when necessary.

What about Mom?

While your newborn is adjusting to life outside the womb, your body must also recover from labor and delivery. Though most women's recovery following the birth of their baby is uneventful, there are risks, such as excessive vaginal bleeding or infection. If you experience any warning signs, contact your doctor.

Red flags for mothers

- Very heavy bright red bleeding that soaks through a pad in an hour
- Clots larger than a golf ball
- Blood with a bad odor
- Fever greater than 101°F (38°C)
- Difficulty passing urine or burning when passing urine
- Increased pain or swelling in your stitches
- Redness, swelling, increased tenderness, or drainage from an abdominal incision

Bleeding

It is normal to have vaginal discharge, called lochia, for several weeks following your baby's birth. Initially, it will be bright red, like a heavy period, so come to the hospital prepared with a supply of overnight maxi pads. The discharge will gradually decrease in quantity and lighten in color. If you are breast-feeding, you may initially notice menstrual-type cramps and an increase in your discharge while your baby feeds. This is normal and will decrease with time.

Perineum care

Following a vaginal delivery, your perineum (the area between the vagina and rectum) will be sore, and you may have dissolvable stitches to care for. To keep the area clean, use a spray bottle to rinse with warm water after toileting, and use toilet paper to gently pat yourself dry from front to back. In the first 24 hours, it is okay to use ice packs to help decrease swelling, but never apply the ice directly to your skin. Your nurse will show you how to use a sitz bath, a portable plastic basin that sits on the toilet bowl, allowing you to bathe your stitches in warm water and soothe the area.

At home, you can continue to use the sitz bath or take regular warm baths. Many women also find it helpful to sit on a ring for the first few days to alleviate pressure on the swollen perineum. Don't hesitate to ask your nurse for pain medication, such as acetaminophen, as needed.

To help strengthen pelvic floor muscles that have been stretched during delivery and to maintain bladder control, be sure to continue the Kegel exercises you were likely advised to do during your pregnancy. These can be described as squeezing muscles to prevent urination, and can be started immediately after delivery, a couple of times per day.

Nutrition and hydration

It is important that you eat well and drink lots of fluids following delivery. You need to regain your strength and energy so that you can properly care for your baby, and, if you're breast-feeding, keeping yourself well fed and hydrated will optimize your milk supply. It is normal not to have a bowel movement for the first couple of days after delivery, but be sure to eat plenty of fiber to decrease the risk of constipation and the accompanying discomfort.

A stool softener may also be prescribed. This will also help alleviate hemorrhoids (swollen veins around the rectum), which can be particularly sore after a vaginal delivery. Hemorrhoids should decrease or disappear within 6 weeks; in the meantime, avoid constipation, lie on your side as much as possible or use a ring to sit down, have sitz baths, and, if needed, ask your doctor for a hemorrhoid cream.

C section

If you've had a Caesarean section, you will generally stay in the hospital longer than those who have delivered vaginally, and your recovery will be longer. Pace yourself and, like all new mothers, ask for help. You will be given pain medication and instructions from your health-care team about how to care for your incision.

Warning signs to report to your doctor include fever, increased redness, tenderness or swelling along the incision, bleeding or discharge from the site, and separation of the incision.

Mood changes

At this momentous, long-awaited period in their lives, many mothers are surprised to find that their moments of joy and contentment are interspersed with negative feelings. Tears may flow very easily, and you may experience sleeplessness, loss

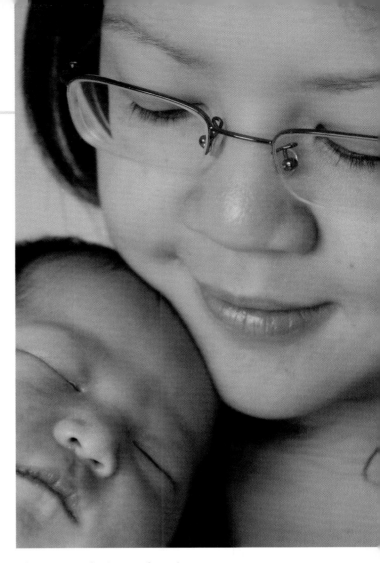

of appetite, feelings of inadequacy, or exaggerated concerns about your baby.

Discuss these feelings with your partner and caregivers. In most cases, the emotions are transient and quite manageable once a new mother catches up on her sleep and sees her baby thriving. But if they persist or intensify, these symptoms suggest that you are suffering from postpartum depression. It's more common than people think, occurring in about 15% of pregnancies, and should not be ignored or viewed as a sign of weakness. In the great majority of cases, postpartum depression is treatable, and it should be treated — for both the mother's sake and that of her baby. This is no time to display a "stiff upper lip."

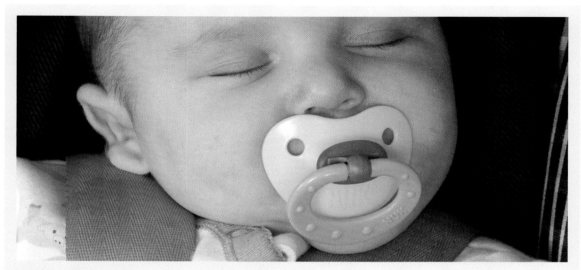

Did You Know?

Pacifiers

Using a pacifier is a controversial practice. Parents will need to assess the pros and cons based on the needs of their own child.

What are the advantages? A pacifier can be used to satisfy a baby's need to suck in between feedings, which may provide comfort and help him to settle. A pacifier is better than a thumb because it is less likely to cause problems with future tooth development and is easier for the parent to control. Recent medical research suggests that using a pacifier may decrease the risk of SIDS (sudden infant death syndrome, or crib death).

What about the disadvantages? Not using a pacifier properly (starting too early or using it for too many hours of the day or for too long) can lead to problems with breast-feeding, dental cavities, overbite, and, possibly, ear infections.

If you choose to use a pacifier, limit the time you allow your child to suck on it.

Allow it at sleep time and to give comfort until 12 months, then plan to give it up. If your older child still wants a pacifier, give him the choice of swapping it for something (a reward) or throwing it away. A reward chart may be helpful as positive reinforcement. Praise your child when he has given it up. Do not give in to his requests for the return of his pacifier.

Pacifier use guidelines

- Don't start using one until breast-feeding is established.
- See if your baby is hungry, tired, or bored before resorting to the pacifier.
- Sterilize it in boiling water before first use and clean with soapy water after each use.
- Don't dip it in sugar or honey.
- Don't tie it around the baby's neck (this can cause strangulation); instead, use a clip with a short thread.
- Don't use it all day long.

The newborn exam

While your baby will be assessed several times between birth and hospital discharge, at least one complete examination should take place before he is sent home. This exam is done by a physician or a nurse practitioner. If you already have a doctor picked out for your baby, and your doctor has privileges at the hospital where you are delivering, she will likely come herself to meet and examine her new little patient. Otherwise, the hospital will have the on-call doctor perform the exam; you don't need to worry about making the arrangements.

Ask questions

Your baby's first physical exam can, in most circumstances, be carried out with you present, right in your hospital room. Many parents appreciate this opportunity, because the doctor can explain any findings and offer guidance about what the next few days will bring. It's also a great time to ask questions about your baby, so make a list ahead of time if you get the chance!

Don't be alarmed if it seems like your doctor has missed an essential part of the physical exam. Much can be accomplished via keen observation; as he walks into your room and begins to talk to you, your doctor will already be observing your baby and taking note of his condition. If you're at all concerned, don't hesitate to ask questions. This exam is just the first of many that will take place in the infant period.

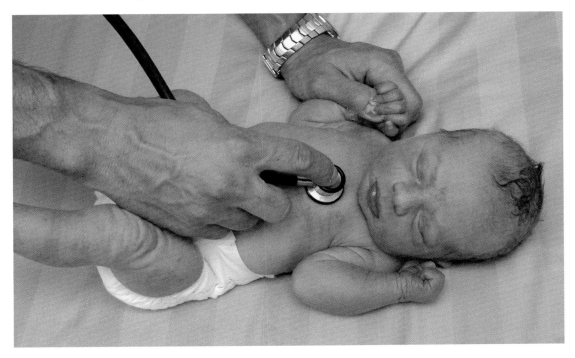

Procedure

As you might imagine, the examination of a newborn infant is much different from the adult exam you are likely familiar with. Don't be surprised if the physician first asks you questions about your own medical history, as well as your pregnancy and delivery. Since your health and that of your baby are directly linked, these questions are all relevant.

A "head to toe" examination is very rarely performed on an infant; rather, a flexible approach is taken to work around the ever-changing state of the baby. When the baby is sleeping, it is an ideal time to listen to his heart and lungs, while crying provides a perfect opportunity to examine inside his mouth! Regardless of the order in which it is performed, the health-care professional will be certain to cover each part of the physical exam.

Growth

Your doctor will note your baby's weight and measure his length and head circumference. She will plot these measurements on a graph that shows how big your baby is in comparison to other newborns. How your baby compares with others is not in itself important, but rather provides a reference point from which your child's growth can be followed over time. You should make a note of these initial measurements and keep a record of them.

Head and neck

Babies are born with two soft spots, or fontanelles — one on top of the head and a smaller one at the back of the head. The physician will feel for these fontanelles and for the suture lines, or small spaces, that separate the skull bones. These soft spots and spaces are necessary to allow for

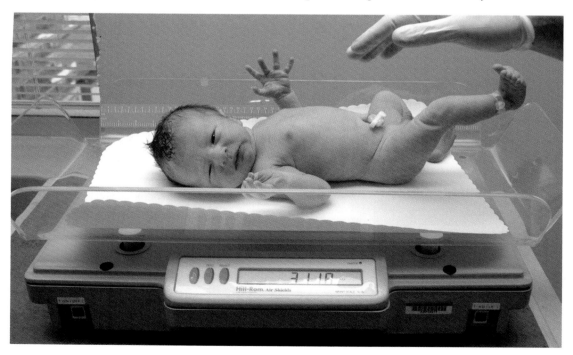

your baby's head to grow, and will all close naturally over time.

Your doctor will also observe your baby's eyes and look into them with an ophthalmoscope, examine his ears and nose, and look into his mouth. Don't be surprised if she puts a clean finger into your baby's mouth, making sure that the palate, or roof of the mouth, is intact, and checking that he is able to suck. Finally, the neck will be checked for any unexpected lumps or bumps.

Chest

Your doctor will watch your baby breathe, listen with a stethoscope to the heart and lungs, and feel for his pulses. Important pulses to check for, called the femoral pulses, are found in the creases in the groin, so you will notice your doctor feeling these with the tips of her fingers.

Abdomen

With the palm of her hand, the physician will feel for the organs of this region — in some newborn babies, the kidneys and the edge of the liver and spleen are palpable. She will also examine the umbilical stump and inspect the anus to ensure that it is open. It will be helpful for her to know if your baby has already passed meconium, the initial newborn stool.

Genitalia

The doctor will examine the genitalia of both boys and girls to ensure that they appear normal. In boys, the testicles will be palpated to check that they have descended from the abdomen (where they start off in fetal life) into the scrotum.

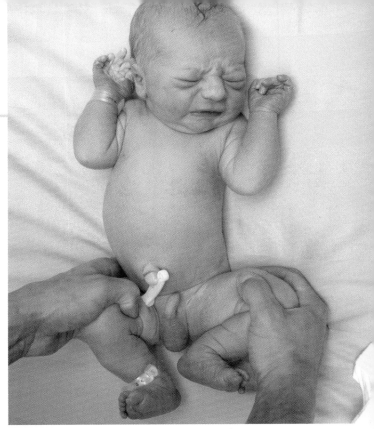

■ Examining the hips for dislocation.

The genitalia are often a bit swollen and/or pigmented in the first few days. This is entirely normal.

Skeletal system

Your baby's arms and legs will be checked, and he will be turned over so that his back and spine can be properly examined. His legs will be rotated to ensure that they are properly in their sockets. While this is often uncomfortable for your baby and can make him cry (and, therefore, is usually left to last), congenitally dislocated hips (also known as developmental dysplasia of the hip, or DDH) are not uncommon and, if detected early, are easily treatable.

Skin

Your baby's skin will be examined for birthmarks or rashes. Many rashes are normal in the newborn period, and your doctor will usually be able to reassure you during the examination.

Reflexes

Babies are born with several reflexes that will gradually disappear over time. Your doctor will elicit some of them, checking your baby's neurological system. They are often fun for parents to watch!

A few examples include the "Moro" reflex, in which the physician will gently support your baby's head while letting it drop, which will result in both arms quickly extending outwards and then coming back together; the palmar and plantar grasp reflexes, in which the baby's fingers or toes will curl around your finger when it's placed on the palm of the hand or the sole of the foot; the rooting reflex, in which the baby's head will turn toward you and his mouth will open (looking for food) as you stroke his cheek alongside his mouth; and the tonic neck reflex, in which the baby takes up a traditional fencing posture when you turn his head to one side, with one arm extending toward the side of his gaze and the other arm flexing.

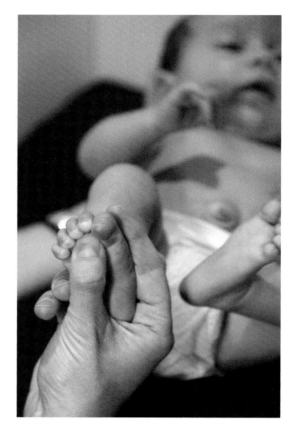

■ (Above) Plantar grasp reflex; (Below) Palmar grasp reflex.

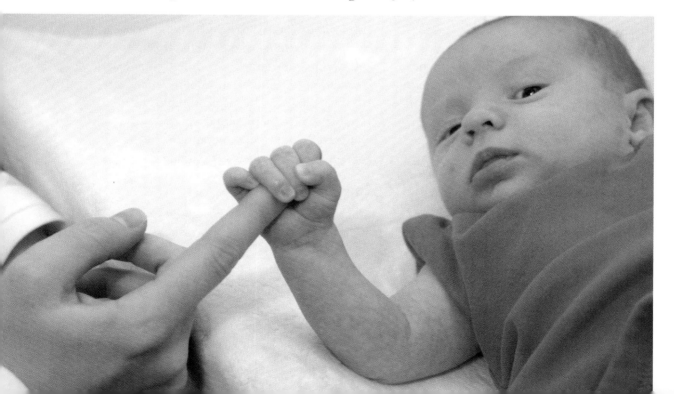

Did You Know?

Ear care

Your baby's ears require very little specific attention. The outer ear can be cleaned along with the rest of the body during the baby's bath. There is no reason to stick any object, be it your finger or a Q-tip, into your baby's ear canal. In fact, this is a dangerous practice.

You will see earwax in your baby's ear: it's natural and is the body's way of protecting the eardrum. It does not need to be washed out, but rather will make its own way to the outside of the ear and fall out on its own.

There has been wax in children's ears for a lot longer than there have been cotton swabs on the ends of sticks. If you're worried that your baby's earwax is blocking his ear, speak to your doctor about your concern rather than attempting to remedy the problem yourself.

Did You Know?

Penis care

The penis is made up of the shaft and the rounded end, called the glans, which is covered by the foreskin. Some parents choose to have their son circumcised, others don't.

UNCIRCUMCISED

At birth, the foreskin is attached to the glans. The two will gradually separate naturally, usually within 2 years, but sometimes over a longer period of time.

You should not try to separate the foreskin from the glans; this could be harmful to your baby. At this age, pulling the foreskin back to expose the glans will probably cause more problems than it prevents. Rather, simply wash the penis externally during your baby's bath, using soap and water just as you would the rest of his body.

CIRCUMCISED

If you choose to have your baby circumcised, the penis will require some attention for a few days following the procedure. The health care provider who performs the circumcision will provide you with specific instructions for care. Generally, petroleum jelly is all that is needed. It is applied directly to the penis with every diaper change until the wound is healed. A small amount of bleeding is normal within the first day or two and is not usually a cause for concern. If there is a large amount of blood or the bleeding is not stopping, see your baby's doctor. Sponge baths are recommended for the first 4 or 5 days, until the scab falls off. After this, when the wound is healed, the circumcised penis is simply washed with soap and water along with the rest of the body in the bath.

HOW TO
Bathe your baby

Newborn babies are small, squirmy, and slippery. It's no wonder that the thought of bathing one is enough to make a new parent's heart race! Relax. Before you know it, giving your baby a bath will be just one of many new tasks at which you are an expert. Your nurse will give your baby his first bath before he leaves the hospital. This is a wonderful opportunity for you to watch, learn, and ask questions.

How often should newborns be bathed?

Once you get home, you do not need to bathe your baby every day. Before he begins to crawl and get really dirty, two to three times a week is adequate. Of course, the diaper area should be cleaned well with each diaper change, and, if your baby tends to spit up, it is helpful to use a damp washcloth in between baths to clean the baby's neck folds.

With time, you may find that your baby's baths have become a part of his routine, enjoyed by you both. In this case, feel free to bathe your baby as often as you like. However, if your baby's skin is sensitive, try limiting the use of baby wash, a very mild soap, to two to three times per week. The rest of the time, simply bathe with water.

What schedule is best for bathing?

There is no right or wrong time of the day to give your baby a bath, though many parents find that the warm water helps to relax their baby before bedtime and also helps to establish a bedtime routine. Try to avoid a bath time when your baby is likely to be hungry, because he will inevitably be upset. It is also not a good idea to bathe a small infant immediately after a feed because he will be more likely to spit up.

What equipment is needed?

Have everything prepared before you undress your baby, to minimize the time that he is undressed and potentially cold.

- Baby wash (milder than soap; avoid dyes and perfumes)
- Washcloth
- Towel (a hooded one is not essential but is nice to have)
- Clean diaper
- Fresh clothing or sleepers

How do I give my baby a bath?

You may wash your baby by giving either a full bath or a sponge bath. Both are fine right from the beginning, though if your baby boy is circumcised, sponge baths are recommended until the wound is healed.

Remember that this is a new experience and possibly frightening for your baby. Don't be put off if he cries the first few times you give him a bath. Provide comfort by keeping both the room and the water warm, and have his towel ready to wrap and cuddle him immediately after. Reassure your baby by keeping a firm hold on him the entire time and talking or singing to him in a calming voice. Feel free to introduce safe toys to help make bath time fun — bath books, rubber ducks, or plastic stacking cups are just a few good options!

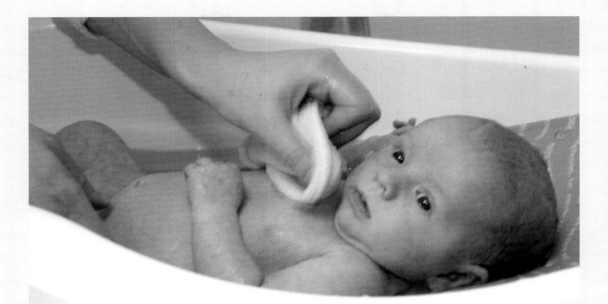

Sponge baths

1. Choose a stable surface to set the baby down on, such as a change table, counter, or bed.

2. Cover the surface with a waterproof pad or towel.

3. Make sure your water supply — either a sink or a basin filled with warm water — is close enough that you can keep at least one hand on the baby the entire time.

4. In the newborn period, you may be more comfortable holding your baby in your arms while you give him a sponge bath rather than setting him down. In that case, you might wish to wear an apron to help keep you from getting too wet.

5. Depending on the temperature in the room, either undress your baby completely or keep him loosely clothed, removing one item of clothing at a time and washing and drying each area before moving on.

6. Put some baby wash on a damp washcloth, soap up one area at a time, rinse with clean water, and pat dry.

7. While there is no magic order in which to wash your baby's body, the general rule is to wash from "clean to dirty," so you don't contaminate the cleanest areas of the body.

8. Wash your baby's eyes by gently wiping the washcloth across the closed eye, from the outside in toward the nose.

9. Wash girls' genitalia from front to back.

10. Remember to wash your baby's fingers and toes and to dry well in between each digit.

11. Be sure to get into the skin folds and turn your baby on his side or tummy to wash his back.

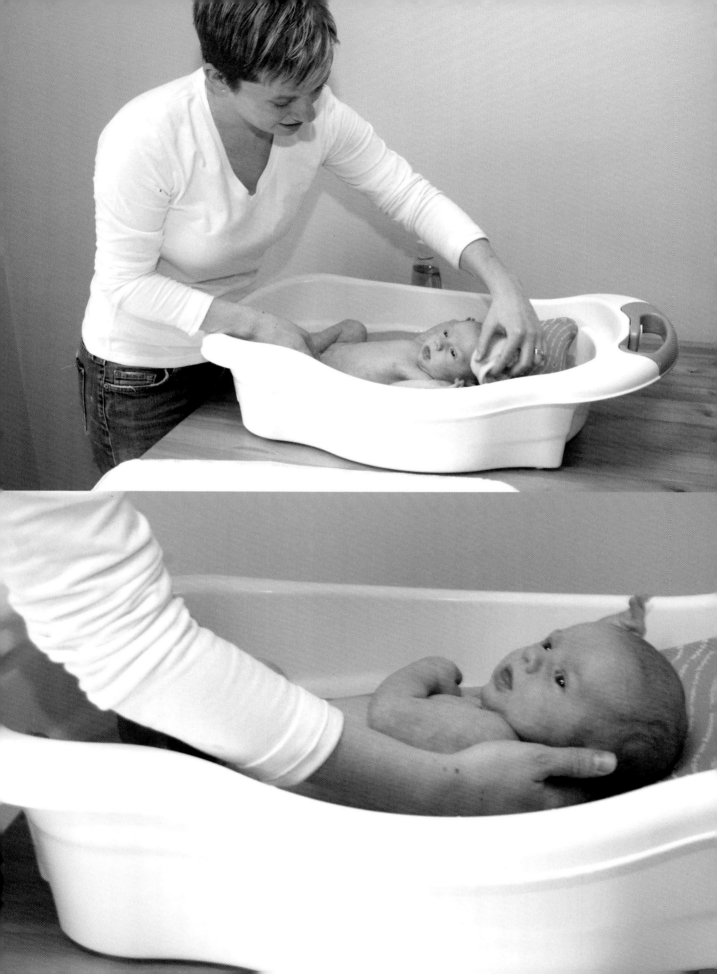

Full baths

1. You can bathe your baby directly in the sink or use a small portable tub. Given the need to fully support the baby at this early stage, the sink is often easiest because it puts the baby at a comfortable level.

2. Ensure that the sink is well cleaned and its bottom is covered with a towel or rubber mat to prevent the baby from slipping.

3. Fill the bath with warm water — a few inches or centimeters is all that is needed.

4. Undress your baby and gradually slip him into the water.

5. Wash him using the same principles as for sponge baths, soaping up and rinsing the whole body.

6. Pay particular attention to holding your baby's head steady until he gains more neck control.

7. To wash his buttocks and back, turn him over so his tummy rests on your arm.

Safety tips

Although there are very few "rights" or "wrongs" in caring for your baby, there are some safety rules that must be followed when giving him a bath. By staying relaxed, keeping your baby warm, and following the safety rules, bath time will soon become a treasured part of your baby's routine.

1. Always test the water temperature with a sensitive part of your body — your elbow or the underside of your wrist. The water should be warm to the touch, but not hot.

2. Never run the water directly from the tap while your baby is in the bath because unexpected temperature changes may occur.

3. Never leave your baby alone in the bath — even for a second. Babies can drown quickly in even a few inches (centimeters) of water.

4. Always empty the water immediately after the bath is finished.

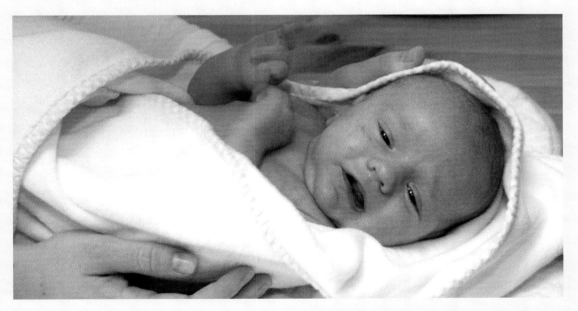

HOW TO
Care for your baby's nails

A newborn baby's hands and feet are so small and cute that you might not even consider that the tiny nails require care. But they do! Some babies are even born with long nails, and although their nails are initially very soft, they will very quickly scratch their own face, not to mention scratching you. Babies' nails grow quickly, so even if your baby's don't start out long, they too will soon require a trim.

Invest in an inexpensive nail clipper or scissors made especially for babies, or a small nail file. These clippers or scissors have rounded tips designed to lessen the chance of injury.

Most parents find the process nerve-wracking at first, given a baby's tiny fingers, delicate skin, and squirmy disposition! You'll find, though, that if your baby is relaxed, his nails are so soft and small that the process is actually very quick and easy.

1. If you need a quick solution to your baby's scratching before you are prepared to cut his nails, placing mittens or socks over his hands will do the job.

2. The best time to trim your baby's nails is when he's relaxed or even asleep. This time may often follow a feed, when he is lying content across your lap.

3. Make sure you have a good light source and two free hands. It's a job you can do either by yourself or with your partner's help.

4. With one hand, pull the fleshy tip of the finger back, away from the nail, to avoid snipping the skin.

5. With the other, simply clip the nail straight across.

6. If you do accidentally clip the skin, your baby may cry out, and there may even be a small amount of blood. Simply apply pressure to the cut with a clean tissue for a few minutes, and give your baby a cuddle. It's rarely serious. Rest assured that, at some point, it happens to every parent.

7. Don't forget about the toes! They're trimmed the same way, though you'll find that they don't grow as quickly as fingernails and thus need to be cut less often. Watch for redness or discharge at the outer corners of the toenails. Sometimes a nail becomes ingrown and inflames the surrounding tissue. If warm soaks and topical antibiotic ointment don't solve the problem in a few days, have your doctor check it out.

8. Trim your baby's nails routinely, every week or two. The frequency with which you'll need to care for your baby's nails is variable, as some nails grow faster than others.

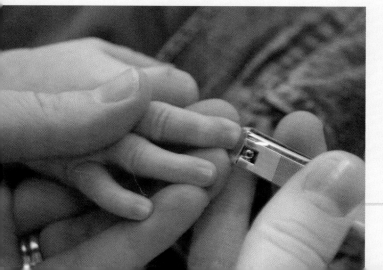

Newborn screening

Many disorders are, unfortunately, not apparent at birth, even with a complete newborn physical exam. Though most of these conditions are rare, significant strides have been made in managing them if they are detected in a timely manner. With this in mind, all babies born in developed nations are screened for certain conditions.

Blood tests

Most of these diseases are related to a problem with genetics, metabolism, blood, or hormones. They can be tested with a blood sample. Your nurse or midwife will take the sample by pricking your baby's heel, then squeezing out a drop or two of blood into a small vial or onto special paper. Many babies cry when the blood is being taken, but the pain is short-lived and worthwhile. There may be a small amount of redness and possibly a bruise at the site, all of which will resolve in a few days.

Most tests are accurate only if the blood sample is taken after the baby is 24 hours old. If you and your baby are discharged from the hospital before this time, make sure that arrangements are made to have your doctor or midwife do the testing at the appropriate time. The results often take several weeks and will be sent to your doctor, who will notify you if there are any concerns.

There is considerable variation among countries and states or provinces in what is tested. Some areas are now employing techniques to test for many disorders (for example, homocysteinuria and maple syrup urine disease) with just one small blood sample. These conditions are individually quite uncommon, but, cumulatively, they add up to a lot of babies whose lives can be immeasurably improved by early detection and treatment.

Conditions screened

Babies are typically tested for three conditions: phenylketonuria (PKU), congenital hypothyroidism, and hearing disorders.

Phenylketonuria (PKU)

PKU is a metabolic disease that affects approximately one in 14,000 babies. When affected by PKU, the body cannot metabolize, or break down, a protein called phenylalanine. If untreated, PKU can lead to mental retardation. When it's detected early on, careful regulation of the child's diet can prevent this consequence and lead to a relatively normal life.

Congenital hypothyroidism

This is a hormonal condition affecting approximately one in 3,000 babies in which too little thyroid hormone is produced. The baby's thyroid-stimulating hormone (TSH) level will be tested in the blood obtained by a heel prick. If congenital hypothyroidism goes untreated, developmental problems and poor growth will be the result, a condition called cretinism. However,

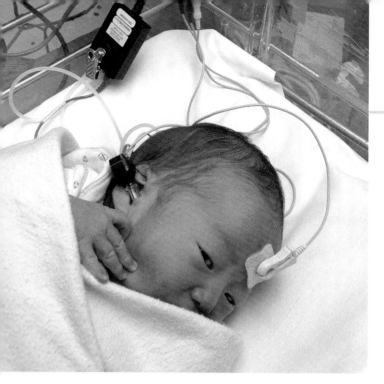

■ Newborn screening for hearing loss.

simply by providing thyroid hormone replacement, these outcomes can be completely prevented.

Hearing

Simple non-invasive methods are available to test a newborn baby's hearing. Hearing loss is one of the most common congenital conditions, affecting approximately three in 1,000 babies. Furthermore, up to half of all babies with hearing loss have no known risk factors that will alert caregivers to an increased probability of hearing deficit. It is vital to detect hearing loss before 6 months of age because intervening from this early stage markedly improves the chances that the baby's speech and language will develop normally. This makes screening all babies particularly important. Most communitites in the United States and Canada offer universal screening. Ask about hearing tests during your prenatal classes or in the hospital after your baby is born, so that, if it is offered, you and your baby can benefit from this fast, simple test.

Jaundice

Your baby's routine assessments in the first days of life by his nurse, doctor, or midwife will include monitoring for signs of jaundice. This will entail physical assessments noting the presence of the yellow color that indicates jaundice and checking for signs of hydration, as well as tracking your baby's weight. While jaundice is easiest to see in Caucasian babies, it is evident in darker-skinned babies by looking at their eyes as well as the palms of their hands and soles of their feet.

Jaundice facts

"Jaundice" is a medical term familiar to many parents. It refers to the yellow pigment on the skin or in the whites of many newborns' eyes. Jaundice is caused by excess bilirubin — a product of the natural breakdown of red blood cells. Normally, bilirubin is processed through the liver and excreted primarily in the stool. In newborn babies, several aspects of bilirubin metabolism are not yet fully developed, resulting in the common appearance of jaundice as part of a physiologic, or normal, process.

Jaundice typically begins in a full-term infant after the first 24 hours of life. The bilirubin level — or degree of jaundice — peaks at 3 to 5 days, and then gradually decreases over approximately 2 weeks. If your baby is healthy, and the bilirubin level is not too high, the jaundice is harmless and will resolve naturally. Since bilirubin is excreted in the stool, an important component of clearing jaundice is to ensure that babies are well hydrated and passing meconium stools, which is generally accomplished by establishing feeds.

Jaundice begins by affecting the whites of the baby's eyes; as the bilirubin level increases, the yellow appears to spread downward, from head to toe. An experienced clinician may be able to predict the bilirubin level based on the extent of jaundice affecting your baby's body, although this is definitely not reliable.

Testing for jaundice

If your health-care provider is concerned, he will check your baby's bilirubin level by taking a blood sample — usually a simple heel prick. While most babies' jaundice is harmless, very high bilirubin levels can affect the brain, a consequence thankfully avoided by monitoring and treatment. The majority of babies whose bilirubin levels are high must simply have subsequent levels checked until your doctor is confident that the jaundice is decreasing.

Toward the end of the first week of life, breast-fed infants have higher levels of bilirubin than those who are bottle-fed, a condition called breast milk jaundice. This type of jaundice begins slowly, peaks at approximately 2 to 3 weeks of age, and may persist for more than a month. Though the reasons for this phenomenon are unclear, the resulting bilirubin levels are very rarely dangerous. While being monitored by your doctor or midwife, it is best to continue to nurse your baby, letting the jaundice resolve on its own.

Red flags for jaundice

There are several other reasons for jaundice to persist, or to be more significant than physiologic jaundice. Prematurity and blood group incompatibility are two of the more common scenarios. In general, there are a few red flags that would indicate that your baby's jaundice is more than just a routine case:

- Jaundice that is apparent within the first 24 hours of life
- Baby is not feeding well
- Baby is not voiding
- Baby is not passing meconium
- Fever
- Lethargy

Treatments for jaundice

Some babies require special ultraviolet lights, a treatment called phototherapy, to help bring the jaundice level down. If phototherapy is needed, your baby will be placed in an incubator with lights surrounding it, with his eyes covered for protection. Although this generally requires hospitalization, it is a very effective therapy that is harmless and commonly used. Given that the lights may be dehydrating, and that hydration is an important part of clearing bilirubin from the body, your baby

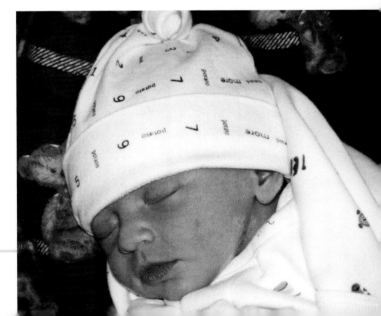

may require additional fluids if his feeding is not yet established. These fluids may be in the form of supplementation with milk by various methods (cup, syringe, lactation device) or even through intravenous fluids.

In rare circumstances when the phototherapy fails to work quickly enough, a special blood transfusion (exchange transfusion) may be required, whereby the baby's blood is exchanged for blood that is low in bilirubin. This treatment takes place in the neonatal intensive care unit. This is almost never required for routine cases of jaundice, but rather in more complicated circumstances.

Weight loss

Surprising to many parents is that most babies lose weight after birth, before they start gaining again. Newborns may lose up to 10% of their birth weight over the first few days of life. This is due to the loss of fluids and the elimination of meconium after birth. Babies also have minimal intake initially, particularly if they are breast-feeding. This is nothing to be worried about. In fact, it's very normal.

Your baby's weight should be followed closely at the beginning, to ensure that he does not lose too much and that he begins to appropriately gain it back, both signs

that your baby is getting enough milk and is not dehydrated. Your baby should regain his birth weight by 2 weeks of age, and then will gain about 1 ounce (30 g) per day over the first 3 months. It's no wonder that parents feel their babies are growing before their eyes!

Subconjunctival hemorrhage

A vaginal delivery is hard work not only for the mother, but for the baby, too! Increased pressure in the vessels of the baby's eye during delivery can cause some bleeding, appearing as a red streak in the white of the eye. This is frequently seen in newborns and is completely harmless. You don't need to worry or do anything special; the blood will disappear on its own within a few days.

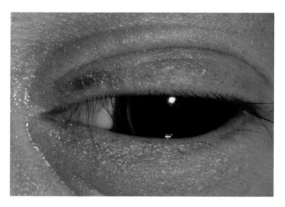

Did You Know?

Lip blisters

Another common occurrence in the first few week of a newborn's life is the formation of a blister, or callus, in the middle of the upper lip. This is due to the baby's vigorous sucking, and is completely harmless. There's no need to try to stop your baby from sucking to deal with the blister; sucking is a natural reflex in babies, and the blister will heal on its own.

Did You Know?

Rashes

Several types of rashes may affect your baby's skin as early as the first day of life. Most are harmless and resolve on their own. There are four common rashes: milia, baby acne, *Erythema toxicum*, and Mongolian spots.

MILIA

Milia are tiny white bumps on the skin, most prominent over the bridge of the nose and the cheeks. They are small sebaceous glands containing a buildup of natural oils. They require no treatment and will disappear within a few weeks.

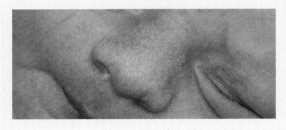

BABY ACNE

As the name implies, your baby may get pimples long before puberty hits! Just wash the skin normally and pat dry. The acne will resolve within a few months and should not leave any lasting marks.

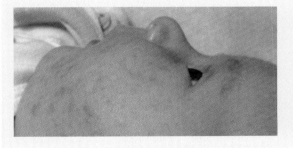

ERYTHEMA TOXICUM

This is an extremely common rash, often noted in the first couple of days of life. The rash consists of a red flat base with a tiny white or yellow pustule in the center. You may see just a few such markings or several over your baby's body. They seem to come and go in different areas, almost before your eyes. Once again, this rash is harmless and no treatment is required.

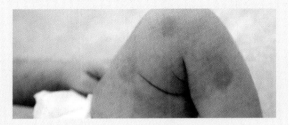

MONGOLIAN SPOTS

These are deep blue lesions found over the buttocks or lower spine of Asian, African-American, South Asian, and sometimes darker-skinned Caucasian babies. To an untrained eye, these markings may be mistaken for bruises. However, a bruise will undergo color changes over the course of a week, while Mongolian spots stay the same. Many babies are born with these spots. They are harmless and are usually gone within the first few years of life.

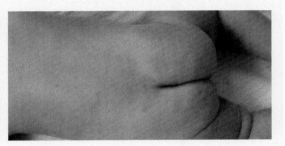

HOW TO
Dress your baby

No doubt you've gazed at rack upon rack of adorable baby clothes in the months leading up to your baby's birth. But now that your baby's here, knowing what is practical to buy, what your baby will be comfortable wearing, and how to fit your squirmy munchkin into these little clothes can be overwhelming! Here are some handy guidelines.

1. First, remember that your baby's initial couple of months will consist largely of feeding, sleeping, and being held. From a clothing standpoint, this translates to one thing — sleepers! They are comfortable for the baby whether he is awake or asleep, can be layered with an undershirt or "onesie" (short- or long-sleeved) underneath depending on the season, and snap open at the crotch to make for easy diaper changes.

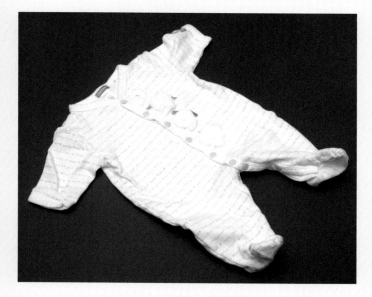

2. If you buy one-piece sleepers with feet, you won't need to worry about socks that are always falling off their little feet. Of course, it is always fun to take our babies out of sleepers and dress them in a little outfit once in a while. You'll find that you'll do this occasionally at first, and increasingly as your baby emerges out of the newborn period, until you're in a routine of dressing your baby in regular clothes during the day, with sleepers reserved for nighttime wear. With this in mind, and remembering that babies grow fast, don't stock up on too many clothes in the "0–3 month" size.

3. Regardless of the type of clothing you buy, look for items that are easy to put on and take off your little one. With tops or sleepers that have snaps all the way up, you won't have to pull clothing over your baby's head — something no baby enjoys. If you do buy items that pull over his head, make sure there are snaps at the shoulder or overlays of material on either side of the neck, designed to stretch easily. Pants or overalls with snaps at the crotch make diaper changes possible without pulling your baby's pants off and on again — a struggle with kicking feet!

4. In terms of keeping your baby warm but not overheated, a simple rule of thumb is to dress him as you would dress yourself, adding one thin layer in colder weather. Babies' heads are a major source of heat loss, so it's a good idea to use a cotton hat, even indoors, in colder weather, especially when your baby is sleeping. If you live in a colder climate, appropriate outdoor gear, such as a snowsuit or bunting bag with feet, mittens, and a warm hat, are essential. One-piece snowsuits that zip the entire length will make your life considerably easier. Remember that scarves are a strangling hazard; avoid them for babies and small children.

5. As with diaper changes, try to change your baby's clothes in a spot that is both comfortable for you and safe for the baby, such as a change table or crib, or the floor. Toys to visually stimulate your child and ongoing interaction with you will again help to calm and distract your baby.

6. For items that snap or zip all the way, simply lay out the open piece of clothing and lay your baby on top, slipping his feet into place and his arms through the sleeves, then fasten the snaps or zipper.

7. Try reaching up through the sleeve to retrieve your baby's little hand and assist it through, rather than struggling to get it through from the top end.

8. For clothing that fits over the head, first stretch the neck in your hands, then place either the front under the baby's chin or the back at the back of his head and lift the shirt up. This method will prevent the baby from feeling trapped or smothered by the clothing, and will minimize the amount of time his face is covered.

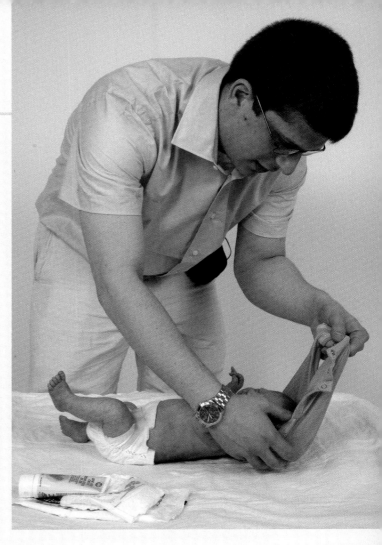

Gifts

You might receive many baby clothes as gifts, undoubtedly all well-intentioned and given with love. While you may want to keep some, keep the tags on the clothes until your baby is ready to wear them. That way, you can sort through what you have bought or received in each size and make note of duplicates, unnecessary items, or clothing for the wrong season.

Many gifts come with gift receipts that make returns easy, but even without a receipt, many stores will accept returns for credit. As your baby grows, you'll have lots of opportunity to buy him new clothes — and your credit note will be much appreciated.

HOW TO
Carry your baby

If you're like many new parents, yours may be the first newborn baby you've held. It can be intimidating — they seem so small and fragile. But like everything else, it will very quickly become second nature to both you and your baby.

Support

The most important thing to remember when handling a baby is that you need to support his head and neck during the first few months of life until he gains better head control. When lifting a baby lying on his back, place one hand under his head and neck and the other under his bottom. Babies feel comforted when they're close to your body, so lean down, bringing yourself close to your baby as you lift him up to you. By the same token, lean down with him as you set him down, keeping your hands in place until he is settled, and then gently slip them out from under him.

Holds

There are several ways to carry your baby. As long as you have control over his head and neck, and you are both comfortable, go with whatever hold you both prefer!

1. Shoulder: Many newborn babies are comfortable being carried over your shoulder. One of your hands will be on your baby's bottom, with the other hand supporting his head. Depending on your baby, he might prefer to curl up against your chest

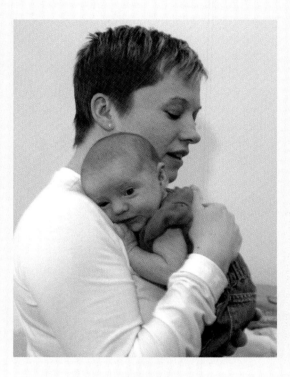

or to be placed farther up, with his head over the top of your shoulder.

2. Front-facing: Some babies enjoy looking out at the world, achieved safely with a front-facing hold. With your baby's back against your front, keep one hand under his bottom so he is "sitting" on you and place your other arm across his chest, supporting his neck with your hand. As your baby gets older and has better head control, you'll be able to accomplish this with one arm, bringing your arm either over or just under your baby's shoulder and across his body, supporting him with your hand under his crotch.

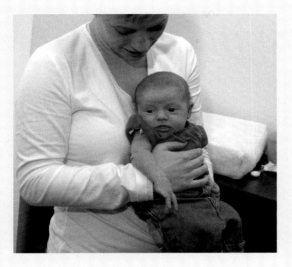

4. Hip: As your baby gets older and has better head control, you may find that he is comfortable with his bottom resting against your hip and one of his arms tucked in around your back. Depending on how heavy your baby is, you will be able to use either one or two arms to support him, often leaving one hand free for other things. This position is convenient, but can be hard on your lower back. Get into the habit of bending at the knees when lifting your baby up — it will save your back some hardship!

3. Tummy: Some babies, especially gassy ones, are comforted by resting on their tummies. Depending on the size of your baby (and your arm), you can hold your baby along the length of your forearm, with your hand supporting his chin and neck. Or you can hold him with one hand around the diaper area, and the other across the chest and supporting his head.

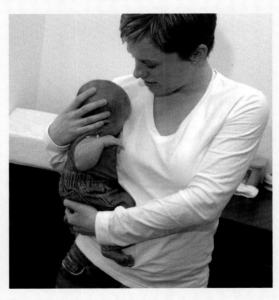

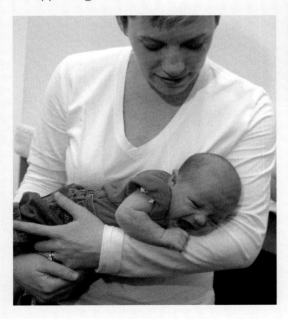

Baby carriers

Many parents find that baby carriers or slings designed to hold a baby vertically against your front are invaluable for the first few months. Babies are snug up against you, and often fall asleep in this position. These carriers allow your arms to swing freely by your sides on a walk, to push a stroller with an older child, or to do things around the house.

Leaving the hospital

Many parents remark that, upon hospital discharge, they feel as though they are being "let loose" with a new baby to care for — and no idea where to begin. What will hopefully be one of the most wonderful periods of your life will also, undoubtedly, be physically and emotionally challenging. Every new parent requires support, so don't be afraid to accept offers or ask for help.

Don't forget to take care of yourself as well! You will have a scheduled postpartum visit with your obstetrician, family doctor, or midwife, but don't hesitate to make additional visits if you have questions or concerns about your own physical or emotional health. Friends, relatives, and your public health department can all be of assistance.

Establishing supports

If your partner is available, and his workplace allows, take advantage of the opportunity for the two of you to be home together, even for a few days, with your new baby. This will allow him to begin bonding with his newborn, will enable you to provide each other with emotional support, and will contribute an extra set of hands around the house.

Relatives and friends

Grandparents, other relatives, and close friends are all supports to be drawn upon at this time. You will find that the first few days fly by and are consumed largely by feeding your baby, changing diapers, and sleeping when the baby does. Enlist others to do laundry, cook food (freeze leftovers for the coming weeks), hold the baby, care for older siblings, and run errands.

Support groups

Apart from household chores, caring for the baby is a new challenge. Reference books and friends or relatives who are parents themselves can be invaluable. Mother's groups are helpful sources of advice, company, and peer support.

Public health care

Don't hesitate to take advantage of services offered through your local public health department. Public health nurses will often make home visits, during which they can provide reassurance and guidance about your baby's care. Your baby will also be visiting with his doctor or midwife in the first few days, so begin to keep a list of questions to ask at your next appointment.

Lactation consultants

If you're nursing your baby, breast-feeding can be a rewarding but challenging task. Check with your public health department to see if they offer breast-feeding help, or access a lactation consultant by contacting either your birth hospital or La Leche League (a breast-feeding support group).

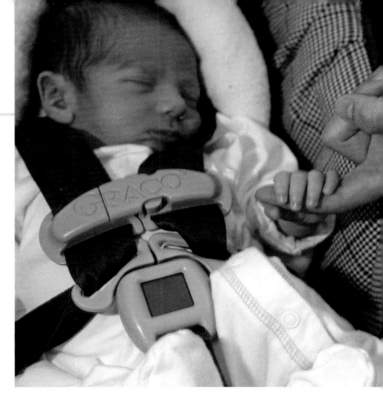

Visitor caution

Newborn babies quickly become star attractions! Well-intentioned family and friends are likely already discussing their plans to visit you and your little one after the birth. While visitors can be wonderful, supportive, and even helpful, keep in mind that they don't all need to descend on you immediately; thoughtful visitors will discuss with you the best time to visit, will offer to help, and won't overstay their welcome.

In the hospital

Labor and delivery is hard work. New mothers need some time on their own to recover. Hospital limitations on visitors are usually set with the best interests of both you and your neighboring families at heart. Most hospitals allow you to designate one individual who is allowed to remain with you throughout your stay. While most women ask their partner to be with them, don't hesitate to think creatively and do what works best for you. If there's an older sibling at home, for example, your partner may remain with him to ease the transition while your mother or best friend is at your side. While you remain in the hospital, it's wise to check the visitor policy to prevent disappointed guests from being asked to leave.

At home

Each of us feels differently about the involvement of family and friends during and following the birthing process, so be sure to discuss your feelings with your partner beforehand. The period following the delivery will be the first time that the three of you (or more, if you have older children) will be together as a family. Some couples want to "nest" and spend the majority of this time alone, while others welcome having lots of family and friends around. Whichever route suits the two of you is fine, but be sure to relay your wishes to the relevant parties.

Infection risk

Whether in the hospital or at home, keep in mind that, like all newborns, yours will be prone to infection. Anybody who is ill should stay away until fully recovered; if visitors do not display this common courtesy, don't hesitate to politely ask them to delay their visit until they are no longer sick.

By the same token, all guests should wash their hands before holding the baby. Toddlers who visit should be supervised and guided to gently touch the baby if they wish, but should avoid touching his face and hands.

Did You Know?

Documentation

Before leaving the hospital, you will receive a few important documents that need to be filled out in a timely manner.

The newborn record

This document reports your baby's condition at delivery, his initial physical examination, and his condition prior to discharge, including APGAR scores and newborn screening blood work. Be sure to bring a copy to your baby's health-care provider at your first visit to be kept as part of your baby's chart.

Birth registration

In the United States, you usually start the paperwork for a birth certificate and social security number for your baby before leaving the hospital. Mail in the application, and you should receive these documents a few weeks later. In Canada, you need to submit an application for the Registration of Live Birth; in turn, a Notice of Birth Registration will be sent to you, which you will use to apply for your baby's birth certificate.

Health insurance

In the United States, be sure to enroll your baby in your state or private health insurance plan. In Canada, an infant registration form will be processed by the Ministry of Health, and a temporary health card will be provided until you receive a permanent one in the mail. Remember to take your baby's health insurance information to your first doctor's visit.

Parental leave

In the United States, people eligible for protection under the Family and Medical Leave Act (FMLA) are guaranteed 12 weeks of unpaid leave for the birth or adoption of a child. In Canada, if you have paid for Employment Insurance (EI) as part of your income taxes, you are eligible for maternity and paternity leave benefits. You will need a Record of Employment from your employer in order to apply for benefits. If you are not eligible for benefits, speak to your employer or your professional association.

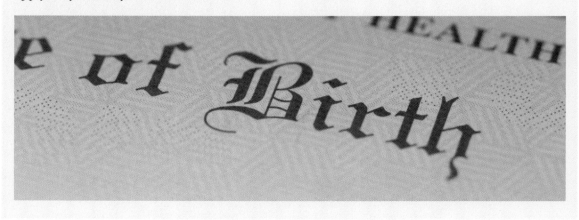

What about Dad?

When so much attention is focused on a mother during her pregnancy, labor, delivery, and breast-feeding, fathers sometimes seem unsure of their own role. It's understandable. But fathers need to feel like an equal part of their new family. They are true partners in parenting. Of course, some of the concerns and feelings that new fathers experience are unique to them.

Adjustments

Before birth

Before their baby is due, fathers should find out what their particular workplace policy is and determine whether they can take off a week or two once the baby is born. This time is valuable for them to adjust to being dads and to enable them to provide help — physically and emotionally — to their partner. If a father can't be at home during the baby's early days, try organizing a team of supporters, whether family, friends, or visiting nurses, to help out. Many fathers discover that they truly enjoy being at home with their baby. Taking a paternity leave once their partner goes back to work has become an increasingly popular option.

After your baby is born

Nursing a newborn takes a considerable portion of a mother's day and night. During this time, the mother and baby have a chance to bond with one another. However, fathers can sometimes feel left out of this process; they may feel a little resentful and then guilty about this resentment.

Fathers need to be reassured that they have a huge parenting role to play; there is no need for them to feel excluded from bonding with their baby. Though many men may not be immediately comfortable handling such a tiny being, they inevitably adjust with time. Caring for their baby soon becomes second nature. There is simply no point in them shying away from caring for their baby.

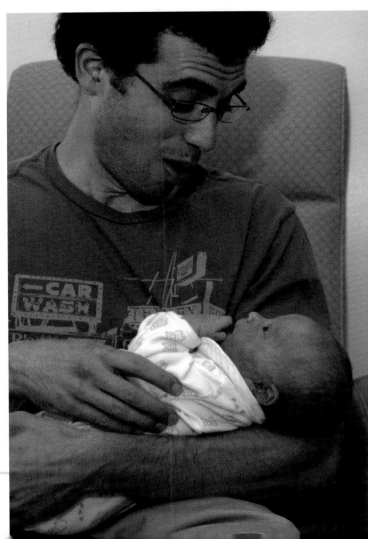

Dad's role

The list of things fathers can do is exhaustive: bathing, diapering, cuddling, taking the baby for walks, singing, and playing. If the baby is bottle-fed or gets an occasional bottle, fathers can cuddle with their baby during feeds. Once breast-feeding is established, some families choose to have Dad give the baby a regular nighttime bottle, whether of formula or pumped breast milk. This routine enables mothers to get at least one long stretch of sleep, while also giving a father more opportunity to bond with his little one.

Many fathers experience a protective instinct toward both their new baby and their partner, who has undergone the physical toll of labor, delivery, and now sleepless nights. Such feelings are a reflection of love. Fathers should convey the important message that they are committed to support and helping out with the baby. This is a step in the right direction toward maintaining a relationship as a couple, as distinct from a paternal role.

Challenges and rewards

It can be difficult for a new father to work all day and then come home just in time for the baby's evening fussy period. Whatever happened to those carefree days before children? There is simply no denying that the newborn period is a physically and emotionally demanding time for everyone. This is a time for partners to support each other and offer one another some respite.

Although at first it may be difficult for couples to find time for each other, it's important for them to make sure they have time together, be it for a regular walk, dinner out, or a movie. Parents should talk about things other than the baby!

With the baby's first smile and increasing interaction, fathers will feel well rewarded and happy that this new magical family relationship has a solid foundation.

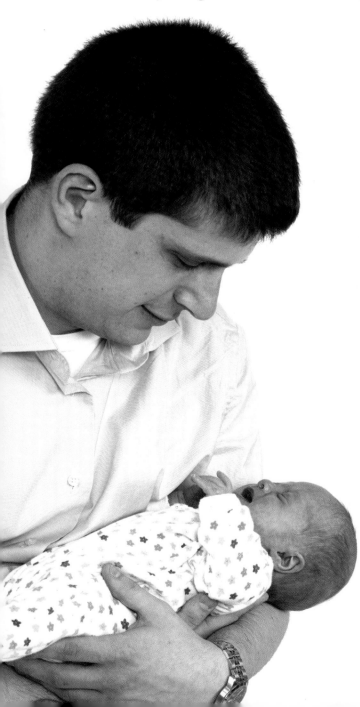

Premature arrivals

Some things in life just don't go as planned. Under normal circumstances, a baby grows in the mother's womb for about 40 weeks. However, for a variety of reasons, many infants are born prematurely. When this happens, the already stressful newborn period gets even more complicated. And if the baby is extremely early, the experience can become immensely challenging for both the infant and the family. Fortunately, this generation of premature babies has benefited from the dramatic progress that has been made in the management of prematurity.

Emotional impact

The parents of premature babies, especially very small ones, have lots to think about. Although prematurity is usually associated with several specific medical issues, the biggest problem for parents isn't the actual medical concerns but the emotional impact of having a premature baby.

When parents see their tiny infant struggling to survive, it's understandable that they wonder if they are somehow responsible for the premature birth. Could they have done something differently to prevent the prematurity? In most cases, early labor just happens. If there is some reason to explain the early labor, it is invariably no one's fault. While there are many emotions that parents might legitimately feel in these circumstances, guilt should not be one of them.

All kinds of questions come to mind. If my baby is in the neonatal intensive care unit (NICU), how often can I visit? Can I hold him, or can I at least touch him? How do I feed him? Are all these tests really necessary? Why is that monitor beeping? When can he come home? Will he be okay? These are all legitimate questions. Ask them.

Parenting a premature baby is more stressful than looking after a full-term infant. You're allowed to feel stressed. In fact, you would be abnormal if you didn't. Try not to feel inadequate when you experience these troubling emotions. Most parents, supported by the NICU staff and their own loved ones, quickly adjust to the situation and successfully take up their parenting duties.

Mildly premature infants

For those infants who are born just a few weeks earlier than expected (greater than 34 weeks' gestation), the first week of life is, in many ways, similar to that of the full-term baby. It's just that the usual newborn problems become somewhat amplified.

Feeding problems

Many newborns, especially very small babies, have some difficulty breast-feeding during the first few days. Premature infants tend to tire at the breast more easily than term babies. They often suck poorly, feed erratically, and seem to prefer sleeping to nursing on schedule.

Did You Know?

Definitions

Prematurity is defined as a gestation of less than 37 weeks. This overlaps the term "low birth weight (LBW) infant," which refers to all babies with a birth weight of less than 5.5 pounds (2.5 kg). About 7% of all births in North America are low birth weight babies, of whom 70% are premature. The rest are small full-term infants, many of whom have an underlying medical reason to account for their low birth weight.

Not all premature infants have a low birth weight: many are sufficiently developed to weigh as much as full-term infants and, fortunately, behave like them too. A few infants are very premature, however, and weigh less than 3 pounds, 5 ounces (1.5 kg) at birth. These "very low birth weight" (VLBW) infants tend to have a much more turbulent beginning to their lives.

For several reasons, infants of African descent and children in the developing world have a much greater chance of being born weighing less than 5.5 pounds (2.5 kg).

These difficulties are more than minor irritants for parents; they can sometimes lead to serious problems. Inadequate nutritional intake can result in dehydration, excessive weight loss, and low blood sugar (hypoglycemia). Fortunately, the nursery staff, which usually includes a lactation consultant, can assist you with nursing advice and monitor your baby's progress. Still, there are times when supplemental nutrition in the form of expressed breast milk or infant formula will be needed for a few days. Depending on how your baby is doing, these supplements are given by bottle, sippy cup, feeding tube, or even intravenously.

Hypothermia (cold stress)

Normally, an infant's subcutaneous fat provides insulation to help retain body heat. Premature infants tend to have less fat under their skin; therefore, preemies often have more difficulty maintaining a normal body temperature.

To avoid cold stress, or hypothermia, low birth weight (LBW) infants must be carefully dried right after birth and then warmly bundled. If their temperature drops too much, an overhead heater or incubator will be used to prevent hypothermia. Although incubators separate mother and child, this necessary barrier shouldn't prevent you from holding your baby's hand or physically comforting him.

Once the LBW infant is stable enough to come out of the incubator, he must still be kept warm. The nursing staff will guide you on how to dress your baby and bundle him. A cold infant will often have cool hands and fingers, and his skin may appear mottled. Conversely, an overdressed baby may appear flushed and sweaty.

Jaundice

Because their livers are still immature, many newborns develop temporary jaundice in the first week of life. Preemies

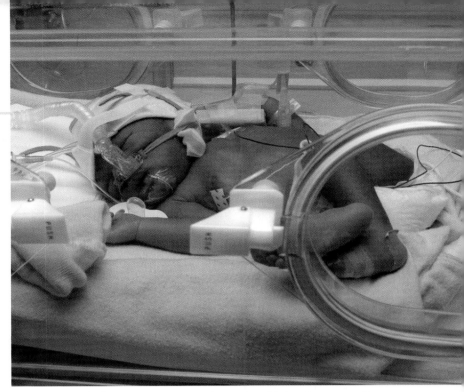

■ A premature baby on a respirator in the neonatal intensive care unit.

possess even less developed liver function, so they are much more likely to develop neonatal jaundice.

Usually, this jaundice is no great problem, merely producing a temporary yellow-green discoloration of the skin. However, if bilirubin levels are allowed to rise sufficiently, this may lead to permanent brain damage. To avoid this, a preemie's bilirubin level will be monitored closely and, if necessary, phototherapy — essentially, increased exposure to light — will be used to lower the bilirubin.

Very low birth weight infants

When babies are born very prematurely, they enter a world they are not yet prepared to handle. As a result, the first weeks of life can be very turbulent, often a difficult struggle for survival, filled with unique challenges. The site where this takes place is the neonatal intensive care unit.

It's remarkable how very tiny a human being can be. Two or 3 pounds of baby weight doesn't seem like much, yet it is usually enough to survive. There's not much fat on a small preemie either. The skin looks thin and very pink. Nor are there many skin folds on the soles of the feet, and the baby's little ears lack much cartilage. The elbows and knees aren't as flexed as with a full-term infant. Nor is the cry very loud. Yet, invariably, inside this frail little frame is a human being willing to fight long and hard for survival.

Did You Know?

The neonatal intensive care unit (NICU)

The NICU is a place where miracles occur. But miracles don't come easily. It's no simple matter to replicate the womb and treat the many potential complications associated with prematurity. The skills required to keep tiny babies alive and healthy are truly remarkable.

The modern NICU is a very high-tech place, whose monitors, respirators, tubes, and incubators can be overwhelming to parents already shocked by a premature birth. But thanks to the typically attentive staff serving in the NICU, parents soon become familiar with it.

HOW TO
Parent your child in the NICU

Parents of premature infants often feel as if they have no control over the scary first few days of their baby's life. The doctors and nurses seem to be the decision-makers, and life in the NICU seems to have a routine of its own. But parents can be, should be, and usually are an integral part of the caregiving team, helping their baby face his early challenges. Tiny babies need their mothers and fathers too.

Communicating with your baby

At first, parents might feel that their baby is too immature to communicate his needs, but even very little babies can send a definite message. Because parents tend to spend so much time with their preemie, they usually become quite expert at recognizing their baby's subtle signals.

Signals

What types of signals do premature infants communicate? The contented baby might assume a calm, relaxed posture; have no wrinkles on his brow; display a reflexive smile; or even suck on his fingers. A distressed infant might tense up his arms and legs; seem restless; grimace; or have an elevated heart rate. Over time, parents can even distinguish a contented and relaxed baby from an exhausted one.

Comforting your baby

Parents also quickly learn how to comfort their child by gently massaging and stroking him; how to soothe him with a gentle voice; how to settle him by placing an index finger in his little hand. Later, when their baby becomes more stable, they can experience the immense joy of cuddling their tiny child. A parent's love can be very healing.

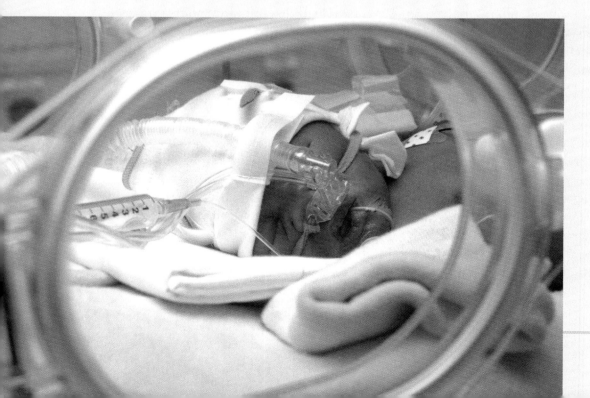

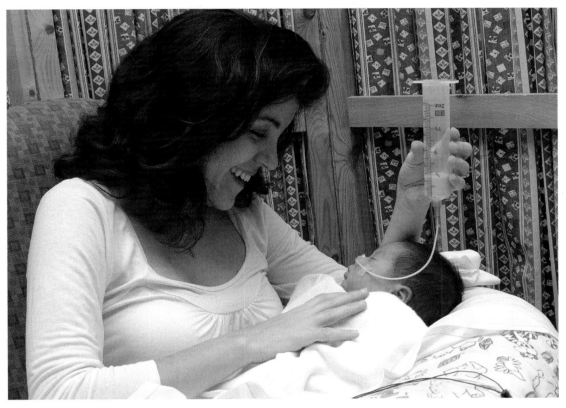

Feeding very low birth weight infants

Premature babies can be fed in a number of different ways. Remember that providing adequate nutrition is the important issue; the actual method of feeding is merely a technical matter.

Intravenous feeding

Although the larger, more mature premature baby can attempt to nurse at the breast, VLBW infants need extra help. Efficient sucking, effective swallowing, and a protective gag reflex are just too much to ask of a child born 12 weeks earlier than expected. Very sick preemies will be fed intravenously. Initially, the IV fluid is a mixture of water, sugar (glucose), and salts (electrolytes). Later, if needed, amino acids, fats, minerals, and essential vitamins can be added to provide total nutrition.

Nasogastric feeding

If a premature infant can digest food but is unable to suck and swallow adequately, the preferred method of feeding becomes the nasogastric (NG) tube. A fine plastic catheter is passed, usually through the nose, into the baby's stomach. Then fortified expressed breast milk or specially prepared formula can be given to the baby, satisfying his nutritional needs. It's important for tube-fed preemies to continue to develop their sucking skills by frequently practicing on a pacifier or mother's breast.

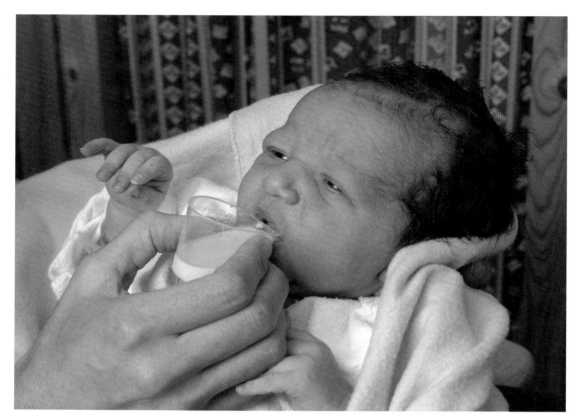

Cup feeding

One effective way to offer expressed breast milk or infant formula to a premature baby is the feeding cup. With the baby comfortably swaddled, a small medicine cup of breast milk or formula for preemies is lifted to the mouth. Tilting the cup gently allows a small amount of milk to touch the lips, allowing the baby to taste it. Soon this tasting progresses to licking and then effective lapping.

Breast- and bottle-feeding

Parents will sometimes decide that bottle-feeding their baby is the best option for them. And, in many cases, it is. There's no need for guilt or a sense of inadequacy because you're not breast-feeding. The nursery staff will instruct you on the best way to bottle-feed a small infant. Small, soft, flexible nipples will be used. Special formulas designed specifically for premature infants will likely be recommended by the hospital nutritionist. The nursery staff will also assist in developing an optimal feeding schedule for your baby.

Special problems

Very low birth weight infants may experience special health problems, including intracranial bleeding (hemorrhage in the brain), metabolic instability (particularly, low blood sugar and calcium), cardiac problems, and hernias. More commonly, they may be prone to apnea and other breathing problems, as well as anemia and infections. Fortunately, these potential difficulties can be addressed in the NICU. Most babies will meet these difficult challenges successfully.

Apnea of prematurity

Newborn infants, even full-term ones, often pause for a few seconds between breaths. This is called periodic breathing, and is quite normal. Sometimes, the pause between breaths can be longer, more than 15 to 20 seconds. Known as apnea, this is very common in premature babies. In fact, the more premature an infant is, the more frequent and prolonged apneic spells are likely to be. If an apneic episode is long enough, the baby's heart rate will slow excessively, and he might turn bluish, or cyanotic.

Most of the time, an apneic infant will resume breathing spontaneously, but sometimes some gentle stimulation, such as stroking the baby, is needed. If the episode is severe, the infant may require help breathing, and oxygen will be given using a bag and mask. When premature babies have repeated episodes of significant apnea, they may require ongoing assisted ventilation using a respirator, or they might be given medication, such as caffeine, to stimulate breathing. A sudden increase in the duration or frequency of a preemie's apnea can occasionally be a sign of a new problem, such as infection.

Respiratory distress syndrome

The lungs of the very premature infant have fewer air sacs than those of full-term infants, and their airways lack a special substance, called surfactant, that helps keep them open. These poorly inflated lungs result in respiratory difficulty. Small premature infants often must work very hard to get enough oxygen, sometimes to the point of exhaustion.

Fortunately, this respiratory distress can be treated and even prevented. Synthetic surfactant can be instilled (dropped as a liquid) in the airway to help keep the lungs inflated. If a baby does develop respiratory distress syndrome, the infant's oxygen levels will be closely monitored, supplemental oxygen will be given, and ventilators will be used to help the baby breathe adequately.

Did You Know?

Bronchopulmonary dysplasia

Because of recurrent apnea or respiratory distress syndrome, some very premature infants will need supplemental oxygen and ventilator support for extended periods. There can be a price to pay for these life-saving measures. The ventilator pressures needed to deliver enough air to the baby and the extra oxygen used may result in damage to the lungs, which might take weeks or even months to resolve. This lung injury is called bronchopulmonary dysplasia. It produces prolonged oxygen dependency, cough, and wheezing. The chest x-ray shows smallish lungs with a distinctive bubbly appearance.

Anemia

Premature babies are prone to anemia — a reduced amount of the oxygen-carrying molecule known as hemoglobin. There are two main reasons for this. First, preemies aren't in the womb for much of the last trimester and therefore miss the opportunity to store essential nutrients, such as iron. Second, the close monitoring that VLBW babies require necessitates frequent blood tests, which, collectively, add up to a lot of blood.

Mild anemia is not much of a problem, but when anemia is more severe, a VLBW infant might feed poorly, experience increased apneic episodes, or need more respiratory support.

To prevent anemia, premature babies are given essential nutrients, such as folic acid and iron. To treat it, a blood transfusion might be necessary, or even injections of a hormone called erythropoietin, which stimulates the bone marrow to produce more red blood cells.

Increased risk for infection

The immune system of premature babies is immature. Serious infection is much more common in VLBW infants. The signs of infection can be very subtle in these tiny babies, so they must be watched closely for any deterioration in their status. Because infection can spread quickly in this age group, prompt treatment with intravenous antibiotics is necessary even when infection is suspected but not yet proven.

Necrotizing enterocolitis

Like most systems in the VLBW infant, the gut is fragile and prone to injury. Necrotizing enterocolitis (NEC) is a condition in which the bowel of tiny babies is damaged due to impaired blood supply, hypoxia (reduced oxygen in the blood), or infection. The problem can be relatively minor, treated simply by resting the bowel, or it might be major, causing the death of large sections of the bowel and requiring surgical management.

Did You Know?

Bringing baby home

Sooner or later, the premature baby is ready to go home. What a wonderful milestone in a family's life!

There is no fixed age or weight that determines when a LBW infant can go home. Rather, your baby must be stable and meet the following medical criteria:

- The child can feed adequately at the breast or bottle.
- The child is gaining weight steadily.
- The child no longer needs support to breathe properly.
- The child no longer has apneic episodes.
- The child can maintain his temperature without needing an incubator.
- The parents are able to care for their child at home.

HOW TO
Care for a premature baby at home

The first few days at home can be a bit overwhelming. Getting into a successful routine might seem a utopian dream — hour-to-hour survival is often the only initial goal. Eventually, though, things will settle down.

Here are a few important points for parents of preemies to remember:

- **Behavior:** Premature babies generally behave differently than full-term ones. They might sleep more and appear more sensitive to household noises and activities. They also tend to have less regular sleep and eating patterns.

- **Corrected age:** A premature baby's development is measured on his "corrected age," not the actual time since birth. The corrected age is calculated by subtracting the number of weeks of prematurity from the actual age. For example, a 30-week-old baby who was born 10 weeks early has a corrected age of 20 weeks. That baby should be expected to reach the developmental milestones of a 20-week-old infant. Any progress beyond that is considered a bonus.

- **Immunizations:** Although development is based upon corrected age, childhood immunizations are best given according to chronological age. Some premature infants should also receive special monthly injections in their first winter of life to help reduce the serious effects of a highly infectious virus called respiratory syncytial virus (RSV).

- **Hypothermia protection:** Larger premature infants don't need excess clothing or an overheated home, but smaller preemies, say those less than 4 pounds (2 kg), will need to be kept a bit warmer. The NICU staff will provide parents with advice on preventing hypothermia in their baby.

- **Infection protection:** Premature infants are prone to infection. The baby's handlers should wash their hands carefully before picking him up or feeding him. Avoid crowded, enclosed places where germs can be transmitted, especially in winter. Although not every runny nose needs to be examined by a doctor, any signs of infection in a premature baby's first months should be medically evaluated.

- **Neonatal follow-up:** Preemies need to be carefully followed even after their discharge from hospital. A number of problems related to prematurity may become apparent only after leaving the NICU. The neonatal follow-up clinic and your baby's doctor will be on the lookout for conditions such as cerebral palsy (abnormal muscle tone), hearing loss, crossed eyes (strabismus), eye damage (retinopathy of prematurity), nutritional concerns, and possible developmental delay.

- **Support systems:** Family, friends, physicians, spiritual advisers, home-care nurses, and neonatal follow-up clinics can all serve to lessen the burden and stress that are part of parenting the very premature baby.

Frequently asked questions

As family doctors and pediatricians, we answer many questions from parents. Here are some of the most frequently asked questions. Be sure to ask your health-care providers any other questions that arise. If they don't have the answers, they will refer you to a colleague who does.

Q: My baby has blue eyes. Will they remain that color?
A: Brown eyes invariably remain brown, but blue eyes may gradually change color over the first 8 or 9 months. Usually, deeply blue irises will remain blue permanently, while greenish blue irises are more likely to darken over time. Considerable discussion revolves around eye color, but remember, the issue is merely a cosmetic one.

Q: I have noticed a pinkish-orange stain in many of my newborn's diapers. Should I be concerned? Is it blood?
A: This pinkish stain is quite common during the first week of life. Known as pink diaper syndrome, it is not caused by blood; rather, it results when crystals in the urine are deposited onto the diaper. Although it is usually a completely normal phenomenon, it is often present in the concentrated urine that accompanies dehydration. Ask your health-care provider to weigh your baby; this is the best way to evaluate his state of hydration.

Q: My newborn boy seems to have little breasts. Is that a sign of a hormonal or genetic problem?
A: Breast tissue is noticeable underneath the nipples in many boys and girls during the newborn period. This phenomenon is normal, caused by maternal hormones that were circulating around the time of your delivery. Don't worry: the "breasts" will eventually go away on their own.

Q: My son is tongue-tied. Will this interfere with his ability to feed? Will I need to do anything about it?
A: "Tongue-tied" refers to a situation in which the tongue seems excessively tethered to the floor of the mouth by a thin strand of pinkish tissue, called the frenulum. It doesn't usually cause any problems unless it is so marked that the baby cannot protrude his tongue beyond his lower lip. In the rare case that treatment is truly needed, a simple release of the tongue can be achieved by snipping the frenulum. If your son is nursing well, it's best to leave things alone.

Q: My baby has a small bony lump in the middle of his chest. What should I do?
A: The lump is likely the slightly upturned triangular tip of the breast bone, called the xiphisternum. There isn't much fat or subcutaneous tissue at this site, so it often appears to be pushing up against the skin. Show the lump to your health-care provider at your next visit. If it's the xiphisternum, nothing further needs to be done.

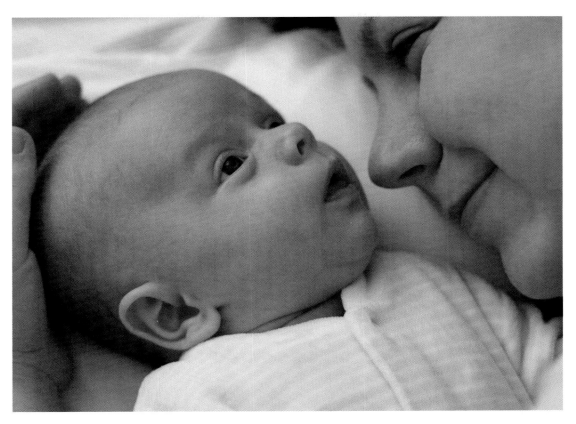

Q: My 1-week-old daughter sometimes seems to breathe very quickly, and then she actually stops for a few seconds. Does she have a breathing problem?

A: Not necessarily — or even likely. The normal breathing patterns of a newborn can seem quite irregular at times. What you are describing sounds like "periodic breathing," which is entirely normal. The breathing speeds up, then slows down, and sometimes even stops for a few seconds. Your daughter will outgrow this.

If, however, your daughter has to work very hard to breathe — sucking in the skin below or between her ribs, flaring her nostrils, or grunting with each breath — or if she stops breathing for more than 10 seconds or seems to be going a little blue around the mouth, you should definitely be concerned. True respiratory difficulty warrants immediate medical assessment.

Q: My baby boy is uncircumcised. Should I be retracting the foreskin to clean around his penis?

A: Most people are unaware that the foreskin doesn't usually retract fully until a few years after birth. Many boys even have incomplete retraction of the foreskin into early adolescence. Washing the genital area with soap and water should be more than adequate cleansing. It is unwise to forcibly pull back on a foreskin that still naturally adheres to the underlying head of the penis.

Sam's Diary

February 9 (you are born)

When Dr. Barrett came to see us at about 9:00 p.m. last night, he was surprised to find that Mom was already fully dilated. Dad was absolutely fantastic during our labor, rubbing Mom's back and looking after us.
Dr. Barrett found that you were lying in a position called occipito-posterior, with your head facing the opposite direction from the way most babies come out, which made your birth a little more tricky. He tried to turn you, but you weren't having any of it!

Mom had an epidural and, after trying to push for a bit, we were told you would need a little help to be born. The nurses wheeled Mom into the OR, and very soon you were on your way. Dr. Barrett tried forceps but didn't want to hurt you, so he elected to do a Caesarian section. In a short time, at 2:48 a.m. on February 9th, you were born.

What a wonderful experience! Dad cut your cord, the nurses cleaned

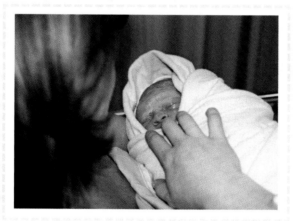

you up, and you came to meet your mom. You were covered with sticky white stuff and a bit of blood, and your head was all swollen and cone-shaped, but we were so happy to see you at last. You weighed 6 pounds, 9 ounces (3.2 kg) and measured 20 inches (50 cm) from the top of your head to the tip of your heel. Your Apgar scores were 9 and 9, which meant that you came out breathing and crying beautifully. We put you straight onto Mom's breast, and you seemed to know what you were supposed to do.

We spent some time in the recovery room, then the nurses wheeled us up to our hospital room and placed you in a bassinet right beside Mom's bed. We organized a pullout bed for Dad and are now settled in for the first few days of your life. We have been really busy, with lots of visitors and phone calls — everybody wants to hear all about you.

February 12 (4 days old)

You've been attending breast-feeding classes with Mom, where we've met lots of other mothers and babies. It's not quite as easy as you would think, but thanks to the helpful nurses and lactation consultant we are starting to get the hang of it. You are latching on much better and are staying awake for your feeds.

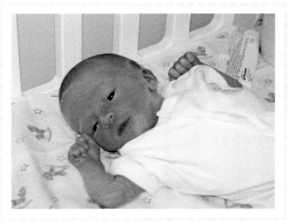

We are keeping a record of everything that comes out of you! Your poops are changing from a blackish green color to a more watery brownish yellow. You are wetting lots more diapers, which hopefully means you are getting enough to drink.

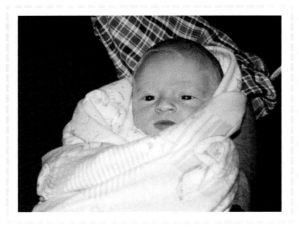

Dad stayed with you when they poked your heel to do some blood tests. Apparently, you gave quite a loud cry!

The nurses taught us how to bathe you. You really like to be tightly swaddled in your blanket — maybe it reminds you of being in Mom's tummy — so Mom and Dad have learned how to do this.

You are a little jaundiced, but Dr. Murphy decided you were well enough to go home. So we dressed you up warmly and put you in your car seat for your first drive.

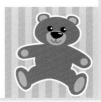

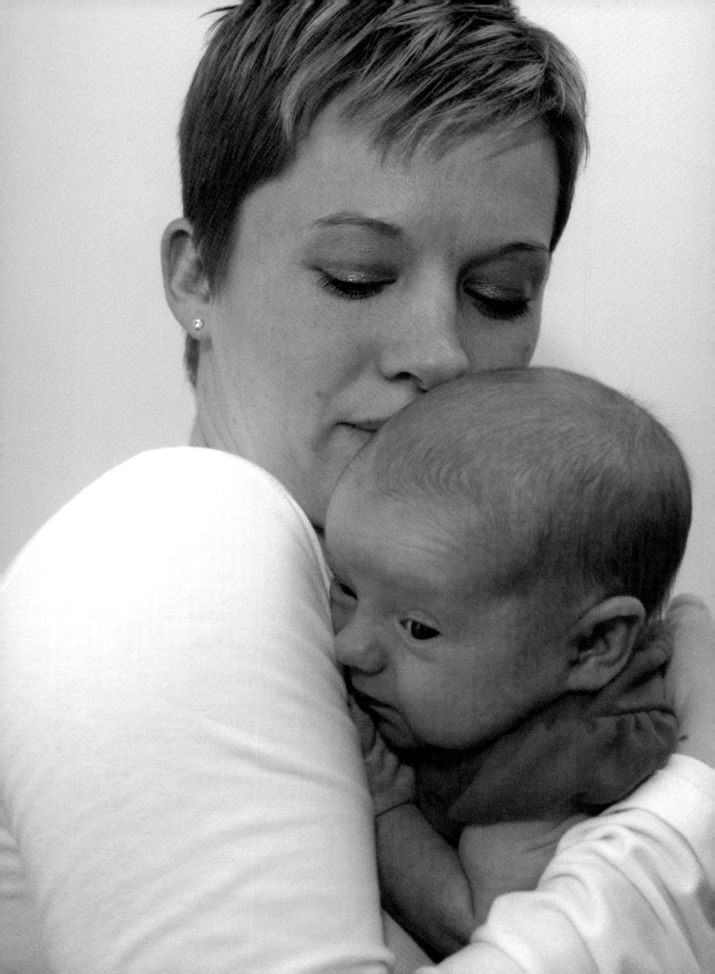

Feeding
Your Baby

Breast-feeding or formula-feeding

One of the first decisions you will need to make as a new parent is how to feed your baby — whether to breast-feed or formula-feed. Although exclusive breast-feeding until 6 months of age is recommended by most health agencies, both breast-feeding and formula-feeding are safe and nutritious ways to feed your baby. There is no "right" decision that applies to every family, but do try to make your decision before your baby arrives. If you start by formula-feeding, it will be very difficult to change to breast-feeding if you wait too long, although you can switch from the breast to the bottle at any time.

Personal preference and social pressure

There was a time when formula-feeding was preferred by the majority of families in North America. Today, the tables have turned: breast-feeding has become popular, largely because medical research has shown that this method of feeding has greater advantages for the baby and the mother.

In a society that expects all mothers to breast-feed, the decision to formula-feed may be an emotional one. You may have concerns about how people will react when they see you feeding your baby formula. You may be anxious that they will make critical comments or ask why you aren't breast-feeding. While breast milk is undoubtedly the best milk for newborn babies, infant formula is the next best thing. Formula is nutritionally sound, even though it does not offer the protective antibodies contained in breast milk. Infants will grow and develop appropriately and will be generally healthy when fed formula. You should not be made to feel guilty if breast-feeding is not your preferred option or is not possible for you.

There are many factors to consider when you're choosing a feeding method. What works for one family may not work

Did You Know?

Medical opinion

Breast-feeding is recommended by the World Health Organization, the American Academy of Pediatrics, and the Canadian Paediatric Society as the preferred method of infant feeding. In fact, breast-feeding exclusively is recommended until a baby is 6 months old, and breast-feeding as an ongoing source of fluids and nutrition is often advised until 2 years of age and beyond. Any amount of breast-feeding is considered to be better than none at all.

for another. Weigh the advantages and disadvantages in relation to your personal situation before making a final decision.

Recommended feeding options

Ideally, babies should be fed breast milk exclusively, with no other foods, until the age of 6 months. At that point, solid foods can be introduced. While the introduction of solid foods at 6 months is ideal, some parents start solids as early as 4 months.

Continue to feed your baby breast milk or formula until she is about 1 year of age, at which time, if you are feeding her formula, you can switch to homogenized, or whole cow's milk, which contains sufficient fat (3.25%) for the baby's growth. Of course, if your baby is known to have a specific allergy to cow's milk, non-dairy products will be needed: consult your doctor on which to try.

Cow's milk or any other kind of milk, such as pasteurized goat's milk, is not an appropriate feeding choice for babies less than 1 year of age. Cow's milk has a significantly higher protein concentration than breast milk or infant formula. This puts undue stress on your baby's kidneys. The iron content in cow's milk is also low, which can place your baby at risk for iron deficiency anemia. In short, breast milk and infant formula are the only appropriate feeding choices for your baby.

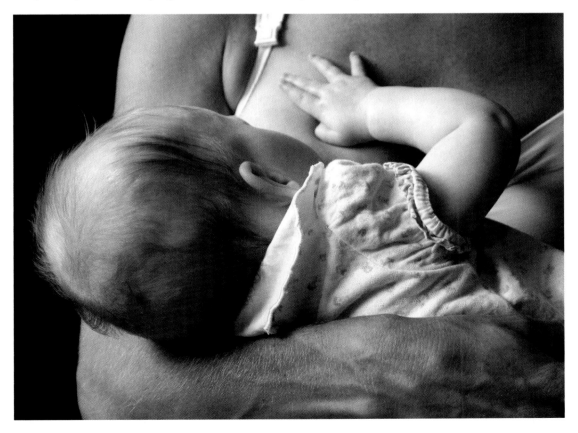

Breast-feeding Option

New scientific evidence is surfacing on a regular basis that supports the benefits of breast-feeding for your baby, for you, and for the environment.

For the baby

The most important advantage of breast-feeding is the positive effect breast milk will have on your baby's immune system. Newborn babies' immune systems are immature, lacking the ability to fight off infections. Not until 4 months does your baby's immune system really begin its maturation process; it reaches more effective levels by about 2 years of age.

Breast milk provides your baby with *your* antibodies to help fight infections. As long as you are breast-feeding, your baby receives these antibodies. As a result, breast-fed babies have lower rates of gastrointestinal illness (such as diarrhea), ear infections, blood infections, meningitis, respiratory infections, and urinary infections.

For the mother

UTERINE CONTRACTIONS
Immediately following your baby's birth, breast-feeding will stimulate your uterus to contract. These contractions, much milder than the painful contractions of labor, decrease the risk of postpartum bleeding and help the uterus return to its original size. At the same time, your risk of breast and ovarian cancer also decreases.

WEIGHT LOSS
Breast-feeding burns approximately 500 calories a day. Studies show that mothers who breast-feed have an earlier rate of return to their pre-pregnancy weight.

LACTATIONAL AMENORRHEA
Breast-feeding also leads to lactational amenorrhea, increasing the time it will take for you to menstruate post-pregnancy and decreasing your chances of getting pregnant again soon after giving birth. But be aware that breast-feeding is by no means a reliable method of birth control!

For the environment

Because breast milk is produced naturally by the human body, there is no need to process your baby's food, which can be taxing on the environment. Formula use also produces waste. Bottles need to be washed with soap, and cans need to be disposed of.

Other considerations

Depending on what formula you choose, you will spend a significant amount of money on feeding your baby; breast-feeding is free.

It takes more time and effort to prepare formula than to breast-feed. If you plan on going out, you will need to put some thought into formula preparation while "on the road."

Human breast milk is made specifically for human beings, so there is no perfect substitute. Its design is so good that, as your baby grows and develops, its composition changes to meet her needs. Formulas are made from animal or vegetable products and do not change as your baby grows and develops, although you can switch to the one recommended for the next stage.

Breast-feeding Issues

While breast-feeding does have some minor drawbacks, the advantages still far outweigh the disadvantages. With the proper support and guidance, breast-feeding can be a very enjoyable experience — and a wonderful time to bond with your young baby.

For the baby

For the baby, breast-feeding usually has no disadvantages; however, there are many myths that might lead you to believe otherwise. Some women are concerned that their breast milk isn't as nutritionally sound as formula and that their baby won't gain weight as well. Breast milk may look watery, but it is very nourishing. Other women are concerned that they don't or won't have enough breast milk. In most cases, a mother is able to produce as much breast milk as her child needs. In the rare instances where this is not true, supplementing with formula will allow you to continue breast-feeding.

For the mother

Breast-feeding may raise other concerns for the mother, but there are usually easy ways to accommodate them.

ANXIETY

In the first week or two, a nursing mother may experience significant anxiety about her ability to feed her baby. An encouraging partner and a skillful lactation adviser can provide invaluable reassurance that she, like most women, will succeed at nursing.

ISOLATION

Breast-feeding requires a mother to be with her baby most of the time, which can be limiting at times. One way you can overcome this issue is by expressing breast milk, which can be fed to your baby in a bottle, allowing other care givers an opportunity to feed the baby. This can be initiated after breast-feeding has been established.

PUBLIC ATTENTION

Some women may be uncomfortable with the idea of breast-feeding in public. This may, indeed, be challenging at first, but many women become comfortable with it, finding ways to breast-feed discreetly. There are "privacy" drapes you can purchase that help you cover up when feeding, or you can simply fold a receiving blanket under your bra strap to cover yourself and the baby. Some stores and restaurants consider themselves "nursing

Did You Know?

Disease and disorder protection

Some literature has shown that breast-feeding may decrease a child's risk of allergic disorders, notably asthma, as well as the risk of obesity, diabetes, cancer, high cholesterol levels, and sudden infant death syndrome (SIDS). More research in these areas is needed to determine the full extent of the benefits. From a growth and development standpoint, there is some evidence that breast-fed babies perform slightly better on cognitive development tests.

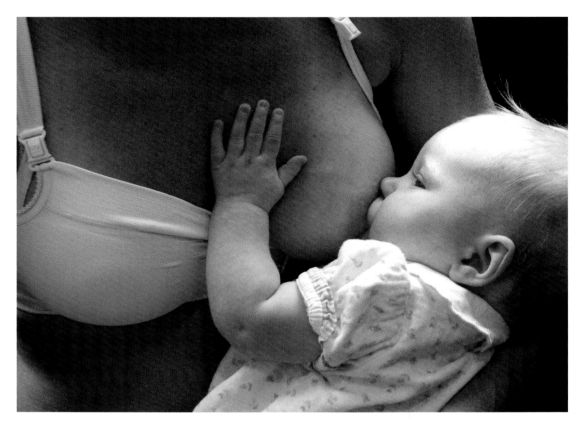

friendly" and may even have a private room where you can feed your baby.

COMPLICATIONS

Breast-feeding mothers may experience certain complications, such as sore nipples or yeast infections. These are generally easily treated.

REDUCED SEX DRIVE

Breast-feeding causes changes to vaginal secretions and to breast tissue, which may affect a woman's sex drive. These changes are not permanent, lasting only as long as you breast-feed.

Did You Know?

Breast surgery

For women who have had breast surgery, including augmentation, reduction, or biopsy, breast-feeding is often still possible. Depending on the surgical procedure, the mother's ability to produce milk may or may not be affected. The only way to know if you will be able to breast-feed is to try. Be sure to consult with your health-care provider to evaluate your baby's weight gain and to determine if you are producing enough breast milk. If not, you may need to supplement with formula.

Contraindications to breast-feeding

In a few rare situations, it is not recommended for a mother to breast-feed her child.

- **The mother has active untreated tuberculosis:** For 2 weeks after treatment begins, the infant should be separated from her mother because of the risk of infection. The mother can pump breast milk for her baby during this time. After the initial 2 weeks, she can breast-feed directly.
- **The mother has an active herpes simplex lesion (cold sore) on her breast:** She should refrain from breast-feeding from the affected breast until the lesion resolves. In the interim, she can pump and discard milk from that breast to maintain supply. She may continue to nurse on the other side if no lesions are present.
- **The baby has galactosemia:** This condition is the result of a congenital deficiency of a galactose enzyme, possibly leading to nutritional failure, mental retardation, and other serious illnesses.
- **The mother is HIV-positive:** In developed countries, such as the United States and Canada, HIV-positive mothers should not breast-feed their babies because of the risk of HIV transmission. (In less developed countries, with high infant mortality rates secondary to common infections and malnutrition, the risk of transmitting HIV via breast milk is less than the risk of death secondary to infection or malnutrition.)
- **The mother has been exposed to radiation:** Mothers who are being treated with or have been exposed to radioactive materials should not breast-feed for as long as their milk is radioactive.
- **The mother tests positive for human T-lymphotropic virus type I or II.**
- **The mother is being treated with chemotherapy.**

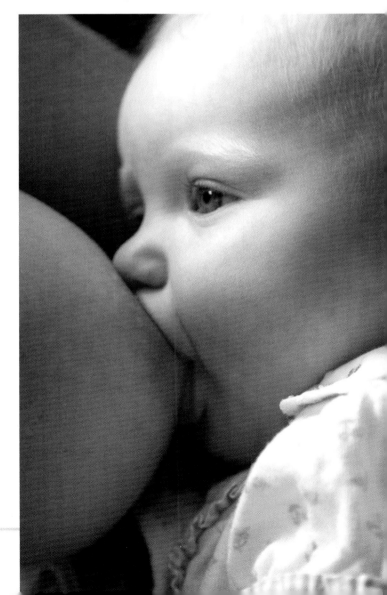

Formula-feeding Option

Despite the clear benefit of breast-feeding for children, formula-feeding has several possible attractions.

Family Support

Formula-feeding may promote involvement of fathers, grandparents, other family members, and close friends who can help feed your baby formula from a bottle.

Flexibility

Formula-feeding offers a little more flexibility for the mother because she does not need to be present for every feeding. Some mothers may need that "space," either just to have a break or to do other activities, such as returning to work. This can also be achieved by pumping breast milk after breast-feeding is well established.

Privacy

Mothers do not usually feel uncomfortable when formula-feeding in social situations, nor do they feel limited in their outings with their baby.

Regularity

Because formula takes a little longer to digest, formula-fed babies may not need to be fed as frequently as babies who are breast-fed. You are also able to tell exactly how much formula your baby is getting in a 24-hour period. While this may be interesting information, remember that the best way to ensure that your baby is receiving appropriate nourishment is to monitor her growth in consultation with your health-care provider.

Formula-feeding Issues

Decreased immunity

The biggest disadvantage of formula-feeding is that your baby will not receive the protective immunoglobulins found in breast milk, which help a baby fight infection. Babies who are fed formula have an increased risk for infection, especially respiratory and gastrointestinal tract infection.

Less convenience

Because it requires advance planning and preparation, formula-feeding is generally not as convenient as breast-feeding. At home, you need to ensure that you have both formula and clean bottles and nipples on hand. If you plan on going out, you will need to bring formula and clean bottles and nipples with you.

Did You Know?

Higher cost

Formula-feeding can be expensive. While some formula preparations are less expensive than others, it will cost $1,500 to $2,000 dollars a year ($125 to $165 a month) to feed your baby a regular formula. If your baby requires a specialized formula for digestive or allergic problems, it will cost considerably more.

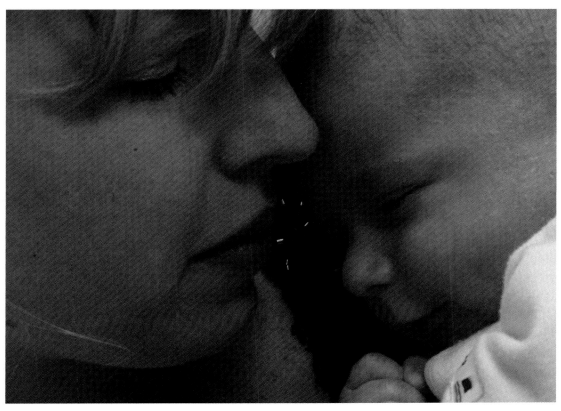

Depending on the kind of formula you use, you may be able to prepare it ahead of time and keep it in a cooler, or you may need to mix it on-site. If you plan on traveling, you will need to think about how you will clean your bottles and nipples, and where you will find a clean water source.

Conditioning

Formula-feeding may affect how long it takes your body to return to its pre-pregnancy state. Menstruation is often delayed for women who are breast-feeding; this is not usually true for women who formula-feed. Breast-feeding also burns up extra calories and causes your uterus to return it to its original shape in less time.

Bonding

Whether you choose to breast-feed or formula-feed your baby, take advantage of your opportunity to bond with her. Mothers who are breast-feeding have to hold their babies close when they feed, which often leads to eye contact and interaction. Those who are formula-feeding should do the same thing — but in this case, both parents can participate.

Infancy is a very special time in your baby's life — and in yours. Interaction with your child is so important now. Hold your baby in a loving way while feeding her, stroke her cheek or head, make eye contact, talk or sing to her, and even rock her if you like. All this attention will lead to a special bond between parent and child.

Getting started with breast-feeding

So you have decided to breast-feed. Congratulations — it's a wise decision. To be successful at breast-feeding, there are a few things you will need to know. If you have spoken with any first-time mothers, they may have told you that breast-feeding is anything but natural at first. Both you and your baby will need to practice to get good at it. To make the process as effortless as possible, you need the proper support, knowledge, and equipment. With these three things in place, breast-feeding should be a lot easier.

Support

If all goes well at the delivery, your baby will be breast-fed shortly after birth. Of course, you may not be at your best. Luckily for you, your baby will probably be quite alert. Studies have shown that a baby who is placed on her mother's tummy following birth will instinctively move up to the breast and latch on. Still, you will likely want help with breast-feeding. Prior to delivery, determine what breast-feeding classes and resources are available in your community; once you have your baby, you may not feel up to doing this.

Breast-feeding classes

Ideally, you'll be able to attend a class on breast-feeding before your delivery. Your midwife, obstetrician, local hospital, public health unit, or La Leche League can provide information on beginner's classes being held in your neighborhood. Encourage your partner to attend. Directly following birth, and for the next few days, you may have difficulty remembering exactly what you learned in class. A supportive partner can help you remember all the little tips and help you with positioning.

Lactation consultants

Specialized support from a professional lactation consultant can be an invaluable resource when you start breast-feeding. Look for an International Board Certified Lactation Consultant (IBCLC) or a Registered Lactation Consultant (RLC).

Postpartum wards

If you deliver in a hospital, your nurse should be able to help you with breast-feeding. Many hospitals offer classes on breast-feeding and employ lactation consultants. Even if you have attended a class prior to delivery, a refresher course may be helpful once you are actually breast-feeding. Some hospitals have breast-feeding clinics, where you can get assistance after you go home.

Family

In addition to professional support, you may be able to call on your family for help.

However, this support is not always forthcoming. Well-meaning relatives who are not fully aware of the benefits of breast-feeding may not understand why you chose this feeding method. If you are concerned that your partner or your parents may not know how best to help you, you may want to provide them with written information outlining the benefits of breast-feeding. Alternatively, have them speak to a supportive health-care provider who can update them on current recommended practices.

Breast-feeding equipment

You may choose to breast-feed sitting in a comfortable chair or lying on a favorite couch, your bed, or even the floor. Wherever you end up, you should be completely relaxed so that your breast-feeding experience is as comfortable and enjoyable as possible.

Did You Know?

Breast milk basics

Breast milk is based on "demand and supply" economics — the more your baby drinks, the more your breasts produce. Most women are able to produce more than enough breast milk to feed their baby, even if they have twins.

Your breasts are able to produce milk by the middle to end of your second trimester of pregnancy. You may notice your "first" milk, called colostrum, coming out of your nipples even before your child is born. Once you deliver your baby, your body releases a hormone called prolactin, which signals the glands in your breasts to start milk production. These milk glands both produce and store your breast milk.

The "letdown" reflex is triggered when your baby suckles at your breast, stimulating nerve endings that send a signal to your brain, which releases a hormone called oxytocin. (Pain, stress, and anxiety may decrease oxytocin levels.) Oxytocin signals your milk glands to release milk into your milk ducts, which lead out through the nipple and into your baby's mouth. Many women feel tingling or an unusual sensation in the nipple as this happens; others do not feel the reflex at all. In some women, the letdown reflex can be stimulated by other signals, such as hearing a baby cry or even looking at a picture of a baby.

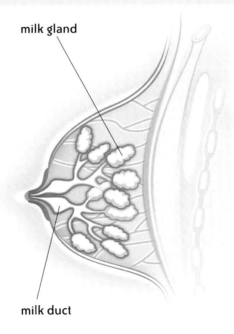

milk gland

milk duct

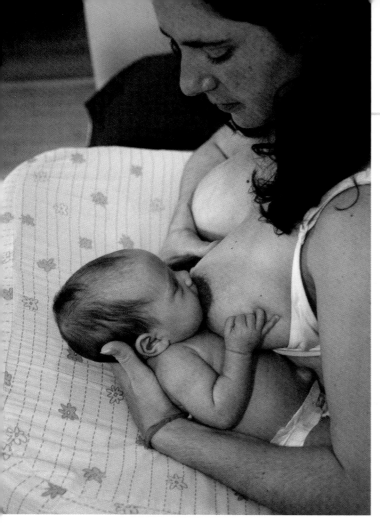

Pillow

If you are sitting up to feed, you will likely need a pillow. People have different and often quite strong opinions on the need for a special breast-feeding pillow, which can range in price from $30 to $100. Before you purchase one, try supporting your baby with a king-size pillow. If this does not feel comfortable, invest in a breast-feeding pillow. These pillows may require you to use a chair with low or no armrests.

Nursing stool

Once you are sitting in your chair, with your baby on the pillow, you may need to bend toward your child or even slouch, and one shoulder may lean forward more than the other, all of which can make you very uncomfortable over time.

The solution is a nursing stool. Most women, unless they are tall or are sitting in a short chair, require a footrest. You can purchase a specialized nursing stool or simply place a large book, such as a phone book, under your feet to raise your knees, lifting the baby to your breast and preventing slouching.

Nursing bras

Consider buying at least two nursing bras so you don't have to undress when you are feeding. There are many styles, including bras with and without underwire. To prevent undue pressure on the breasts and secondary complications, make sure bras fit properly and are not too tight.

Breast-feeding positions

There are several different positions you can use to hold your baby while she is feeding. Personal preference varies, but the goal is constant: both you and your baby should be comfortable.

Most new mothers prefer to use the cross-cradle hold, and some may continue to use this position for the entire time they breast-feed. Others will transition to a cradle hold once they and their baby get the hang of breast-feeding. The best way to get comfortable with these positions is to practice and to have an experienced person help you. Make sure you have the proper equipment, such as pillows and a footrest, so that you are not slouching or straining.

Whatever position you choose, to prevent improper positioning you should always bring the baby to your breast, as opposed to leaning toward your baby.

Guide to breast-feeding positions

Position	How to ...	Works best for ...
Cross-cradle hold	1. Sit in a chair with your feet supported by a stool so that your legs are perpendicular to the floor, or sit cross-legged on the floor. 2. Hold the baby's back and head with the opposite arm and hand of the breast you intend to feed with. The arm holding the baby should be well supported by a large pillow. 3. The baby should be lying across you, with your abdomens facing each other, and aligned so that the baby's nose is at your nipple. 4. Hold your breast with the hand on the same side. 5. Bring the baby to your breast using the latching technique described on page 137.	• Women learning to breast-feed • Babies who have difficulty latching on • Little babies

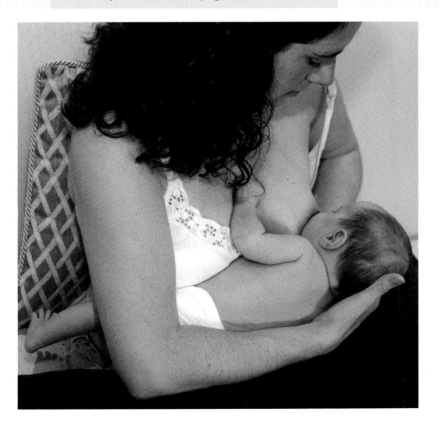

Position	How to ...	Works best for ...
Cradle hold	1. Sit in a chair with your feet supported by a stool so that your legs are perpendicular to the floor, or sit cross-legged on the floor. 2. Hold the baby's back and head with your arm on the same side as the breast you intend to feed on. Your baby's head will lie cradled in your elbow. The arm holding the baby can be supported by a large pillow, but this is not necessary — which makes this a good position to use if you are away from home. 3. The baby should be lying across you, with your abdomens facing each other and with the baby's nose at your nipple. 4. Hold your breast with the opposite hand. 5. Bring the baby to your breast using the latching technique described on page 137.	• Women who are experienced at breast-feeding • Babies who have no difficulty latching on • Feedings away from home, when you are without a pillow

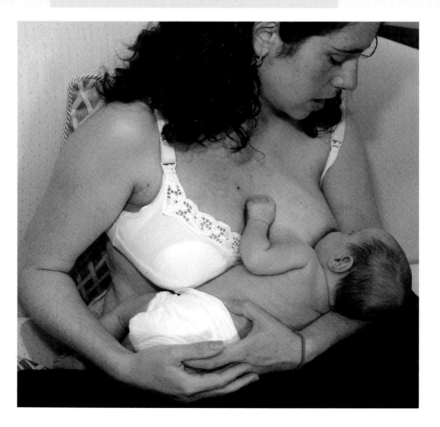

Position	How to ...	Works best for ...
Football hold/ clutch hold	1. Sit in a chair with your feet supported by a stool so that your legs are perpendicular to the floor, or sit cross-legged on the floor. 2. Hold the baby's back and head with your arm and hand on the same side as the breast you intend to feed on. The arm holding the baby should be well supported by a large pillow or two. 3. The baby's head should rest in your hand, and she should be lying somewhat flat on her back. 4. Hold your breast with the opposite hand. 5. Bring the baby to your breast using the latching technique described on page 137.	• Feeding twins • Little babies • Women who have had Caesarean births • Women with large breasts • Women with flat or sore nipples

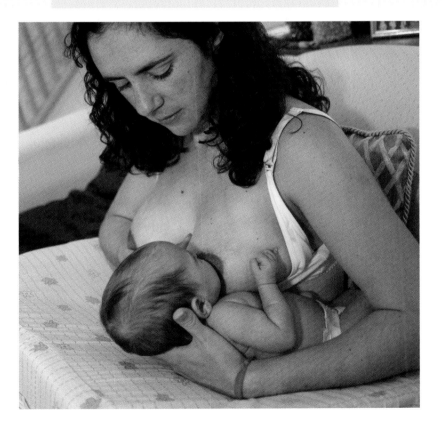

Position	How to ...	Works best for ...
Side-lying	1. Lie on your side with your baby lying on her side, facing you. 2. Draw your baby in toward your bottom breast using the arm on the same side. 3. With the opposite arm, position your bottom breast so that your baby can latch on. 4. Bring the baby to your breast using the latching technique described on page 137. 5. Once your baby is latched, you may move your bottom arm.	• Women who are uncomfortable sitting • Women who have had Caesarean births • Women with large breasts • Woman who want to rest while breast-feeding

Adapted by permission from Toronto Public Health.

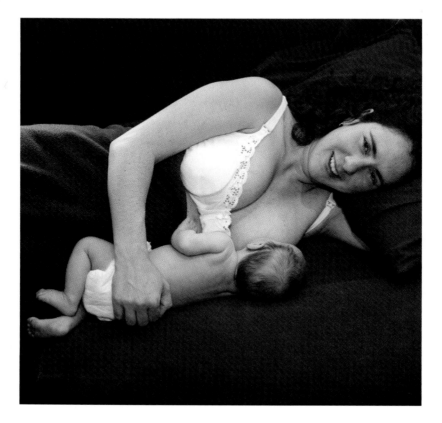

Learning to latch correctly

The latch is one of the most important elements of breast-feeding. An incorrect latch can result in significant breast-feeding problems. It's a good idea to ask for assistance from a trained lactation consultant or someone who has experience with breast-feeding.

There are 8 main steps to latching the baby correctly onto your breast so that both of you are comfortable:

1. Hold your breast between your thumb and forefingers. Ensure that your hand is well behind the areola (the flat, colored part of the nipple) so that your hand does not get in the way of the baby's mouth. Gently compress your breast so that it is flattened out and similar to the shape of your baby's mouth.

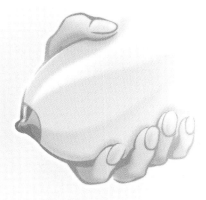

2. Hold your baby so that her nose is at your nipple and her neck is very slightly tipped back.
3. Touch your baby's lip with your nipple to stimulate her to open her mouth.

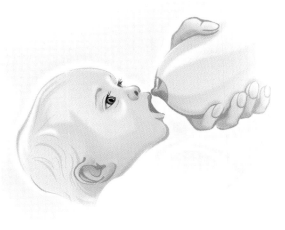

4. Once your baby's mouth is open, pull her to the breast.

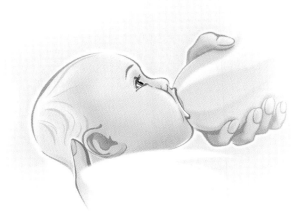

5. Check the latch. If your baby is positioned correctly on your breast, much of your areola should be inside her mouth. Proportionately, more of the bottom of the areola will be in her mouth, and it will look like her chin is up against your breast. Both of your baby's lips should be flanged out — more simply, the baby should have "fish lips."

7. If you feel pain or the positioning does not look correct, pull out the baby's upper or lower lip. If this doesn't rectify the problem, break the latch and try again.

8. To break the latch, slip your finger into the corner of your baby's mouth, tug gently, and break the seal her mouth has formed on your breast. Don't pull the baby off your breast without breaking the latch — this may cause you significant pain.

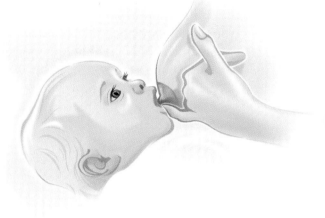

6. If baby falls asleep after a few minutes, squeeze your breast to help your milk to flow. Do not squeeze so hard that it hurts. This will help baby to start sucking again.

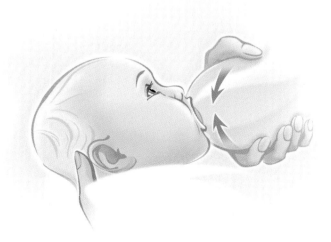

Feeding in the first 72 hours

You will be able to breast-feed your new baby directly following birth. In the first few hours after delivery, your baby is very alert and ready to feed. Initiating breast-feeding at this time will pave the road for success in the future. The American Academy of Pediatrics recommends that the first feeding occur *before* the newborn is weighed and measured, treated with eye ointment, or given vitamin K.

For the first month, your baby will feed about 8 to 12 times every 24 hours. The frequency will increase when your baby goes through a growth spurt or if she is cluster-feeding. As your baby grows, she will likely spread out her feedings and may stop feeding at night. There will be many changes, so be flexible.

Breast engorgement

Most new mothers are able to breast-feed and will produce milk whether or not they intend to breast-feed. As a result, even women who choose not to breast-feed will have some initial engorgement, but this will subside. For women who choose to breast-feed, initial engorgement will subside if the baby is fed frequently from birth.

Colostrum

When you were pregnant, you may have noticed a sticky yellow substance leaking from your breasts. That substance is called colostrum. Colostrum is the "first" milk the breast produces until your mature "second" milk appears a few days later. Colostrum is very rich in nutrients and contains factors that boost your baby's immunity to infections. Colostrum also helps your baby to excrete meconium, the blackish green waste material sitting in her bowels.

Because colostrum is so nutrient-dense, your baby needs only a very small amount at each feeding. In fact, during her first day of life, she needs only about 1 tablespoon (15 mL) of colostrum at each feeding; during her second day, her needs will be about double.

In the first few days, you may be concerned that your baby is not getting enough milk because your breast may not feel different before and after a feeding. Be assured that she is likely getting the

---

Did You Know?

Newborn feeding schedule

A newborn baby will likely require frequent feedings, about every 1½ to 3 hours or 8 to 12 feeds each 24-hour period. Until breast-feeding is firmly established, if your baby is very sleepy, it will be important to rouse her gently every 3 to 4 hours in order to feed her. Once she is gaining well on the breast, your baby will probably fall into an identifiable routine. At this stage, rather than wake her, let her tell you when she's hungry. You don't need a clock to tell you when to feed your baby — after all, no other mammals use one.

appropriate, albeit rather small, amount of food she requires.

Frequent feedings

After your baby's first feeding, she may become very tired and sleep for many hours. Even in these initial 24 to 48 hours, frequent feedings are essential once your baby has had a good rest. These early feedings will not only help your baby to excrete meconium, they will also stimulate your mature milk to come in and prevent engorgement.

Feeding once your milk comes in

You should produce mature milk within 2 to 5 days after the delivery of your baby. Some new mothers have difficulty determining whether their milk has come in. The second milk will look and feel different from colostrum: it will be lighter in color and not sticky. Your breasts will also feel fuller, and, after your baby has

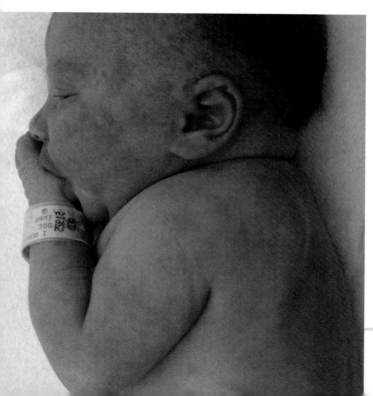

fed, they will seem emptier. When your baby suckles at the breast, you will hear an audible swallowing noise.

Foremilk and hindmilk

During the course of a single feed, the fat and caloric content of your breast milk changes. When your baby first suckles, she gets the "foremilk": watery milk that is lower in fat and calories. Once she has fed for a few minutes, she will start to get the "hindmilk," which has more fat and more calories.

To understand the difference between these two milks, think of a pitcher of orange juice. As it sits unstirred in a refrigerator, the pulp in the juice settles to the bottom of the pitcher. If you don't stir it before you pour yourself a glass, the first pour is very clear and thin. As you pour out more of the juice, the liquid thickens. Breast milk is the same, except that you cannot "stir" your breast milk before the baby drinks it!

The longer a baby feeds on one breast, the greater the chance that she will get hindmilk. The fuller your breasts are, the more foremilk your baby will receive before she gets hindmilk. Although hindmilk is richer in calories, which aid in growth and development, all of your milk is good for your baby.

Scheduled feedings versus demand feedings

One of the questions most frequently asked by new mothers who breast-feed is, "How often should I breast-feed my baby?" Most babies need to be fed 8 to 12 times in a 24-hour period, but some may need to be fed less frequently, and others more.

Guide to

Your baby's hunger cues

Learn to recognize these signs that your baby is hungry:

WAKING

Your baby may wake up or rouse from a deep sleep, stretching and perhaps yawning.

ROOTING

Your baby may start rooting — nuzzling toward your chest or the chest of anyone holding her.

FIST SUCKING

Your baby may suck on her fists or make sucking motions with her mouth.

CRYING

If you don't notice her other cues, your baby may start to cry. One word of caution: a crying baby is not necessarily a hungry baby. When offered the breast, most babies, hungry or not, will suckle, and they will stop crying because suckling is soothing. Learning to read your baby's hunger cues will help you know when your baby is hungry and when she is crying for another reason.

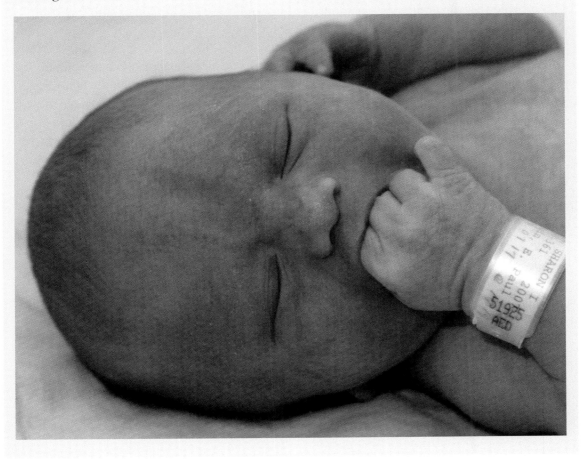

There are two main approaches mothers can use to figure out when to breast-feed: scheduled feedings and demand feedings. With scheduled feedings, you feed your baby on a time-based schedule. For example, after consulting with your health-care provider, you might choose to feed her every 3 hours from the start of one feed to the start of the next feed.

With demand feedings, you feed the baby whenever she indicates that she is hungry. Learn to read your baby's hunger cues so that you can feed her before she starts crying — it can be very difficult to feed a screaming baby.

Regardless of the approach you adopt, be flexible. Breast-feeding is meant to be easy. If you are feeding your child every hour because she demands it, it will be difficult for you to go anywhere or do anything. On the other hand, if your baby is on a schedule where she feeds every 3 hours, but is going through a growth spurt and is crying and rooting 2 hours after a feed, it is not fair to make her wait another hour before feeding her.

Waking your baby to feed

In some situations, babies may be very sleepy and difficult to wake and feed. While you might be ecstatic that your newborn is sleeping for 6 hours in a row at night, you should be waking her up to feed if 4 hours have elapsed since the beginning of her last feeding.

To stimulate a sleepy baby to feed, try changing her diaper, taking off her sleeper, rubbing her back — anything that makes her a little uncomfortable and rouses her.

If your baby is falling asleep on the breast, rub her under the chin to stimulate a suckle or rhythmically compress your breast with your hand to increase milk flow.

Later, once breast-feeding has been firmly established and your baby is gaining weight appropriately, waking her to feed is not necessary.

Feeding duration

Like adults, babies can be fast or slow eaters. Milk supply also varies among mothers: some have a very fast flow of milk, while others have a slower flow, making feeding last longer. Some general guidelines will help you ensure that each feeding is adequate for your baby:

- Let your baby feed for as long as she wants to. You will know she is feeding because you will see her jaw moving and hear her swallow. Once she is finished, she may fall asleep on the breast or she may pull off the breast.
- During a feeding, feed your baby from both breasts. Once she is done feeding on one breast, break her latch and move her to the other. If she is sleepy, you may need to rouse her before she will latch on to your other breast. Alternatively, if she is still hungry, she may latch on eagerly.
- Start each feed on the opposite breast that you last started on. This will help keep your milk supply steady. It is common for babies to drink more from the first breast than from the second. In fact, some babies may not want to feed on the second breast.

Guidelines for the assessment of adequate hydration in breast-fed infants

Day	Frequency of breast-feeding	Urine output	Stool pattern and characteristic	Red flags*
Day 1	• Minimum 6–8 times in 24 hours	• At least 1 wet diaper in 24 hours	• At least 1 meconium in 24 hours	• No voiding • Sore nipples
Day 2	• Minimum 8 times in 24 hours	• 2–4 wet diapers	• Transitional stool to seedy yellow stool	• Decreased voiding • Decreased stooling • Sore nipples
Day 3	• Minimum 8 times in 24 hours	• 4–6 wet diapers	• Transitional stool to seedy yellow stool	• Baby too sleepy to feed • Decreased voiding • Decreased stooling • Sore nipples • Weight loss greater than 7% of birth weight
Day 7	• 8 times per day, every 2-4 hours • Baby satisfied between feeds	• 6 or more wet diapers • Urine pale yellow • No odor	• Seedy yellow stools	• Baby too sleepy to feed • Decreased voiding • Weight loss greater than 10% of birth weight • Sore nipples

*Red flags: When red flags occur, mother and infant should be seen by a health-care provider, as well as by a lactation consultant.

Adapted by permission from Toronto Public Health.

Growth spurts

As your baby grows, you will encounter many changes in her feeding requirements. You will accept most of these adjustments as minor variations and move on. Others, however, will be more noticeable. Making yourself aware of the possibility of these impending changes before they occur will help you manage them.

At 3 weeks, 6 weeks, and 3 months of age, your baby will commonly go through a growth spurt. Growth spurts can last 4 to 5 days. At these times, it will seem like your baby wants to feed constantly. This may be distressing if you have achieved a regular feeding schedule, leading you to question if you have enough breast milk to support your baby's growth. Be reassured that the purpose of these frequent feedings is to *increase* your milk supply. Once this occurs, your baby will go back to feeding less often. During these spurts, resist the temptation to supplement your breast milk with formula; this will not help increase your milk supply.

Cluster feeding

Another common feeding variation is called cluster feeding, when your baby wants to feed more often than usual. This may occur during a growth spurt or on a regular basis at a specific time of day — for example, in the evenings, before bedtime. Not all babies cluster feed, and unlike a growth spurt, it may not stop in 4 to 5 days. All babies are different, so determining your baby's routine is the key.

Milk supply

New mothers often wonder whether their baby is getting enough milk. In almost all cases, a mother produces enough milk for her baby to grow and develop. But unlike formula-feeding, where you know exactly how much formula your baby is taking in, breast-feeding is much less measurable. In fact, it is virtually impossible to know exactly how much your baby is taking in during a feeding, but there are some rules of thumb you can follow:

- **What goes in must come out:** Counting wet and dirty diapers is one of the best ways for new parents to figure out if their baby is getting enough milk. Once you are past the first 5 days, you should expect your baby to have the following urine and stool patterns:
  - At least six urine-soaked diapers a day. The urine should be light yellow or clear in color.

Did You Know?

Weight loss

Following birth, it is common for a baby to lose some weight. A loss of 7% to 10% of your baby's original birth weight is considered acceptable. For example, if your baby weighs 7.7 pounds (3.5 kg) at birth, an initial loss of up to 0.5 pound (0.25 kg) is no cause for concern. When the loss is greater than 7% to 10%, an extensive evaluation of the baby and the feeding method is generally warranted to ensure that the baby is gaining weight appropriately.

- Two to five seedy or pasty yellow stools a day. Once the child is one month of age, stool frequency may decrease to once a day or even once a week.
- **Supply and demand:** Breast milk production follows the rule of supply and demand, so if your baby is not drinking effectively, your breasts will decrease their supply.
- **Latching on:** Fixing an incorrect latch will help your baby to take more milk and your breasts to produce more. If your baby is not latched on correctly, she may not be getting enough milk, even though your breasts are producing it. If your baby is latched on properly, breast-feeding should not hurt. If there is a problem with the latch, there may also be an issue with the amount of milk your baby is receiving. Once your baby is latched and feeding, you should see her mouth moving as she sucks, and you should hear her swallowing.
- **Customer satisfaction:** Your baby should seem satisfied after a feeding.

Possible Problems

If you still suspect that your baby is not receiving adequate breast milk, consult a qualified health-care provider to evaluate your baby's weight gain and general health. If a problem does exist with your milk supply, you may be referred to a lactation consultant or a breast-feeding clinic for additional care to ensure that you have given your body the best "milk-making" setup possible:

- Are you well rested — or, at least, as rested as it is possible to be with a young baby?
- Are you eating a balanced diet?
- Are you nursing exclusively and not supplementing with formula?
- Are you nursing frequently enough?
- Are you nursing long enough?
- Are you nursing on both breasts?
- Have you tried expressing milk after feeding, even though you may get very little or no milk?

If you have addressed these possible sources of the problem, your health-care provider may prescribe a galactagogue, a medication that will stimulate your body to increase its milk production.

Feeding beyond the newborn months

Many mothers wonder how often they should breast-feed their baby after the newborn period (beyond 3 months of age). Many authorities recommend breast-feeding on demand at this stage, but new mothers often want to maintain a feeding schedule and sometimes feel that they can't pick up on all their baby's cues.

For babies who are gaining weight and thriving, it can be helpful to use the recommendations for formula-fed babies as a guide (see table, page 172). Breast milk is digested more rapidly than formula, so it makes sense to breast-feed babies at the upper limit of these recommendations, or slightly more frequently than bottle-fed babies. It is perfectly normal at times for a 1- or 2-month-old baby to breast-feed 10 to 12 times a day. By following these guidelines and assessing your baby's cues for hunger, you should be able to create a feeding schedule that fulfills your baby's needs.

Expressing and storing breast milk

Expressed breast milk allows a baby to feed from a bottle or cup while still receiving the best possible nutrition. In fact, feeding your baby expressed breast milk is a good way to introduce a bottle or cup.

Expressing milk offers many advantages for mothers, too. They are granted some free time to go out alone and can continue breast-feeding after returning to work. Expressing milk may also provide a mother with engorged breasts some relief, even helping to increase milk supply in certain situations. In addition, other family members have an opportunity to bond with the baby while feeding her your breast milk.

Expressing breast milk

There are two basic ways to express breast milk: manually, using your hands; and mechanically, using a pump. While pumps have become increasingly popular, this is an individual decision, and you may find that manual expression works best for you.

Expressing milk manually

Manual milk expression can be done anywhere. It does not require equipment, and it does not make any noise. It is a learned skill — your ability to express milk this way will improve with practice. If you need assistance, contact a lactation consultant or discuss the procedure with a mother who has done this before.

1. Wash your hands.
2. Select a container to hold the milk. A container with a large opening and a pouring spout is best. A large measuring cup works perfectly. Wash it with warm soapy water, then rinse.

3. Hold your hand in a "C" shape and cup the breast closest to the hand. Make sure your thumb is opposite from your index finger and middle finger, about 1 inch (2.5 cm) away from the nipple.

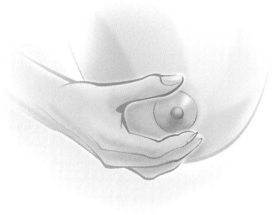

4. Gently pull your thumb and fingers back in toward your chest.

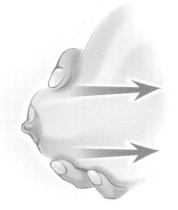

5. Squeeze your thumb and fingers together and move them forward toward the areola.

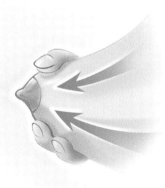

6. Continue to do this until the milk supply slows down (it starts dripping rather than squirting).

7. You may need to change your hand's position, moving it around your breast.

8. Never squeeze the nipple — this will occlude the milk ducts, and milk will not be able to come out.

Expressing milk mechanically

There are three kinds of pumps you can purchase to express breast milk. Each has its benefits and is suitable for a different situation. Wash the pump in hot soapy water after every use. Be sure to check the manufacturer's instructions on cleaning. If you plan on using it while out of the house, remember to pack some cleaning supplies.

Storing expressed breast milk

Once you have pumped breast milk, you will need to store it correctly to prevent contamination and nutrient loss. Expressed milk should be refrigerated or frozen unless you plan on feeding it to the baby shortly after expression.

Storing breast milk safely

There are many different opinions on how to store breast milk — the "best" way has yet to be scientifically determined. In the meantime, here are some guidelines that will help you store it safely:

- Purchase clean glass or plastic containers with tight lids.
- If you choose to store your milk in plastic bags, use breast milk storage bags designed for this purpose. Regular bottle liners or plastic bags may destroy some of your milk's protective antibodies.
- Always date the container so you can keep track of how long you have been storing the milk (see box, page 149, to learn how long it's safe to store it).
- Store milk in small amounts (2 to 4 oz/ 60 to 120 mL) so that you don't end up wasting it.
- Don't add unfrozen milk to previously frozen milk. This may promote the growth of bacteria.
- Never refreeze milk once it is thawed.

Guide to breast milk pumps

Kind of pump	Average cost	Uses and benefits
Hand pump	$30 to $70	• Good for occasional pumping (once a week or less) • Can pump only one breast at a time • Requires small amount of hand strength to operate pump • Easy to travel with • Best results once milk is established (may not work as well immediately following birth)
Small single-breast battery-operated pump	$80 to $130	• Good for periodic pumping (once a week or less) • Can pump only one breast at a time • Battery-operated • Easy to travel with
Large electric (or battery-operated) dual breast pump	$100 to $400	• Good for frequent pumping (daily use) • Can pump both breasts simultaneously, taking less time to pump • Larger than single-breast pumps • More cumbersome to travel with • Best results if trying to establish volume

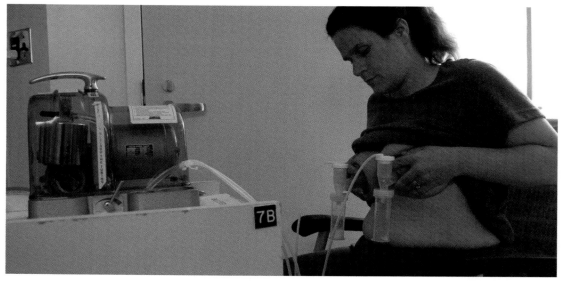

■ An electric pump is the best way to obtain large volumes of breast milk quickly. It is the method of choice for situations that require exclusive feeding with expressed breast milk.

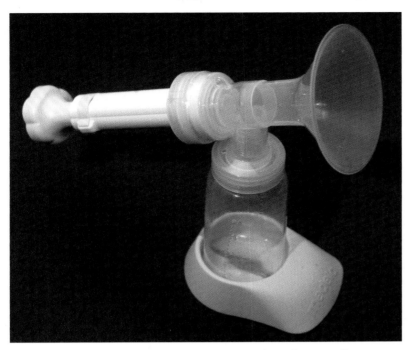

■ A simple hand pump is an inexpensive way to obtain breast milk successfully on an occasional basis.

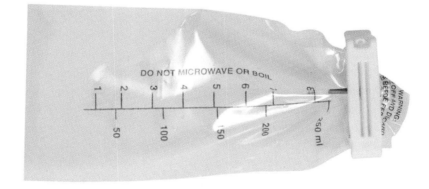

■ A breast milk storage bag.

Did You Know?

Breast milk storage

Store expressed breast milk in the refrigerator for up to 3 days; in the freezer of a one-door refrigerator for up to 2 weeks; in the freezer of a two-door refrigerator for up to 3 months; or in a deep freezer for up to 6 months.

Breast pumping difficulties

For some women, expressing breast milk is very simple. They try it a few times and — voilà — they are able to produce an adequate amount of milk on a regular basis. Other women have more difficulty. Some complain that they are not able to express very much milk; some find pumping very painful. Fortunately, these problems can be overcome.

The first few times you pump, it may seem like you pump forever and get only a very small amount of milk, perhaps just ¼ to ½ ounce (7.5 to 15 mL). While this can be frustrating, it is completely normal. It doesn't mean you have less milk, nor is it at all representative of what your baby is getting during regular feeds.

Letdown

Some women find it difficult to achieve a letdown response using a pump. To make the process more productive, be sure you are in a warm, comfortable place when you are pumping. You may want to put warm compresses on your breasts or take a shower before pumping. Also, make sure you are in a secure environment. If there are others around, you may want to lock the door to ensure your privacy and decrease disruptions. Having your baby present, or a picture of your baby, may help you achieve letdown more easily. You may also want to visualize your baby feeding while pumping.

Take care to choose the best time to pump, coordinated with your regular feeding schedule and your milk supply. Your milk supply fluctuates during the day and night. Most women find their breasts are fullest in the middle of the night and in the early morning, so you could try pumping when you first wake up to get the best volume. By attending to your body's cues and your baby's cues, you will soon determine when pumping works best for you.

Pumping pain

Pumping should not be painful, but if you pump for long periods at a time, you may feel pain. Short, frequent pumping sessions may be more rewarding and less traumatic to your sensitive breast tissue. If you are using an electric pump, you may be tempted to increase the pressure of the pump to shorten the time it takes to

Did You Know?

Nipple confusion

"Give a baby a bottle and she will no longer choose the breast," the old saying goes. While this "nipple confusion" may be true in some cases, the opposite may also be true — give the baby the breast and she will no longer take the bottle. A better term than "nipple confusion" might be "nipple preference." Babies have a tendency to prefer the feeding method they use most often. For women who are breast-feeding, this may be fine, until they realize they can't leave their baby with another caregiver for an extended period of time because their baby refuses a bottle. To prevent this, introduce a regular bottle once breast-feeding is well established.

pump or to pump more milk. Be wary when increasing the pressure: do it very slowly and stop if you feel pain — it may result in sore or cracked nipples. You may end up having more difficulty achieving letdown because you anticipate pain when using the pump.

Introducing the bottle

Once breast-feeding is well established, by the time your baby is 4 to 6 weeks of age, you may want to try expressing your milk and offering her a bottle. How frequently you choose to offer the bottle is up to you. However, infants prefer a routine, so if you don't routinely offer them a bottle, they may not want to take it when you want them to.

Offer your child a bottle of breast milk every few days while you are breast-feeding so she will start to accept the bottle as a substitute. You may have another family member feed her the bottle, depending on your situation. Some babies may not want to take a bottle from their mother because they prefer to breast-feed from her. Now is a good time to let Dad have a hand in feeding.

If you have difficulty getting your baby to take a bottle, never force her. Continue to offer her the bottle from time to time, or have another person offer it to her until she accepts this way of feeding.

Preparing the bottle

If you are feeding breast milk you have just pumped, no preparation of the milk is required. Don't worry if your expressed milk has a slight yellowish or even bluish tinge. This is normal.

Here are some tips for preparing the bottle:

- Clean the bottle before putting milk in it.
- Give the bottle a gentle shake after filling it: expressed milk will separate so that the fat lies on top.
- If you are feeding milk that was frozen, thaw it by placing it in the refrigerator or in a bowl of water.
- Serve the milk at room temperature.
- Do not heat breast milk in a microwave. Too much heat can damage the proteins and vitamins in breast milk. If you choose to warm the milk, do so by placing the container in some warm water.
- Once your baby is finished, discard any milk left in the bottle — it may become contaminated with bacteria.

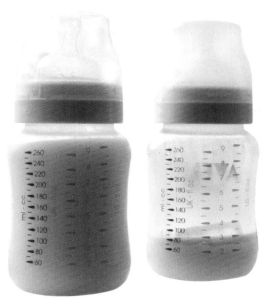

■ A yellowish or even bluish color is normal for expressed milk.

Weaning your child

Most people believe weaning means the process of stopping breast-feeding, but it is more accurately described as the process of starting to feed your child something other than breast milk, such as infant formula or cereal. The current recommendation is to breast-feed exclusively until your baby is 6 months old and then start introducing solid foods along with the breast milk. Be sure to introduce iron-fortified foods, because infant iron stores start to become depleted between 4 and 6 months of age.

While the current recommendation is to continue breast-feeding until a child is 2 years of age or longer, any amount of breast-feeding will benefit your baby.

Natural and mother-led weaning

Children often wean themselves off the breast between 2 and 4 years of age, a process called natural weaning. However, based on your lifestyle and commitments, you may want to wean your baby before then, a process called mother-led weaning.

If a baby is weaned off breast milk prior to 12 months of age, the milk feedings should be replaced with infant formula. At 12 months of age, 3.25% cow's milk may be introduced, and at 24 months, it can be changed to 2% cow's milk.

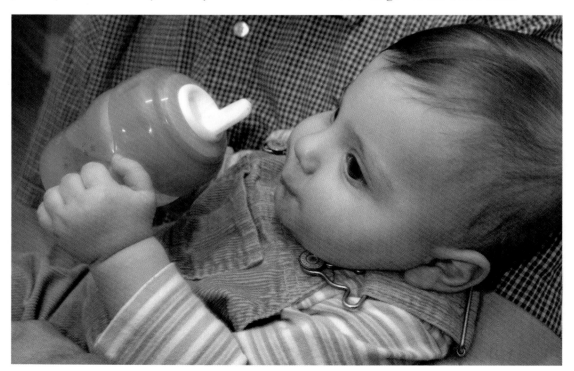

HOW TO
Wean your child

The best way to wean a child off the breast is slowly — it will be easier on both of you. However, there is no "correct" number of days to wait between dropped feedings. You might drop a feeding every few days, weeks, or months. Some women choose only partial weaning, continuing to breast-feed their baby at certain feeding times (for example, morning and night).

To begin weaning, follow these steps:

1. Determine your baby's least favorite feeding. This may seem impossible if she likes breast-feeding — as most babies do. In this event, choose your least favorite feeding or one when your baby doesn't drink very much.

2. For this dropped feeding, give her formula or milk (depending on her age) by bottle or cup.

3. If your child initially refuses the bottle, keep trying, or have another family member try to give this feeding.

4. If you are unsure of how much milk or formula to offer, start with the age-appropriate amount. Your baby will take what she needs; any leftovers should be discarded. If she is still hungry, you may need to offer more.

5. Once this feeding is going well — after, say, a few days to a week — substitute another bottle or cup feed.

6. Continue dropping feedings until you have reached your goal — partial or full wean.

Weaning should not be abrupt unless there is an emergency situation — for example, if a mother needs to start treatment for a disease. If you need to wean your child quickly, you may suffer engorgement, blocked ducts, or mastitis.

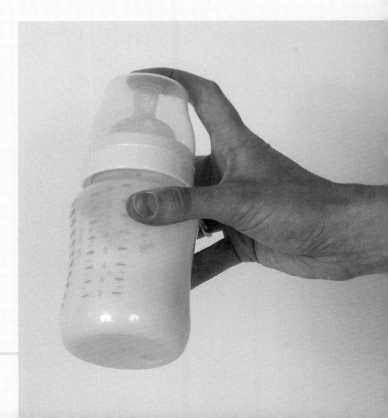

Treating common breast-feeding problems

For many women, breast-feeding is fairly straightforward. If you do encounter problems, knowing how to assess and manage them is important for your health and the welfare of your baby. Listed below are some common problems and their suggested treatments. Seek care from a health-care provider or specialist in breast-feeding if the problem persists.

Treating common breast-feeding conditions

Diagnosis	Signs and symptoms	Common treatment
Sore and/or cracked nipples	• Red, dry nipples • Visible cracks in nipples, bruising • Pain with breast-feeding, usually most severe when baby first starts to nurse • Nipple is "pinched" when baby comes off the breast	• Ensure that your baby is latching correctly — an incorrect latch is the usual cause of sore or cracked nipples. • After feeding, express a few drops of breast milk onto your nipple and let it dry. • Make sure your nipples always have a chance to dry after feeding. • Do not use breast pads that don't allow breast tissue to breathe. • Use a breast shield between feeds if needed. • Apply lanolin ointment to nipples after each feed. • Do not apply creams or lotions that you need to remove prior to feeding. • When bathing, use only water (no soap) on breasts. • Consider nipple shields, but keep in mind that there are many varying opinions and little conclusive research on their use. They can aggravate the problem, so you may wish to speak with your health-care provider to decide if they are appropriate for you.

Diagnosis	Signs and symptoms	Common treatment
Leaking nipples	• Breast milk leaks out of nipples and onto bra or clothing when baby is not feeding or you are not with baby	• None — this is a natural occurrence for some women. • To prevent leakage onto your bra and clothing, use breast pads (cloth is best) to collect milk. • To prevent complications such as dry, cracked nipples, use breast pads that are not lined with plastic.
Engorgement Breasts become too full with milk. Commonly occurs when milk first comes in or if feedings are missed.	• Breasts are extremely full and hard • Breasts may hurt when touched • Breasts are very warm • Areola are hard, difficult for baby to latch on	• Express breast milk frequently to relieve the pressure (preferably with a pump). • Breast-feed more frequently. • Apply warm compresses prior to feeding. • Apply cold compresses for severe engorgement between feeds. • Massage your breasts, starting from your armpit and going down to your nipple, prior to feeding or expressing. • Consider pain medication as required (ibuprofen or acetaminophen). • Consider placing cold cabbage leaves inside your bra for 20 minutes or until the leaves soften — there is no evidence to support this treatment, but some swear by it.
Blocked duct One of the ducts that your milk flows through has become plugged. Usually localized to one breast.	• One section of the breast is red, hard, and often painful • A lump may be felt	• Feed frequently — your baby's suckling will help unblock the duct. • Start feeding on the side that is blocked. • Try feeding your baby in a different position (for example, if you usually feed using a cradle hold, switch to a football hold) and try to position her so that her jaw is on the side of the blocked duct. • Apply moist heat to the affected area. • Massage the affected area. • Monitor a blocked duct very closely — it can lead to mastitis if not treated.

Diagnosis	Signs and symptoms	Common treatment
Mastitis Bacterial infection of the breast tissue, usually localized to one breast. Not a common problem.	• Pain or swelling in the breast, similar to a blocked duct • Fever and other flu-like symptoms	• Try treatments for a blocked duct, but if symptoms persist for more than 24 hours, seek immediate medical attention and treatment with antibiotics. • Continue to breast-feed regularly. This infection does not affect the quality of the breast milk, and feeding may help treat the mastitis — abrupt cessation of breast-feeding will exacerbate the problem. • Start feeding on the affected side. • To prevent in the future, avoid pressure on the breast (from a poorly fitting bra, for example); try to feed your baby regularly; and ensure that she has a good latch and is draining the breast effectively.
Yeast infection May be a new onset when you have not had previous problems with breast-feeding. May follow antibiotic use in mother or baby.	• Deep, shooting pain or burning while breast-feeding that lasts for the entire feed, and even after the feed in some instances • Pain and very sensitive nipples while not breast-feeding — may be worse at night • Breasts may or may not show any physical signs, such as swelling or discoloration, that something is wrong • Baby may or may not have white patches (thrush) in her mouth or a persistent diaper rash	• Ensure that your baby is latching correctly — an incorrect latch will increase your pain. • Continue to breast-feed regularly. This infection does not affect the quality of the breast milk. • Keep breasts dry and, if possible, expose them to the air as much as possible. • Do not use breast pads with plastic lining or wear a bra that traps moisture around the nipple. • Change your bra daily. • If the baby has a pacifier, sterilize it daily. • Seek the services of a health-care provider: topical treatments — such as 1% gentian violet (for 4 to 7 days maximum) or topical antifungals (for example, clotrimazole) — are generally used first. • Treat the baby with gentian violet or a topical antifungal (for example, nystatin). She may have oral thrush.

Diagnosis	Signs and symptoms	Common treatment
Raynaud's phenomenon Vasospasm of the blood vessels — occurs more commonly in other parts of the body (for example, the hands).	• Nipple turns white (vasospasm) after baby finishes feeding — can be very painful and there may be a burning sensation • After some time, color returns to nipple, but pain may persist • Nipple may throb when blood and/or color return to it	• Fix your baby's latch first — pain is often secondary to a poor latch, and this pain increases exponentially when vasospasm occurs. • Apply a warm facecloth to the areola and nipple after breast-feeding and let it cool gradually. • Visit your health-care provider — in severe cases, you may need medication.

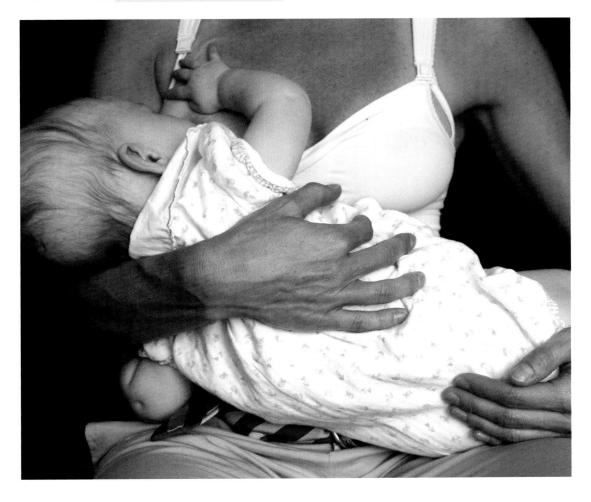

Breast-feeding multiples

While breast-feeding just one baby can be a challenge, multiples can make it even more tricky. Remember that breast-feeding is a learned skill for both you and your babies. The logistics of feeding two babies at one time may seem daunting; however, a mother's body will respond well to the increased demand for milk, producing more as needed. In many situations, mothers can exclusively breast-feed more than one baby without resorting to formula supplements.

Special support

Many obstetrical centers offer breast-feeding assistance for parents of multiples, as well as information on other issues specific to twins and triplets. These centers often facilitate support groups for parents of multiples.

If you are going to be breast-feeding more than one baby, seek out a lactation consultant, who will help you and your babies grow comfortable with latching and show you how to position two babies at one time. While this service may seem expensive, it is much more economical than buying formula for two or more babies. Besides, breast-feeding is beneficial for your babies — especially if they are premature, as multiple babies often are.

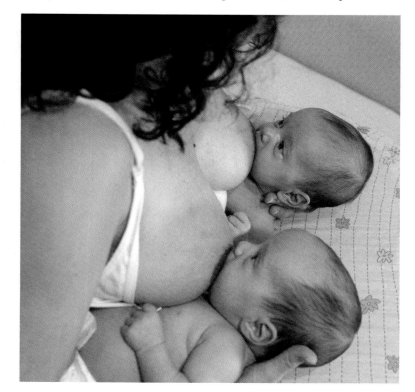

Breast-feeding premature babies

While breast-feeding is recommended for full-term infants, it is highly recommended for premature infants. Never is breast-feeding more important than it is for a premature baby. Premature babies are at greater risk for infection and gastrointestinal problems. Breast milk provides them with immunity factors (immunoglobulins) to help fight infection and reduce the risk of gastrointestinal disease.

Added benefits

Because premature babies need a lot of energy to survive, extra calories may need to be added to your breast milk before it is fed to your baby, but even with this alteration, breast milk is easier for your baby to digest than formula. Premature babies, particularly very low birth weight babies, may spend considerable time in the hospital with many health-care providers — at times, you may feel as if everyone but you takes care of your baby. Providing your child with breast milk will help you keep in touch with your baby and help to shorten her stay in the intensive care unit.

Feeding techniques

How your baby receives your breast milk will vary depending on how premature she is. Your health-care provider will be able to advise you on how to feed your baby depending on her gestational age and condition. If she is very premature, she may initially be fed by a feeding tube through the nose or mouth into the stomach. In this situation, it is best to express breast milk using a large electric dual-breast pump or hospital-grade breast pump to empty the milk from your breasts. Frequent pumping (at least every 3 hours) is essential for building and maintaining your milk supply. If your baby was feeding at the breast, she would likely be feeding every 2 to 3 hours, so it is important to replicate this frequency. A lactation consultant can help you establish the most productive pumping environment and feeding routine. During the tube-feeding period, you will still be able to hold your baby skin to skin (kangaroo care), and she

Did You Know?

Gestational age

The breast milk your body produces is made especially for your baby and her specific gestational age. The milk your body produces for a premature baby will be different from the milk it produces for a 6-month-old baby.

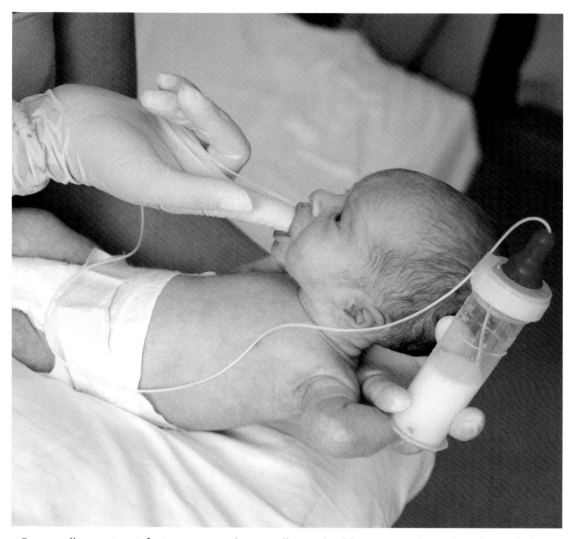

■ Even small premature infants can receive breast milk. Your health-care providers will teach you the best technique for your situation.

may be able to practice suckling at the breast (called a non-nutritive suck).

Once your baby is older and stronger, you will be able to feed her directly from the breast. When she begins feeding at the breast, she may only take a small amount of milk before tiring. She may then need supplemental breast milk by cup or feeding tube. In this case, you will need to pump breast milk after she finishes feeding from the breast to maintain your supply.

Premature babies may also need supplementation with iron because they have not had a chance to fully build their iron stores before birth. Like all breast-fed babies, they will also require vitamin D supplementation.

Getting started with formula-feeding

Receiving more advice on formula-feeding may seem daunting to tired and inexperienced parents. Relax! It doesn't take long to become expert at formula-feeding your infant. Take all the time you need to get things right, then sit back and enjoy feeding your baby.

Extra support

Feeding your baby formula takes additional preparation time, but it means other people can help you. You get a much-needed break while your partner or another caregiver has an opportunity for some bonding time with the baby.

The use of formula also requires extra financial outlay. While regular powdered formula is costly, liquid concentrate or ready-to-feed formula can be even more so, and if your baby requires a special type of formula, such as a hydrolyzed formula, the family budget can go out of kilter.

Formula itself is not the only expense: you'll also need some equipment.

Formula-feeding equipment

If you plan on formula-feeding your baby (or feeding her breast milk by bottle), you will need to buy bottles, nipples, and, in some cases, a sterilizer.

Bottles

There are many types of bottles available on the market — plastic bottles, glass bottles, bottles with disposable liners, straight bottles, angled bottles, venting bottles, and anti-colic bottles. As a new parent, you may be understandably overwhelmed when faced with choosing a bottle for your baby. Should you buy a simple straight bottle or an expensive high-tech bottle with several little pieces that will require cleaning? What size bottles should you buy? How many bottles?

The good news is that most bottles on the market are fine. Many companies make claims about the advantages of their bottles, but the truth is that all bottles work. While some research has been done on the merits of various bottles, there is not enough evidence to recommend one particular type over another. The choice is often one of personal preference. Know yourself: for example, if cleaning out dirty bottles is a hassle for you, go for a bottle with a disposable liner.

Nipples

Once you have chosen a bottle, you face another decision: what nipples should you buy for it? Actually, you may want to make this decision *before* choosing a bottle because certain nipples are meant for certain bottles. Once you choose a nipple, you will be left with fewer bottle choices.

Guide to

Choosing a bottle

Consider these questions when choosing a bottle for your baby:

- Is it made of plastic or glass? If it is breakable, does this concern you?
- What do the instructions say about how to sterilize it?
- Is it microwave-safe?
- Does it have a wide mouth (which makes it easier to clean)?
- Does it have a lot of little pieces to clean?

- Will you need to buy disposable liners?
- Will your baby be able to hang on to it when she gets older?

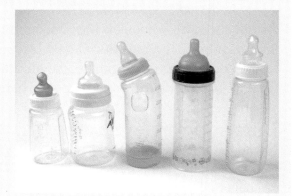

However, in many cases, it is your baby who will end up choosing the nipple. Purchase only a few bottles and nipples before your child's birth in case she does not feed well from your initial choice. While it is not a good idea to introduce different nipples all at once, you need to be open to the idea that the nipple you have chosen may not be right for your baby.

Manufacturers of certain nipples profess that their nipple is more like the human nipple or helps to reduce colic, but there is limited evidence for these claims. Choose a nipple that is easy to clean and that works with the bottle you prefer. If you are breast-feeding as well as bottle-feeding, you may want to choose a nipple that most resembles your own (easier said then done). Your baby should be able to "latch on" to it much as she does to your breast. This kind of nipple often has a round base and a long tip.

Nipples are commonly made of silicone or latex. Silicone nipples are typically (but

not always) firmer than latex nipples; for this reason, new babies may prefer latex nipples. Silicone nipples are clear in color, which makes them easier to clean; latex nipples are usually brown. There are rare cases of children with latex allergies.

Nipples also come in different shapes: standard nipples, long rounded-tip nipples, nubbin nipples, tricot nipples, flat-tipped orthodontic nipples, preemie nipples, and specialty nipples (such as Haberman nipples).

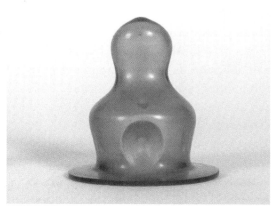

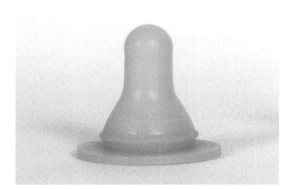

Nipples break down, get worn, and need replacing, so be sure to monitor the quality of the nipples you are using and replace them if they are dirty and cannot be cleaned, if the holes become too large, or if the material starts to break down.

Sterilization equipment

The Canadian Paediatric Society recommends that water and equipment used to feed babies be sterilized until the babies are 3 to 4 months old. This is the age when babies typically start to pick things up and put them in their mouth; it is also when their developing immune system allows them to fight off infections more effectively. Sterilization is no longer warranted by this age.

In fact, many experts feel that, in developed countries with safe drinking water, it is probably not necessary to boil the water used to reconstitute formula. And modern dishwashers do a fine job of cleaning bottles and nipples, especially if the nipples are scrubbed first.

Still, you may choose to sterilize formula water and bottles. The least expensive way to do this is to immerse the equipment in a pot of boiling water for at least 5 minutes. However, many frazzled new parents forget that they have put the bottles and nipples in boiling water — only to return later and realize that they have melted the equipment.

There are faster, safer, and more efficient ways to sterilize equipment. Electric steam sterilizers plug into an outlet and turn off automatically when finished. Sterilizers that you put into the microwave for a few minutes are available, as are containers that hold bottles and nipples in position in the dishwasher.

Did You Know?

Flow rates

Different nipples have different flow rates. Every manufacturer has its own system for grading the flow. Some use numbers, while others grade their nipples as slow, medium, or fast.

- For newborn babies, choose nipples with a slow flow rate. As your baby grows, increase the flow rate (which means purchasing new nipples) according to manufacturer guidelines.

- If you are breast-feeding, you will need to evaluate the flow of milk from your breasts. You will know it is fast if your baby occasionally pulls off your breast and chokes because she has gotten too much milk in her mouth at once. In this case, you may want to choose a nipple with a faster rate because this is what your baby is accustomed to.

Water safety

Even if you sterilize the water you use to reconstitute formula, you need to consider its safety. Some water sources, such as well water, contain substances that may be harmful to small babies, such as nitrites, arsenic, and heavy metals. Before using well water to mix formula, have it tested to ensure that it is safe.

Added fluoride is fine for your baby. In fact, if the water supply in your area does not contain fluoride, your health-care provider may recommend that you supplement with fluoride.

Many older houses contain lead pipes that can leave sediment in your water. Hot water is more likely to contain sediment. It is best to turn on your cold water tap and let it run for 2 minutes to clear any contaminants. Then you can collect the water you will use to mix formula. You should let the water run even if you plan on boiling it.

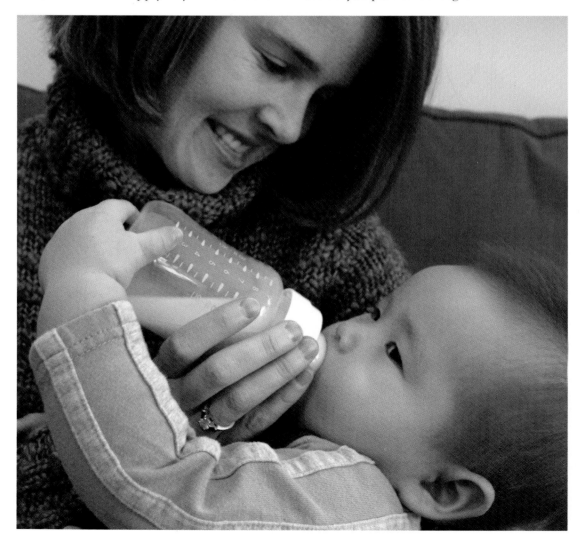

Choosing a formula for your baby

As with so many decisions in the first few months, it can be tough to determine the right formula to choose. When you're standing in the store, all the options you're faced with can be daunting. Relax. Buying formula is like buying a carton of milk: although every company that makes formula claims that their product is unique, they all basically taste the same.

Formula is offered in several different bases — cow's milk, soy, and protein hydrolysate, for example. Once you determine the type appropriate for your baby (formula based on cow's milk will usually do), you just need to choose from one of the many brands. Don't lose sleep over which one to choose.

Iron and fatty acid fortification

Make sure the formula you choose is iron fortified. All soy-based formulas are fortified with iron, but not all cow's milk formulas are. Although regular formulas do have some iron, it is insufficient to meet the baby's needs. Contrary to popular belief, iron-fortified formulas have not been shown to cause constipation, but they will help prevent iron deficiency anemia.

Recently, formula companies have begun to fortify their formulas with the fatty acids DHA (docosahexaenoic acid) and ARA (arachidonic acid), which are building blocks for the brain. These fatty acids are found in the systems of breast-fed babies, but not in those of formula-fed babies. Infants store these substances in their brains and retinas at optimal levels between the third trimester of pregnancy and 18 months of age, during which time the brain undergoes major growth and development. In full-term babies, some DHA and ARA cross the placenta and are stored, but babies born very early do not receive these nutrients. Research has demonstrated that adding these fatty acids to the diet of preterm infants has a positive effect on their visual development.

Further research is needed to determine whether adding DHA and ARA to formula has any effect on infant development or intelligence, but if you can afford formula with added DHA and ARA, it may turn out to be a good choice.

Formula preparations

Cow's milk and soy-based formulas come in three standard preparations: powder, liquid concentrate, and ready-to-feed. All provide adequate nutrition for your baby. Protein hydrolysate formulas come only in powder form, and transition formulas come only in powder and liquid concentrate form.

Guide to formulas

Formula (sample brands)	Characteristics	Use
Cow's milk (Enfamil, Similac)	• Made with cow's milk, but it has been significantly changed so that the composition of fat and protein is similar to that of breast milk • Best taste • Average cost • Not all brands are iron-fortified; choose one that is	• Appropriate for almost all healthy full-term infants, except those with a true allergy to cow's milk protein or a strong family history of allergy to cow's milk protein.
Soy-based (Isomil, Prosobee)	• Made from soybeans • Not currently recommended for routine use unless there is a reason why cow's milk protein formulas are not appropriate • Average taste • Average cost • All brands are iron-fortified	• Not generally suitable for children with an allergy to cow's milk protein, because it is estimated that 50% will be allergic to soy as well (use a casein hydrolysate formula instead). • Recommended for infants with galactosemia (a very rare inherited abnormality of carbohydrate metabolism). • Suitable for infants whose parents wish to maintain a strict vegetarian or vegan diet. • Generally lactose-free, so can be given to infants with lactose intolerance. • Some varieties may be suitable for infants whose parents wish to maintain a halal or kosher diet — check formula containers when purchasing to verify.

Formula (sample brands)	Characteristics	Use
Lactose-free cow's milk (LactoFree)	• Based on cow's milk, but free of lactose • Does not taste as good as regular cow's milk formulas • More expensive than regular cow's milk formulas	• Suitable for infants who are lactose-intolerant (which is quite rare). • Suitable to use for a short period of time following a diarrheal illness (if recommended by your health-care provider because of transient lactose intolerance).
Protein hydrolysate Whey hydrolysate (Nestle Good Start) or casein hydrolysate, also called "hypoallergenic" (Alimentum, Nutramigen, Pregestamil)	• Whey hydrolysates are broken into quite large proteins; casein hydrolysates are broken into very small proteins and can be used in infants with allergic disorders • Casein hydrolysates do not taste good, but are well accepted by younger infants, whose sense of taste is not yet well developed • Casein hydrolysate formulas are more expensive	• *Whey hydrolysate formulas:* Not suitable for children with an allergy to cow's milk protein; sometimes recommended for infants with gastroesophageal reflux disease. • *Casein hydrolysate formulas:* Suitable for infants with a diagnosed allergy to cow's milk protein; casein hydrolysate formulas should be used only if recommended by a pediatric health-care provider. • Used when an infant has one of various conditions that cause damage to the lining of the bowel, making it more difficult to digest and absorb regular formulas.
Amino acid–based (Neocate)	• Made from amino acids • Poor taste • Extremely costly	• Used in special medical situations, such as with severe malabsorptive conditions. • Used only when recommended by a pediatric health-care provider.

Formula (sample brands)	Characteristics	Use
Follow-up formulas Cow's milk or soy-based (Nestle Follow-Up)	• Can be used from 6 to 12 months and beyond • Marketed as good for your baby because they contain higher levels of calcium and iron • Superior to cow's milk for a baby less than 1 year old, but have not been proven superior to starter formulas • Best taste • Less expensive than basic starter formulas	• Suitable for children 6 months and older, if the parent wishes.
Added rice formulas (Enfalac AR)	• Cow's milk formula with added rice starch	• Sometimes recommended for infants who spit up (gastroesophageal reflux) if the reflux is sufficient to cause inadequate weight gain. Medication may be required in addition to thickening feeds and adjusting positioning in some cases.

Note: If you are looking for a halal or kosher formula, make sure you check the packaging or call the company that produces the formula to ensure that it is prepared in the appropriate manner.

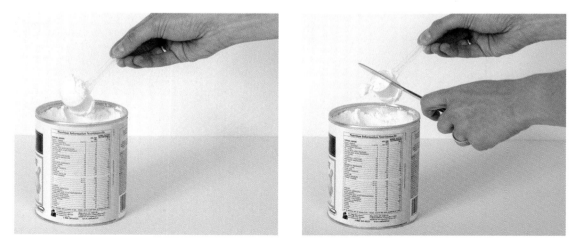

Guide to formula preparations

Preparation	Advantages	Disadvantages
Powder	• Least expensive • Tin of powder lasts for up to 1 month once opened • Tin does not need to be refrigerated	• Can be difficult to dissolve unless you use warm water • Can be messy when out in public — need to have special container to carry it • Need to have clean (or sterile) water to mix with • Risk of incorrect measurement of powder
Liquid concentrate	• Very easy to mix • Very easy to measure • Less expensive than ready-to-feed	• If going out, need to pre-mix bottle • Need to mix more than one bottle at a time; otherwise, you end up discarding and wasting the rest of the concentrate, as it makes more than one bottle • Need to have clean (or sterile) water to mix with concentrate • Once opened, good for only 48 hours and must be refrigerated
Ready-to-feed	• Most convenient: just open, pour into bottle, and feed • No need to have clean (or sterile) water to mix with	• Most expensive

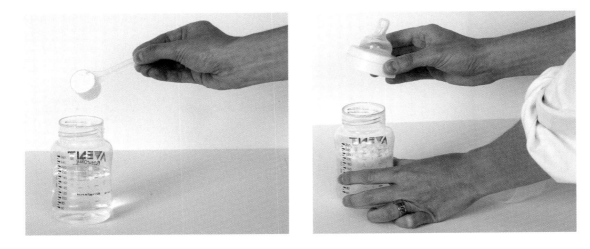

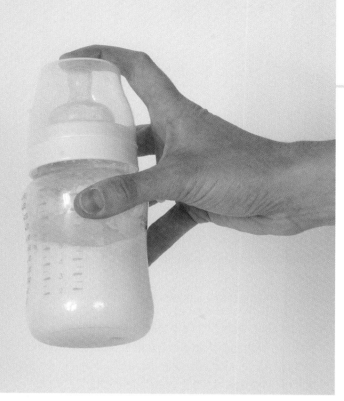

Preparation

The correct way to prepare your baby's bottle is to closely follow the directions provided by the formula company. While most directions are similar, there may be slight differences between companies, so it is important to read the instructions carefully.

Powder and liquid concentrate preparations should be mixed with water prior to feeding. Follow the directions on how much water to add to the letter. Too little water can concentrate the formula, making it difficult for your baby's body to digest and putting undue stress on the kidneys. Too much water decreases the concentration of the formula, as well as the calories, putting your child at risk for failure to thrive (inadequate growth). Unless you are directed by a health-care provider to mix the formula differently, you should follow the directions exactly as they appear on the can.

Warming bottles

The first question you may ask yourself is, Do I need to warm my baby's bottle? The answer is a definite *no*. In fact, incorrect warming of a bottle is much more dangerous than feeding your baby a cold bottle. A room-temperature bottle is appropriate, and most babies will be fine with this. If you do choose to warm the bottle, be cautious about how you do it to avoid burning your baby's mouth.

Storage

Once you have mixed the formula, you may or may not be able to store it. Some formulas can be stored in the refrigerator for up to 48 hours, while others must be used within 1 hour of mixing.

If your baby takes only part of her bottle and you think she may take more, you may feed her the remainder of her bottle within 1 hour of the beginning of the feeding. After this, used formula should be discarded because it is a breeding ground for bacteria. If the formula you choose is one that can

---

Did You Know?

Warm or cold

Babies will drink what they are given and will get used to a warm or cold bottle. If you always warm your baby's bottle, she might not take one that is cold or at room temperature. This may prove difficult if you find yourself with a screaming hungry baby at a time when you are not able to warm the bottle.

be prepared in advance, you can carry it with you in its prepared state, but once it has been out of the refrigerator for more than 2 hours, it should be disposed of.

Cans of formula (liquid and powdered) have expiry dates. Never use formula that has expired. Most formula companies recommend using up a can of powdered formula within 1 month after it is opened. After this time, the remaining contents should be discarded. Liquid concentrate formula can be stored for up to 48 hours once opened, provided it is kept in the refrigerator.

Formula-feeding schedule

Many parents wonder how much formula they should feed their baby, and how often. They worry that they are feeding too much or too little, and aren't sure how to tell when their child is satisfied and when she is still hungry. Parental concern about how much food a child is eating often continues throughout childhood — and sometimes beyond.

Hunger cues

Babies provide cues to indicate that they are hungry, and parents usually learn pretty quickly to recognize these cues. A newborn baby will demonstrate her hunger initially by waking up from a deep sleep, stretching, and maybe yawning. She may start rooting or nuzzling toward your chest. She may suck on her fists or make sucking motions with her mouth. If these cues don't elicit the desired response, she may start to cry. If possible, try to feed her before she starts

Guide to

Warming a bottle

Although it is not necessary, you can warm a bottle by setting it in a container of warm water, which will gently warm the contents. Electric bottle warmers are not neccesary.

- Heat the formula until it is lukewarm. To test the temperature, shake a few drops onto the inner part of your wrist. If it feels neither cold nor hot, then it is lukewarm and should not be heated further. Always mix the contents of the bottle before serving it to your baby to ensure an equal temperature throughout.
- Do not use a microwave to warm a bottle — microwave heat is very uneven. When a bottle of milk is heated in a microwave, it may feel cool to the touch on the outside; however, there may be very hot areas of liquid on the inside. Babies have burned their mouths when drinking from what appeared to be a cool bottle.
- If you feel you must use a microwave to warm your baby's bottle, be cautious about what equipment you are using. Some bottles and bottle liners will degrade in microwave heat. Once you have mixed the formula (post-microwave), check the temperature to make sure it is not too hot.
- Never heat breast milk in a microwave. Microwave heat breaks down the immune factors in breast milk.

crying, as she may be more receptive — it is difficult to calm a frantic baby.

Remember that crying is one of the few ways babies can express themselves, and a crying baby is not necessarily a hungry baby. You will need to assess other factors, such as when she was last fed and how much formula she took.

Once you've finally worked out her cues for hunger, how can you tell when she is full? Babies indicate they are full by falling asleep; by playing with the nipple of the bottle (for example, chewing on it); by stopping sucking; by crying when you try to give them the bottle; or by turning their head away from the bottle.

Never force your baby to eat more once she has indicated that she is full. Even if she takes only 2 ounces (60 mL) of a 4-ounce (120 mL) bottle, resist the urge to try to get her to finish the whole bottle. On the other hand, if your baby still seems hungry after finishing a bottle, give her more. Babies go through many growth changes, and their feeding habits change regularly. A baby knows how much she wants and how often, and she will tell you as much — you just need to learn how to read her cues.

Formula-feeding schedule

The table below is a convenient guide to how much and how often to feed your baby in the first year. Remember, some babies will eat more and some will eat less, so expect deviations from this schedule. If you are concerned that your baby is not taking enough formula, you will need to assess her output from her urine and stool patterns, as well as her weight, which your health-care provider can best evaluate. In the first few months, babies generally gain $3/4$ to 1 ounce (20 to 30 grams) a day.

Transitional feedings

There will come a time when your baby will need to adjust to a different kind of feeding. The transition may be from breast milk to formula or from formula to cow's milk — or you may be instructed by your health-care provider to change formulas. No matter what kind of change you are making, make it gradually (unless you are instructed otherwise) to give your baby a chance to adapt. Slowly increase the amount of the new feed and decrease the amount of the old feed. Wait at least 24 hours after each change to see how your baby reacts. This process may take up to 8 days.

Recommended feeding schedule for formula-fed babies

Age	Feedings per day	Amount per feed
0–1 week	6–10	2–3 oz (60–90 mL)
1–4 weeks	6–8	3–4 oz (90–120 mL)
1–3 months	5–6	4–6 oz (120–180 mL)
3–7 months	4–5	6–7 oz (180–210 mL)
7–12 months	3–4	7–8 oz (210–240 mL)

Adapted by permission from D. Kalnins and J. Saab, *Better Baby Food* (Toronto: Robert Rose, 2001).

HOW TO
Feed your baby with a bottle

1. Before feeding your baby a bottle, be sure that the formula is mixed well, especially if you are using powdered formula. Otherwise, it may clog the nipple, and your baby may seem like she doesn't want the bottle when, in reality, she can't get any formula out of the nipple. Also make sure the nipple size is appropriate, so that the formula drips out easily.

2. To give your baby her bottle, find a comfortable place for both of you. Sitting in a chair or sofa, cradle your baby's head in your arm. You may want to put a pillow under your arm or under your baby so that your arm doesn't get tired from holding the baby and your back doesn't get tired from leaning over.

3. Position your baby so that her head is aligned with but slightly higher than the rest of her body. Never lay a baby flat to feed: because of the angle of the inner ear canal, if a baby is lying flat, formula can flow into her ear when she swallows. If this formula sits inside the ear (the eardrum prevents it from leaking out), it acts as a breeding ground for bacteria, leading to infection. By holding your baby's head higher than her body, you will prevent this backflow of formula.

4. Next, take the nipple and stroke it along your baby's cheek. This should cause your baby to turn toward the bottle and open her mouth. If she is asleep, you will need to wake her up before you do this. Once she opens her mouth, insert the bottle for her to feed.

5. Make sure that you always hold the bottle. Never prop it up with a towel or cloth: this can be very dangerous for your baby, as small babies cannot remove a bottle if they are choking on formula.

6. When you hold the bottle, make sure the nipple is filled with formula at all times to prevent your baby from sucking in air, which can cause discomfort.

7. Look into your baby's eyes when she is feeding, and talk to her or sing to her. This is your special time with your baby — enjoy every minute.

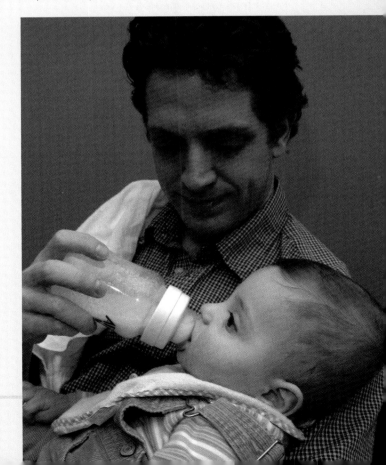

Managing bottle-feeding problems

Parents sometimes run into problems with getting their babies to take a bottle. In some cases, the problems arise when a mother who has been breast-feeding tries to feed her baby formula from a bottle or when another caregiver tries to give a bottle of formula. Parents may fear that they will never be able to leave their child with a caregiver and spend time alone. At times, a baby who has always been bottle-fed may also refuse a bottle. These two different situations need to be treated differently.

Breast-fed babies

If your baby has been breast-fed before being introduced to formula in a bottle, there are different ways to prevent her from refusing the bottle:

- Once breast-feeding is well established, try giving your baby a bottle on a regular basis to ease the transition.
- Check to be sure you have an appropriate nipple. The solution may be as simple as changing nipples.
- Try having someone else offer your baby the bottle, preferably while you are out of the room. Because most babies prefer to breast-feed, they may not take the bottle from their mother.
- Try offering breast milk in the bottle instead of formula. If this is not successful, switch to formula.
- If your baby still refuses the bottle (which is quite possible), you may have to wait until she is hungry enough. A hungry baby will feed eventually, even from a bottle she previously refused.

Patience is very important: ultimately, babies prefer bottle feedings to hunger.
- Never force your baby to take a bottle. This could result in a feeding aversion.

Bottle-fed babies

If your baby has always been bottle-fed and is now refusing the bottle, here is some advice:

- Make sure there is nothing wrong with the bottle or the formula.
- Do not change formulas abruptly without advice from your child's health-care provider. The formula is usually not the issue.
- Remember that a baby's eating habits change as she grows, and her appetite may suddenly increase or decrease. If your child is taking less formula but her urine and stool pattern are the same, this eating pattern may be the new normal for her.
- If your baby is refusing to eat altogether, ask your health-care provider to assess your baby's health.

Burping your baby

Whether you choose to breast-feed or formula-feed your baby, she may need to be burped as part of her feeding routine. Some babies require burping during the feeding (stop feeding, burp, then resume), while others can wait until the end of the feeding.

Although breast-fed babies typically swallow less air than bottle-fed babies during feeding, they may still need burping. The air they swallow collects in their tummies, creating increased pressure and subsequent discomfort. Burping allows this air to be released, relieving discomfort and creating room for more milk.

Burping facts

Different babies require different amounts of burping. Don't be alarmed if your baby won't burp. Not all babies burp at every feeding. There are no strict rules for exactly when they should burp. With practice, you will come to know what works for your baby.

Many babies spit up after a feeding, so don't be alarmed if your baby does. Properly burping her may decrease the chances that she will spit up.

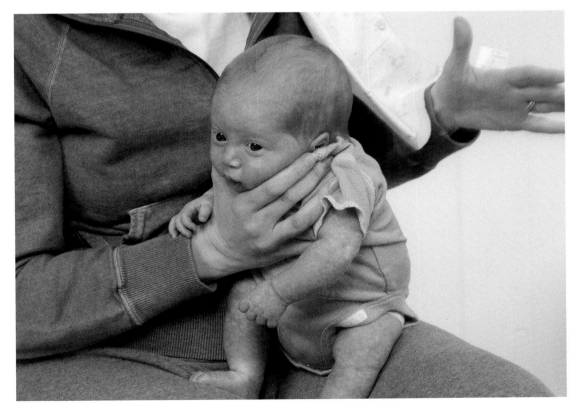

HOW TO
Burp your baby

If you are breast-feeding, burp your baby immediately after she finishes feeding on one breast. If she feeds on both breasts during a feeding, she will need to be burped twice. If you are bottle-feeding, you may need to interrupt the feeding halfway through to burp your baby.

The techniques for burping are the same for breast-fed and bottle-fed babies. A successful technique requires that you apply mild pressure to the baby's abdomen and hold her head elevated above her stomach. Some babies will even burp on their own when brought from a lying to an upright position. You can use one of the following three techniques, or you may find another one that is comfortable for you and your baby.

1. Hold your baby in an upright position with her arms over your shoulder and her tummy resting on your shoulder. Gently rub or pat her back.

2. Hold your baby in a seated position on your lap. With one hand, support her jaw using your thumb and index finger while applying pressure to her abdomen with the heel of that same hand. Gently pat or rub her back with the other hand.

3. Hold your baby so that she is lying stomach down in your lap with her legs hanging off one side. Support her head by holding her chin with your index finger and thumb. Gently rub or pat her back with the other hand.

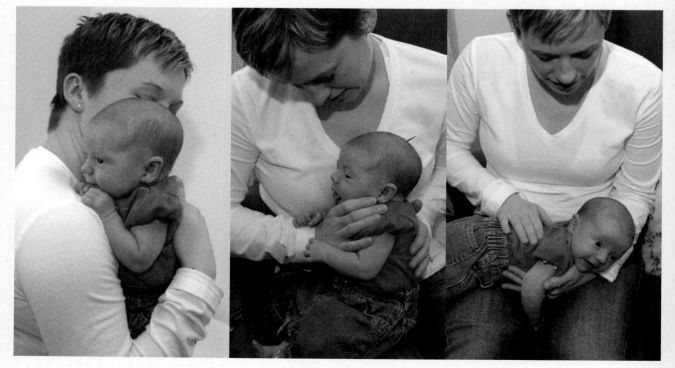

Supplementing breast milk and infant formula

Whether you choose to breast-feed or formula-feed your baby, at some point in the first year she will require nutrient supplements, specifically vitamin D, iron, and perhaps fluoride.

Vitamin D

Children need vitamin D to build strong bones. If they don't get enough vitamin D, infants are at risk of developing rickets, a disease that causes the bones to become soft, weak, and subsequently deformed.

There are several sources of vitamin D. Some foods, such as salmon, contain it, and cow's milk is often fortified with it. The skin can also produce vitamin D when it is exposed to sunlight. People with darker skin require more sunlight exposure to create the same amount of vitamin D as people with lighter skin.

Children at greatest risk of getting rickets are those who live in colder climates, where they may not be exposed to enough direct sunlight. This is especially true for children with darker-colored skin, particularly if their mother has a vitamin D deficiency or if they are exclusively breast-fed. Breast milk contains vitamin D, but only in minute quantities (15 to 40 IU per quart or liter).

Exposing children to sunlight is one way to ensure that they get enough vitamin D, but this is not always practical and carries the long-term risk of skin cancer. Sunscreen prevents the skin from making vitamin D. Therefore, leading pediatric health-care agencies recommend that babies take vitamin D in supplemental form.

Recommended dosage

The current recommendation by the American Academy of Pediatrics and the Canadian Paediatric Society is that breast-fed babies be given a vitamin D supplement starting in the first 2 months of life. Children who are partially breast-fed and receive supplemental formula do not require extra vitamin D, provided they drink over 18 ounces (500 mL) of formula a day. Formulas are fortified with vitamin D.

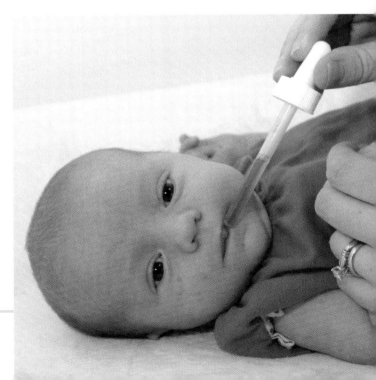

If your child is taking both breast milk and formula, you will need to calculate the total amount of formula your child takes in a 24-hour period. If it is less than 18 ounces (500 mL), your child will require a vitamin D supplement.

In the United States, the recommended dose of vitamin D is 200 IU (international units) a day. In Canada, the recommended dose is 400 IU a day, and in very northern communities, 800 IU a day.

Older children who do not drink milk or who live in northern communities may continue to need vitamin D supplementation. This should be discussed with the child's health-care provider.

Iron

Babies are born with good iron reserves, received from their mothers during pregnancy. When these reserves are combined with the iron provided by breast milk, most babies have enough iron in their diet until they are 6 months of age. However, if iron-containing solid foods or iron-fortified formula and cereals are not introduced at that time, your baby could become iron-deficient, resulting in anemia, irritability, and decreased activity. Iron deficiency may also adversely affect development, as well as other behavior.

Recommended dosage

Meat, green vegetables, and iron-fortified cereals are all high in iron. In general, if any of these are introduced to your baby's diet when she is around 6 months of age, no further iron supplements will be required. If your baby is premature, she may need to have iron drops from the time she is 8 weeks of age until her first birthday.

Fluoride

Fluoride is important to the development of healthy teeth. Children may require supplemental fluoride if their water supply does not contain a sufficient amount.

Recommended dosage

Children who are 6 months to 2 years of age need fluoride supplementation if their water supply contains less than 0.3 ppm (µg per L) of fluoride. Parents should consult with their baby's health-care provider to discuss whether supplementation is advisable.

Caution

Ingesting too much fluoride can result in staining of the teeth, also known as fluorosis. In severe cases, this can lead to serious mottling of the teeth, making them more prone to decay. To prevent fluorosis in babies, use toothpaste that is not fluoridated, because they tend to swallow their toothpaste. For older children, use just a pea-sized amount of toothpaste containing fluoride and encourage them to spit it out rather than swallowing it.

Supplemental juice

Children under 1 year of age do not need to drink any fluids besides formula or breast milk and water. Although many companies sell juice for infants — advertising its vitamin C content, for example — your baby does not need it. Vitamin C is also present in breast milk and formula, which are much more complete sources of nutrition. The healthiest option is to avoid giving your baby juice in the first year.

Supplemental water

Given in a volume that offers sufficient nutrients, formula will generally provide all the water an infant needs. Extra water is seldom necessary. Still, when it is very hot outside, formula-fed infants can be given supplemental water.

Babies who are breast-fed do not require extra water. A mother's milk contains enough fluid to satisfy the baby. The breast milk produced in a mother's body actually changes based on the climate. In warmer climates and seasons, the breast milk will be more watery, in order to meet the baby's hydration and caloric needs. If your baby is growing and gaining weight, it is not "wrong" to give her water, but it is certainly not required.

Supplemental formula

Babies who are breast-fed and who are growing well do not need supplemental formula. Breast milk provides all the calories and protein a baby requires in the first 6 months. Contrary to the old wives' tale, your baby will not sleep any longer if she is given formula or cereal at night.

However, supplementation may be appropriate if your baby's weight gain is poor. If you are concerned about your baby's growth, discuss it with your health-care provider. The goal should always be to ensure a healthy, thriving baby.

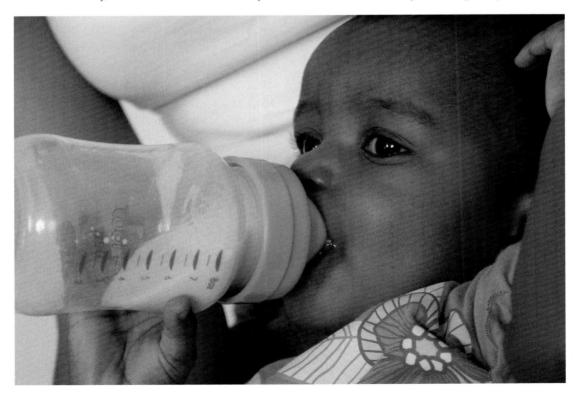

Frequently asked questions

As family doctors and pediatricians, we answer many questions from parents. Here are some of the most frequently asked questions. Be sure to ask your health-care providers any other questions that arise. If they don't have the answers, they will refer you to a colleague who does.

Q: Perhaps it was because I was so exhausted immediately after my son was born, but I found myself getting very upset when the night-shift nurse's advice on breast-feeding seemed to be quite different from the information I was given during the day. Can't they at least get their facts straight?

A: Breast-feeding is as much art as it is science. There are many different ways to successfully do it, and even more ways to explain it. As a result, the advice you get can often seem to differ or even conflict with what you've already been told. Everyone on the ward really does want to help you, and their suggestions are generally consistent; sometimes, it just doesn't seem that way.

In the first postpartum days, most first-time mothers are exhausted and insecure, and are not really ready to critique all the advice they are given. So it is easy to understand their frustration those few times that the health-care providers "don't seem to have their act together."

Trust your own instincts and follow the plan that makes you feel most comfortable. In a month or so, you and your baby will be the real authorities on what works best for you.

Q: My 5-month-old-son has been solely breast-fed, yet this week he came down with a very bad cold and developed an ear infection. I thought breast-feeding was supposed to prevent him from getting sick. What happened?

A: There is no doubt that breast-feeding provides your baby with protective antibodies that measurably reduce the chances of various infections, such as gastroenteritis, colds, and serious blood-born illnesses. Unfortunately, breast-feeding does not guarantee complete protection for all the common infections of childhood. Breast-fed babies will still get sick sometimes. In fact, they need exposure to the common viruses to stimulate their immune systems.

Q: I chose to formula-feed my baby. I considered my options carefully and, because of my personal circumstances, decided not to breast-feed. Maybe it's my own guilt that is troubling me, but I can't help feeling that my friends, my relatives, and even my colleagues at work disapprove of my choice. Did I make a mistake?

A: No one but you walks in your shoes. Without a thorough knowledge of your

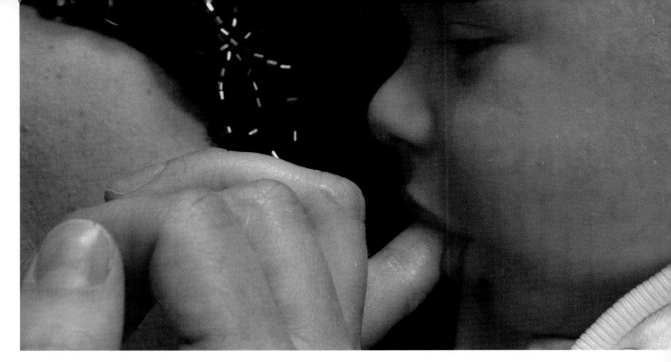

situation, no one has the right to judge you. No one should. Yet, it is very easy for a vulnerable individual to become upset by the opinionated and judgmental. Although breast-feeding does have definite advantages and is recommended as the preferred form of infant nutrition, it is not for every mother. There are medical contraindications to breast-feeding. There are practical reasons that might preclude breast feeding as an option. You said that you considered your options carefully. So trust yourself and your decision. If you remain troubled, discuss your feelings with your health-care provider.

Q: My partner and I want to do things the natural way. If breast milk is the perfect food, why must we supplement it by giving our baby commercial vitamin D drops?
A: If you lived in the tropics and didn't wear sunblock, vitamin D supplementation would not be necessary for your baby because the small amount of vitamin D

in your breast milk (15 to 40 IU/l) would be augmented with vitamin D produced by the skin. So far, humans haven't fully adapted to living in northern climates. Until we do, you would be wise to provide your baby with vitamin D drops.

Q: Some authorities recommend scheduled feedings for young breast-fed infants, while others advise feeding on demand. Which should I choose?
A: Some parents, especially first-time mothers and fathers, need structure and routine to feel confident in their parenting skills. Others are comfortable recognizing their baby's cues and prefer to feed on demand. No single method is superior, so choose what works best for you. In practice, there is not much difference between feeding schedules. Young infants naturally feed 8 to 12 times a day, which is what they tend to get by routine or by demand. Besides, few mothers will continue to let a hungry baby cry without feeding her, even if it is earlier than her schedule suggests.

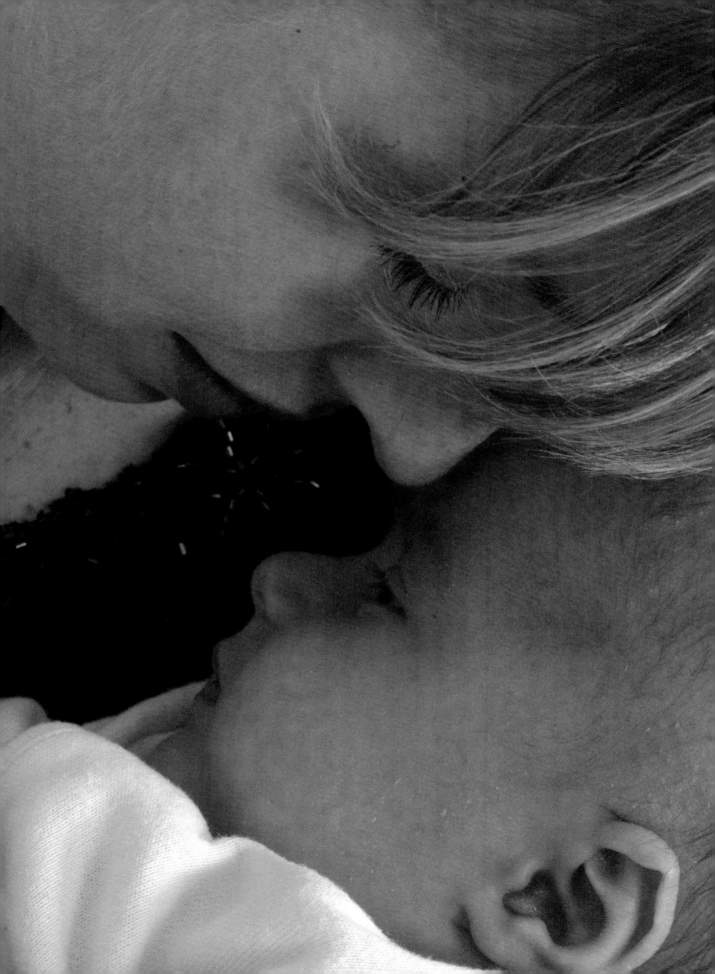

Your Baby's
First Month

Getting to know your baby and yourself

Congratulations! By now, you have mastered the important skills of holding, bathing, dressing, and feeding your baby. Don't underestimate your achievement. You are back at home and likely in the process of moving on from the chaotic first few days following your baby's birth and establishing routines. The first few weeks of your baby's life are a time for nestling in, getting to know your baby, and adjusting to your new family.

Communicating with your baby

Allow yourself some time to just sit back and observe your baby. Even in the first weeks of life, babies can communicate their needs even if they cannot talk. You will begin to learn your baby's cues and cries: rooting for hunger, showing fatigue, crying for food, or having wet diapers. Learning these cues will help you to tend to your baby's needs and may help guide you in developing a routine.

However, there will be many times in the first few months of your baby's life when, despite trying to decipher his cues, you will feel unable to understand and address his needs. Be assured that there are only a few things that cause a baby to cry. In these situations, trial and error is a good approach.

If it has been a while since his last feeding, your baby may be hungry. Try to feed him. Does he need a diaper change? Change his diaper. Does he seem tired? Try to get him to sleep. Does he just want some comfort? Try holding him, talk to him, perhaps sing him a song. Many babies love motion — try taking him for a walk.

You will soon develop your own methods of soothing and calming your baby — but this takes time.

All new (and not so new) parents have times when they feel inept, inadequate, and overwhelmed — these are very normal feelings. When they happen, take a break. If you have someone who can help, take a few minutes for yourself. If you don't have help at that moment, put your baby in a safe place — his crib, for example — and take a few minutes to collect yourself. You can try drinking or eating something, taking a shower, or flipping through the newspaper. Later, you may want to reflect on any particular events that led to your feeling overwhelmed … other than the obvious lack of sleep, possible episiotomy, and hormone shifts! That way, you can try to anticipate and avoid them as much as possible.

Schedules

As the initial crowds of visitors start to thin a bit, and your energy starts to wane, you may be starting to think about what life with your baby is going to be like. What will you "do" all day? Will you have a schedule or routine? For "goal-oriented" parents, routines give a sense of accomplishment at the end of the day.

Transitions

The first month of your baby's life is a sharp transitional stage. Prior to delivering your baby, you may have held down a job and been involved in sports, with an active social life. You had plenty of time to do the things that *you* wanted to do. This is still achievable, but probably not in the first month. This time is all about getting to know your baby and discovering what works best for him and for you.

Routines

In the first month of life, you should not expect your newborn to display the regularity of a clock, feeding every 3 hours or sleeping precisely every 2 hours. If you are, like many others, someone who takes comfort in having a routine, you can imagine your schedule as follows: your baby will eat, then sleep, then have quiet awake time. The amount of time in each of these periods may vary for different babies and even in your own baby as he grows older and has more awake time. For example, a 3-week-old may feed for 30 minutes, sleep for 2 hours, be awake for 20 minutes, and then feed again.

You may want to use that sleep interval to catch up on your own sleep or do some necessary household activities. Also try to take even a few minutes for yourself. You could spend your baby's awake period reading to him, showing him objects and shapes, listening to music, or taking him for a walk. This approach breaks up your day (and night) into manageable segments.

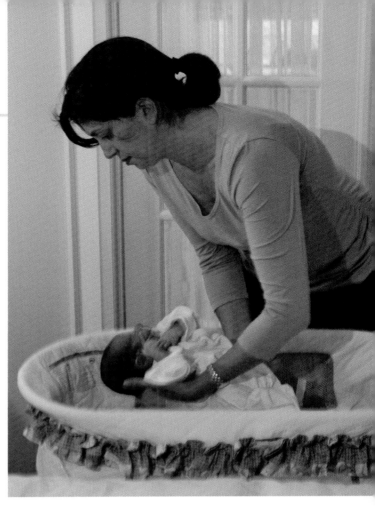

First visit to your baby's doctor

Part of your routine will be regular visits to your baby's doctor. The first visit is usually a few days after your baby is discharged from the hospital. This early follow-up visit enables prompt detection of significant feeding issues, dehydration, or excessive jaundice.

This will be the first of many health maintenance visits for you and your baby, designed to address any concerns or questions you have, review your baby's growth parameters and developmental milestones, discuss age-related safety tips, examine your child from head to toe, and provide immunizations when needed. During these visits, you and your doctor will to get to know one another: the doctor-parent relationship can be very important if significant problems arise.

Guidelines for

Visiting your baby's doctor

There are some things you can do to make the most of your regular visits to your baby's doctor, starting with the first visit in the first month:

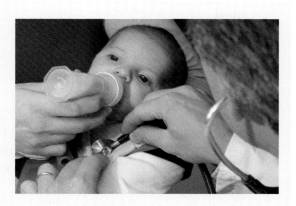

- Ideally, both parents should attend these visits. If only one parent can attend, try to have a friend or trusted relative accompany you to help with the baby so you can concentrate on the discussion at hand. This may be the first time you have left home with your baby, and an extra adult can be very helpful, if only to carry the diaper bag and hold open the doors.

- Some parents like to prepare a written list of questions ahead of time. This will help you remember all the questions you seem to have the minute you walk out of the office. Don't forget that your doctor is an expert on general child-care issues, parenting, and health promotion. Ask your doctor to recommend any additional resources for you if you feel that you need further information.

- Most family doctors or pediatricians have busy waiting rooms; you may have to wait a while. Be prepared to amuse, comfort, and feed your baby while you wait.

- After going into an examining room, you will likely be asked by a nurse to undress your newborn. Your baby may first be weighed and measured by the nurse. Let the nurse know of any questions or concerns you have —

nurses are often very experienced at dealing with these issues.

- Your doctor will likely inquire about your baby's feeding, sleeping, number of wet and dirty diapers, and how you as parents are coping with your newborn. Be prepared to answer these questions. The doctor may also ask about your own health and the health of your family, because some illnesses in children can run in families.

- The doctor will then examine your baby in detail from head to toe. Afterwards, you should have an opportunity to discuss any questions or concerns you have. Ensure that all of your questions are addressed and that you are comfortable with the answers. If you don't understand something, your doctor should be happy to review it with you or suggest an alternative source for the information you need.

- Before you leave the office, make sure that you learn the procedures for scheduling new appointments, whom to call after hours and on weekends with questions, and whether your doctor provides any telephone advice.

Understanding growth and development patterns

From the moment your new arrival is placed on the scale, your baby's growth will be the focus of much attention for you and your health-care provider. Your baby's weight, length, and head circumference will be measured at birth and before discharge from the hospital. Keep a record of these measurements and bring them to your child's checkups.

Infants grow and change rapidly throughout their first year. If you need any proof of this, just think about their constant need for new and bigger clothes! Adequate growth — in particular, weight gain — means that your baby is obtaining sufficient nutrition to support the amazing development he will undergo in the upcoming months.

Charting your baby's growth

Just like adults, babies are quite different from one another. Some begin life smaller, some larger, some leaner, and some chubbier. Your baby's size at birth may be affected by his mother's health, nutrition, lifestyle, and weight gain during pregnancy, his parents' sizes, and blood flow through the placenta. Certain medical conditions during pregnancy, such as diabetes, may lead to a higher birth weight. Smoking, high blood pressure, health problems during pregnancy, or some medical problems in newborns may be associated with lower birth weights.

What will be most important over the upcoming months is the rate at which your child gains weight and grows.

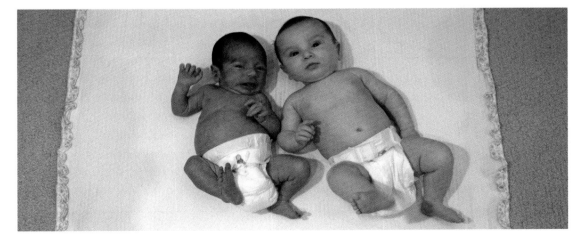

Measuring your baby

Health-care providers will periodically measure your baby's weight, height (or length), and head circumference to ensure that he is growing normally.

Weight

At every visit with your doctor, weight will be measured using a special infant scale until your child is big enough to stand on a scale alone.

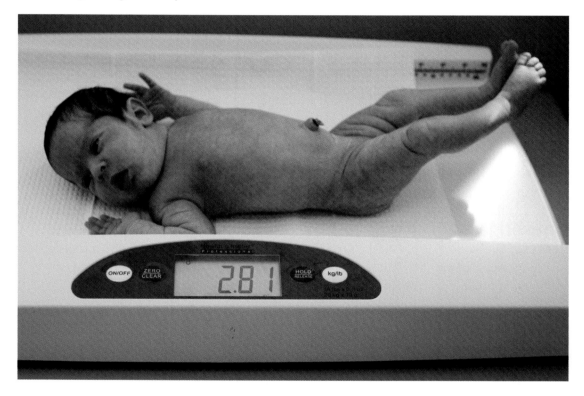

Did You Know?

Growth facts

On average, newborn babies weigh 7.5 pounds (3.5 kg), are 20 inches (51 cm) long, and have a head circumference of 14 inches (35 cm). In general, your baby's size at birth does not predict his ultimate size as an adult. Many other factors, such as nutrition, family genetics, and disease, contribute to that. Still, growth and weight gain in the first few months of life is an important indicator of your baby's overall health.

Babies tend to lose 5% to 10% of their birth weight during the first few days of life and usually regain this weight by 7 to 14 days.

In the first 3 months of life, babies gain an average of 0.5 to 1 ounce (15 to 30 g) per day. However, many healthy babies will gain less. Your doctor and nurse will help you to determine how well your baby is growing and gaining weight.

Length

An infant's length is most accurately measured using a special measurement board.

Head circumference

A measuring tape wrapped around the largest part of the head (above the eyebrows and ears to the back of the head) is used to measure your baby's head circumference.

Growth curves

Growth measurements are recorded on standard growth curves, which describe the range of normal weight, length, and head circumference for a given age, with expected changes in those measurements shown. The curves shown on pages 190–93 are based on measurements from a North American population.

There are separate growth curves for boys and girls, as girls tend to be smaller than boys and change in size at a slightly different rate. The normal values presented here are for Caucasian populations. Children of other ethnic backgrounds may have slightly different growth patterns.

Reading the curves

The 50th percentile on these growth curves describes the average weight, length or head circumference measurement per age. The range of normal measurements falls between the 3rd and the 97th percentiles. For example, the average weight for a Caucasian newborn baby born within 2 weeks of the expected due date is 7.5 pounds (3.5 kg), average height is 20 inches (51 cm), and average head circumference is 14 inches (35 cm). However, any weight between 5.5 and 9 pounds (2.5 and 4 kg) would be considered within the normal range. Similarly, birth length between 18 and 22.5 inches (46 and 55 cm) is considered appropriate.

By plotting growth measurements on a growth curve, your doctor will determine whether they fall within the typical range, whether your baby is growing proportionately (weight is appropriate for his length), and whether he is growing at the expected rate (typically following along one of the curves).

Deviations from these expectations may mean that your child is simply expressing his own unique growth pattern. However, poor growth can sometimes indicate a problem, such as insufficient nutrition or a medical disorder. Such a finding may lead your doctor to recommend adjustments to feeding or to do some tests to look for a medical explanation while following your baby's growth more closely.

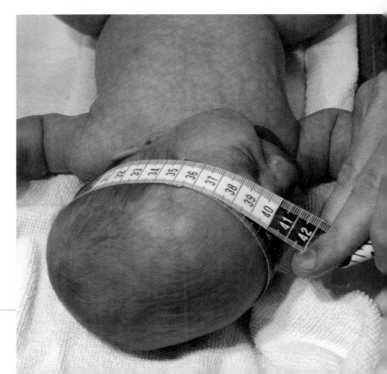

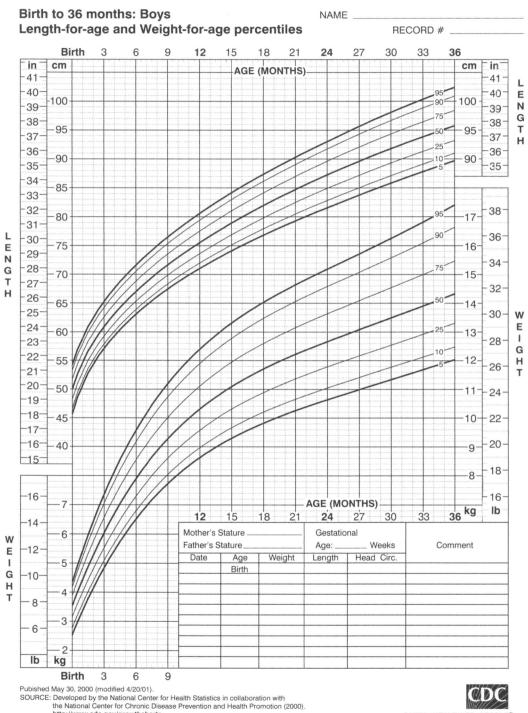

Birth to 36 months: Boys
Length-for-age and Weight-for-age percentiles

NAME _____

RECORD # _____

Pubished May 30, 2000 (modified 4/20/01).
SOURCE: Developed by the National Center for Health Statistics in collaboration with
the National Center for Chronic Disease Prevention and Health Promotion (2000).
http://www.cdc.gov/growthcharts

CDC
SAFER · HEALTHIER · PEOPLE™

Birth to 36 months: Girls
Length-for-age and Weight-for-age percentiles

NAME _____

RECORD # _____

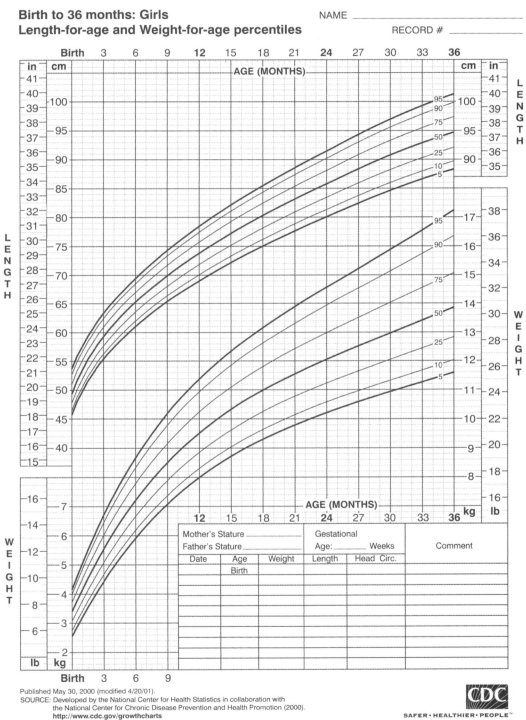

Published May 30, 2000 (modified 4/20/01).
SOURCE: Developed by the National Center for Health Statistics in collaboration with
the National Center for Chronic Disease Prevention and Health Promotion (2000).
http://www.cdc.gov/growthcharts

CDC

SAFER · HEALTHIER · PEOPLE™

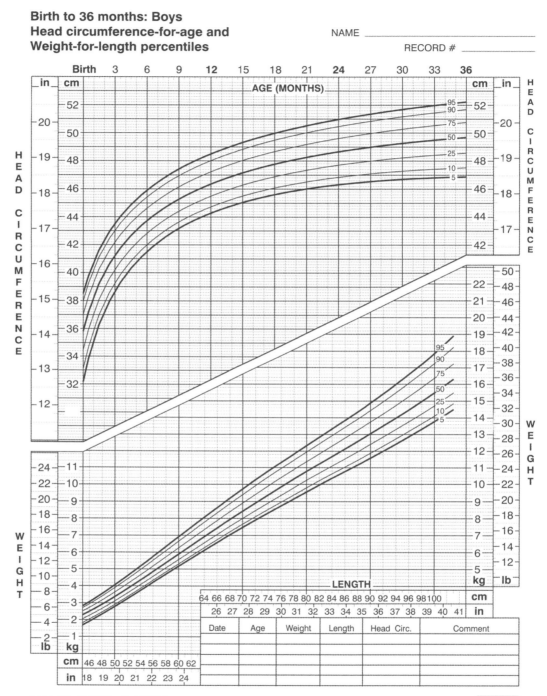

Birth to 36 months: Boys
Head circumference-for-age and
Weight-for-length percentiles

NAME _____

RECORD # _____

Published May 30, 2000 (modified 10/16/00).
SOURCE: Developed by the National Center for Health Statistics in collaboration with
the National Center for Chronic Disease Prevention and Health Promotion (2000).
http://www.cdc.gov/growthcharts

SAFER · HEALTHIER · PEOPLE™

Birth to 36 months: Girls
Head circumference-for-age and
Weight-for-length percentiles

NAME _____

RECORD # _____

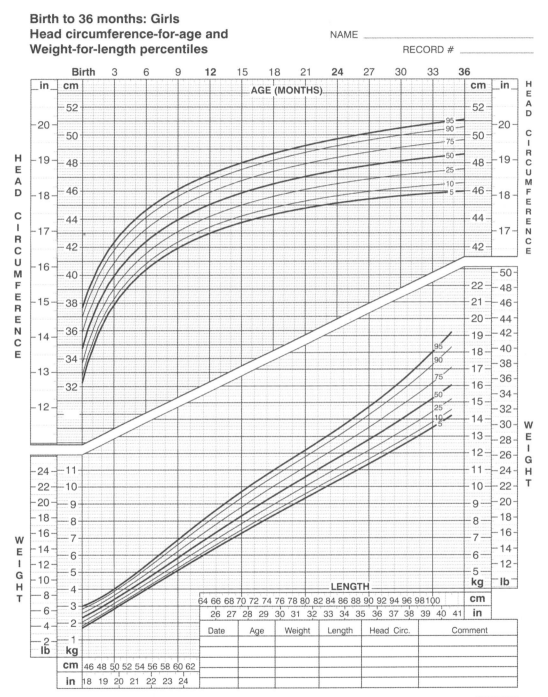

Published May 30, 2000 (modified 10/16/00).
SOURCE: Developed by the National Center for Health Statistics in collaboration with
the National Center for Chronic Disease Prevention and Health Promotion (2000).
http://www.cdc.gov/growthcharts

SAFER • HEALTHIER • PEOPLE™

Growth during the first month

Your baby's weight will be followed closely through this period. If weight loss is more than expected or is regained more slowly than usual, you will need to visit a doctor or clinic (for example, a breast-feeding clinic) more frequently to ensure that your baby is getting enough fluids and nutrition.

Weight loss and gain

Although growth and weight gain are important reflections of adequate nutrition, be aware that it is normal for your new baby to lose some weight after he is born. Babies generally lose up to 10% of their body weight following birth. This weight loss occurs as your baby eliminates meconium (fetal stools) and establishes regular feedings.

This weight loss is most common in breast-fed babies because they initially receive a smaller number of feedings. Sometimes, formula-fed babies lose little or no weight after birth. If your baby was born around the expected due date and was of a weight that falls within the typical range, he should generally return to his birth weight within 1 week. Premature and smaller babies may require 2 weeks to return to their birth weight.

After this initial period of weight loss, if your baby is feeding well and is healthy, he will generally gain an average of 0.5 to 1 ounce (15 to 30 g) every day.

By the end of the first month, a baby who begins life at an average weight of 7.5 pounds (3.5 kg) will weigh about 10 pounds (4.5 kg).

At 2 months, an average North American baby weighs between 8.5 and 14 pounds (4 and 6.5 kg).

Length

Growth in length is slower than gain in weight. It is also more difficult to measure accurately. Your baby's height will be measured less frequently than his weight.

During his first month, your baby will grow about 1.5 to 2 inches (3 to 5 cm).

At 2 months, an average North American baby measures 21 to 25 inches (54 to 63 cm).

Head circumference

As for your child's head size, it is often a reflection of your own! If your baby's head appears larger than typical on the growth curve, a doctor should measure both parents' heads to see whether they are also large. It is most important that your child's head grows at the expected rate, following one of the curves on the growth chart. An infant's head usually grows 0.5 inch (1 cm) in diameter every 2 weeks for the first 2 months. If head growth is more rapid or slower than expected, medical tests may be recommended to determine the cause.

Development during the first month

During the first month of life, your baby will spend most of his time sleeping or feeding. Even though it may seem that sleeping and feeding is all he is doing, he is developing a wider range of physical movements and reflexes, as well as exciting new communication behaviors.

Physical movements

Over the course of the month, you may notice some small increases in your baby's quiet awake time. His arms and legs, which are initially held bent up toward his body, will relax soon after birth. He may begin to organize his jerky wiggles into more organized movements and pauses. An infant of this age has very limited ability to hold up his relatively large head with his developing neck muscles and still requires your gentle support.

Moro reflex

From birth through the first month or two, an infant's movements are limited to wiggling and moving his arms and legs. However, if your baby is startled by a loud noise or sudden movement, you may notice his arms and legs stretch out and then bend back toward his body. This is a normal reflex, known appropriately as the "startle" or "Moro" reflex. Your health-care professional may test for this by supporting your baby's head a little off the bed and then allowing it to drop slightly into the other hand. This early reflex will gradually disappear over the first few months as the developing brain masks these primitive responses emanating from the brain stem.

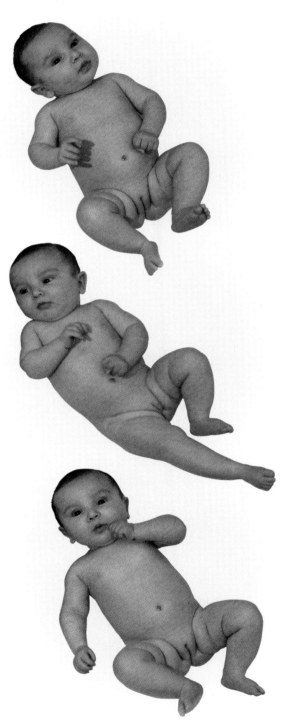

■ Normal baby movements.

Development milestones, first year

Age	Gross motor (how your baby moves)	Fine motor (how your baby uses his hands)	Language	Social development and play
1st month	• Wiggles • Moves arms and legs • Arms and legs stretch out when startled • Little control of head — flops around if unsupported	• Hands held closed most of the time	• Crying • Cooing ("aah" sounds)	• Looks at caregiver's face • Smiles responsively by 5–6 weeks
2 to 3 months	• Kicks legs • Supports head briefly when held upright • Able to lift head briefly when placed on tummy	• Hands open most of the time	• Crying • Cooing	• Quiets when caregiver talks • Looks toward sound • Follows moving object 180 degrees
4 to 6 months	• Turns around when lying on stomach • Rolls over, initially stomach to back and then back to stomach • Good head control when pulled to sitting from lying or held upright • Lifts head and shoulders when placed on tummy	• Reaches for objects • Holds objects in hands and begins to transfer them from one hand to the other	• Cooing in imitation and response to adult sounds • Begins babbling (vowel and consonant sounds) • Makes razzing sounds (gives "raspberries")	• Bats at objects • Laughs • Interested in own image in mirror • Puts toys in mouth • Becomes wary of strangers
7 to 9 months	• Sits unsupported • Crawls • May pull to standing position	• Holds objects and bangs them • Starts to pick up small objects • Can feed himself a cracker	• Babbling (ba-ba-ba, da-da-da)	• Looks for toys that fall or roll out of sight • Plays peek-a-boo • Reluctant to go to strangers

Age	Gross motor (how your baby moves)	Fine motor (how your baby uses his hands)	Language	Social development and play
10 to 12 months	• Pulls to standing position • Walks along furniture (cruising) or with hand held • May start to walk independently (12 to 15 months)	• Holds cup • Picks up small objects • Points • Holds crayon in fist (12 months) • Puts small objects in container	• First words with meaning (12 months) — usually "mama" or "dada" • Imitates speech	• Claps hands • Plays patty-cake • Waves "bye bye" • Rolls a ball • Removes socks

Grasp reflex

Your baby's hands are initially held closed much of the time but now gradually start to open more. If you place your finger in his palm, he will grasp it tightly. This development milestone is known as the "palmar grasp" reflex.

Smile reflex

As the first month progresses, infants start to pay attention to caregiver's faces, watching and following them with their eyes. Infants at this age cannot see details well, but do notice large mouth movements, such as your big smile! Your baby now tends to settle when picked up and watches your face intently when being spoken to or fed. It is heartwarming to see your brand-new baby's smiles, even though they are initially a "reflex." But very soon they should start to become purposeful and responsive, usually by 5 to 6 weeks of age. This is one of the first milestones that many health-care professionals will inquire about.

Communication

Your baby will appear to look around and may respond to noises. This is the time when you and your baby learn to communicate with each other. Your baby is learning to trust you. Your responses to his crying — picking him up, comforting him, and providing him with food, clothing, or warmth — all contribute to this growing bond. You cannot spoil your baby at this age.

Your baby will communicate with you throughout this period mainly by crying and cooing. "Cooing" refers to the "aaah" sounds young infants make: they make your sleepless nights seem worthwhile. If you respond to these noises by imitating them softly, it will help your baby develop early language skills.

Development milestones

Your baby's development will follow a relatively predictable pattern. The achievement of the common developmental milestones usually follows a recognizable sequence, but you must remember that the exact rate will vary a lot from child to child. If you expect your little champ to meet every milestone at the same time as, or even before, his peers in your mothers' group, then you are setting yourself up for unnecessary anxiety and disappointment.

Just like a child's growth patterns, the progression of a baby's development over time is what is most important. We know that some babies will walk at 9 months and others at 15 months, just as some will grow on the 10th percentile and others will grow on the 90th percentile curve. These variations, not unlike facial features or fingerprints, are what make us individuals, but they have little importance in the long term. Developmental variations do not necessarily indicate that one child is "smarter" or more athletic than another. Even siblings can vary in when they start to walk or talk ... or show their temper.

Developmental delay

If your child's development falls outside of the typical ranges shown on pages 190–93, it may reflect a variation of normal or may indicate a problem that needs assessment and intervention. If your child's development plateaus so that he is not progressing over the course of months, or if his development actually regresses and he loses some of his previous skills, he should be carefully assessed by your health-care provider.

Trust your instincts if you are concerned in any way about your child's development, and be sure to mention this to your doctor. Despite the wide variation in normal, a parent's intuition is very important. If you suspect your child may be experiencing a developmental delay, consult with your child's health-care provider.

Warning signs of possible developmental delay

Area of development	Warning sign
Gross motor development	Rolling prior to 3 months Not walking by 18 months
Fine motor development	Holding hands tightly in fists for most of the time at 3 months Preferring right or left hand before 18 months
Expressive language development	No words by 18 months Not pointing by 18 months Words difficult to understand at 3 years
Receptive language development	Not turning when name is called at 18 months Not able to identify body parts by 2 years
Social development	Not interested in other children at 2 years No imaginary play at 2 years

Advancing development

There really isn't much that has been shown to increase the rate of a child's development, beyond what most parents do instinctively. Playing with your children, caring for them, stimulating them, talking, reading, and singing to them, and, of course, loving them is how you can best help your children reach their potential.

Newborn reflexes

At birth, babies demonstrate a number of primitive reflexes — specific involuntary movements brought on by certain stimuli. Each of these reflexes disappears between 4 and 6 months of life as babies start to develop purposeful movements. The most well-known reflex is the grasp reflex. You may not want to mention to your baby's grandmother that grasping her finger is actually a reflex!

Rooting

If you touch the cheek and the corner of your baby's mouth, he will lower his bottom lip and move his tongue to that side. This comes in handy when he's trying to find the nipple. This reflex usually disappears by 3 to 4 months.

Sucking

Placing an object in a baby's mouth elicits strong sucking. This reflex disappears between months 2 and 4.

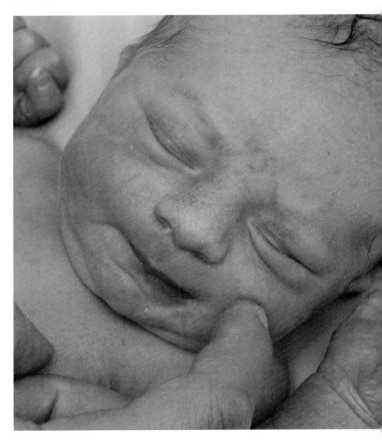

■ Rooting reflex.

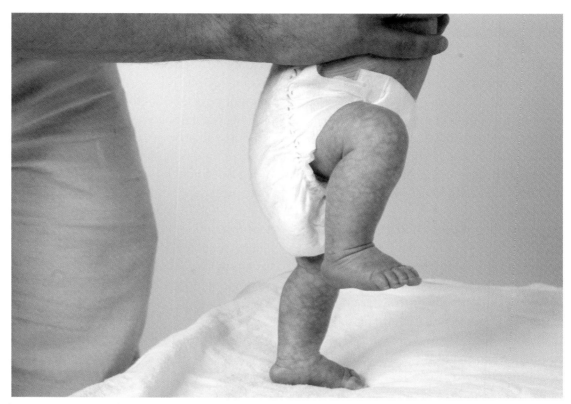

■ Stepping reflex.

Placing and stepping

If you stroke the front of the lower shin just above the foot against the edge of a table, the infant will lift his leg onto the table (placing). If you hold him so that he is leaning slightly forward, he will move his legs as if he is walking. These reflexes disappear by 6 weeks.

Grasping

Placing a finger in an infant's palm or sole will cause him to grasp it by curling his fingers or toes. The palmar grasp is remarkably strong, and one could theoretically lift the baby upwards with your finger, but it is not advised! This reflex disappears by 2 to 3 months.

Fencing

If you turn your baby's head to one side while he is on his back, he will straighten out his arm and leg on the side to which he is looking and bend his arm and leg on the other side. He will look like he is in the fencing position. This asymmetric tonic neck reflex disappears by 3 to 4 months.

Moro, or startle

If the baby's head is lifted slightly and then let go while he is lying on his back, he will move both arms out to his side and then bring them together as if he is catching a large ball. This reflex is also seen in response to loud noises; it disappears by 4 months.

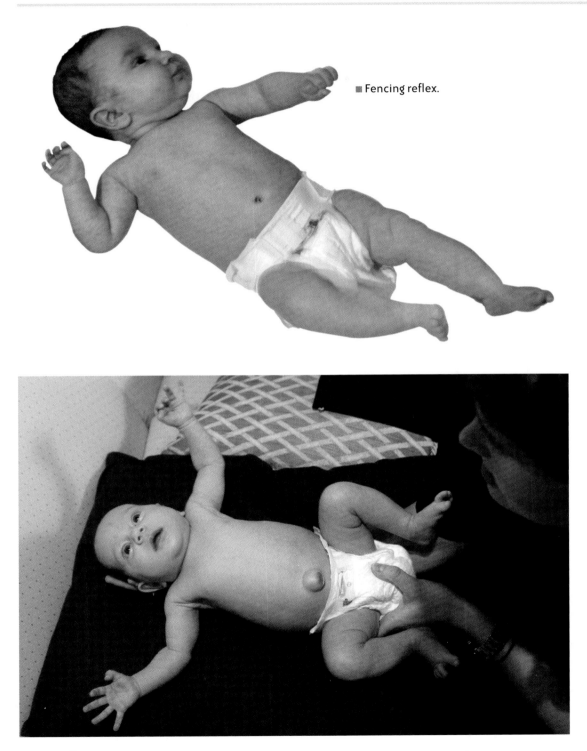

■ Fencing reflex.

■ Moro reflex.

Did You Know?

Postpartum blues

You have waited 9 months for the arrival of your baby, experiencing excitement, anticipation, and elation. Now he has arrived — and seems to need you 24 hours a day. Your feelings may now be tinged with sadness, inadequacy, dread, and fear. In most cases, this is natural, but in some, these feelings can be more serious, leading to depression.

BABY BLUES

Most new mothers have periods of weepiness, unhappiness, anxiety, and mood swings in the first week after delivery. Often called the "baby blues," these feelings can be attributed to changes in hormone levels after delivery, changes in surroundings, and the new expectations of parenting. These feelings usually get better in 1 to 2 weeks and do not interfere with your ability to function.

DEPRESSION

About one in 10 women will have more severe symptoms of depression in the first year of her baby's life. Depression is a mood disorder in which feelings of sadness, loss, anger, or frustration interfere with everyday life for an extended period of time. Women with a previous history of depression or a family member with depression are at increased risk of postpartum depression, but most women with postpartum depression have no such history.

SYMPTOMS OF POSTPARTUM DEPRESSION

Any of the following can be symptoms of depression if they last longer than 2 weeks:

- Feeling restless or irritable, sad, hopeless, or overwhelmed
- Crying often
- Lack of energy or motivation
- Eating too little or too much
- Sleeping too little or too much
- Trouble focusing, remembering, or making decisions
- Feeling worthless and guilty
- Loss of interest or pleasure in activities
- Withdrawal from friends and family
- Headaches, chest pains, heart palpitations (the heart beating fast and feeling like it is skipping beats), or hyperventilation (fast and shallow breathing)
- Fear of hurting the baby or oneself
- Lack of interest in the baby

Very rarely, symptoms can include delusions, hallucinations, or obsessive thoughts about the baby.

TREATING POSTPARTUM DEPRESSION

Some women keep their symptoms secret because they feel embarrassed, ashamed, or guilty about feeling depressed at a time when they are supposed to be happy. They worry they will be viewed as unfit parents.

However, postpartum depression can happen to *any* woman. You and your baby don't have to suffer. There are effective treatments for depression and things you can try yourself:

- Discuss these feelings with someone you trust, such as a family member, a friend, or your doctor.
- Try to get as much rest as you can; nap when the baby naps.
- Ask for help with household chores and nighttime feedings.
- Do not spend a lot of time alone. Get dressed and leave the house. Run an errand or take a short walk.
- Talk with other mothers, so you can learn from their experience.
- Seek medical treatment.

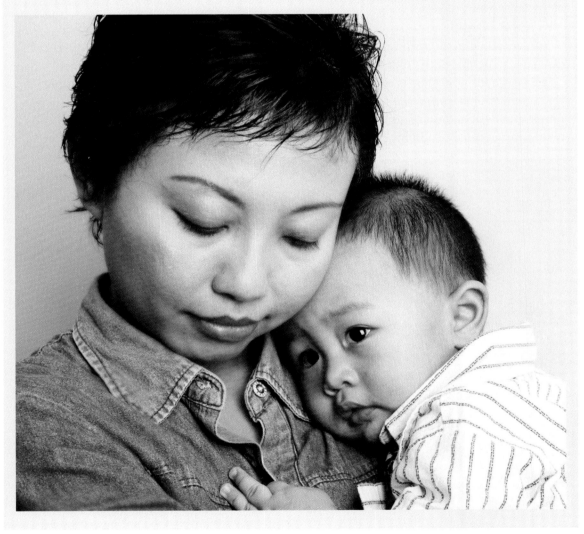

Getting out of the house

Most new parents comment on how helpful it is to get out of the house. This may mean nothing more than a short walk, a visit to a friend, or a trip to the grocery store. If you feel up to it, go ahead and take your new baby out for a while.

The first expedition out of the house is a major step for new parents. Some need a U-Haul to cart around all their supplies. Others forget essentials, such as keys!

Where to go

Wherever you choose to travel, avoid exposure to people with colds or obvious infections. Your new baby is at higher risk for complications from colds that seem minor in older children or adults. Don't take your newborn to a home with a child or adult who has cold or flu symptoms (fever, runny nose, cough, rash, diarrhea, or vomiting). You also may want to avoid large crowds. If you plan on going to a public place, do so in low-traffic times and in wide-open spaces. If strangers approach your baby and try to touch him (as they often do), don't feel embarrassed to say, "Please do not touch the baby. He bites!"

When to go

The timing of your outing is also important. You may want to plan it around your baby's schedule, such as after a feed. Make sure that you have the appropriate safety equipment ready, including an approved car seat, that he is properly buckled into his seat or stroller, and that he is adequately dressed for the weather. Babies can become hypothermic very quickly in winter, and they can sunburn easily in summer. On colder days, bundle your baby in as many layers as you would wear, plus an additional one, and protect him from wind, rain, and snow. In the summer, keep your baby shaded.

The first (or second) venture outside the house may seem overwhelming. But once you have mastered the art, you will feel ready to face the world.

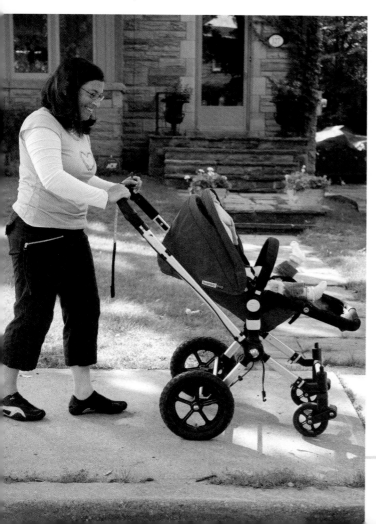

Guidelines for

Your baby's first outing

Initially, try a brief walk, about 10 or 15 minutes in duration, which is unlikely to be a problem. See how your infant

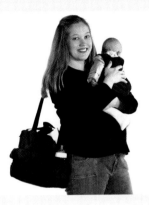

handles that outing and then progress from there.

WHAT TO BRING
Pack a bag with the essentials:

- Diapers
- Wipes (in a refillable pack or zip-lock plastic bag)
- Waterproof change pad
- Change of clothes for your baby
- Bottle and formula if you are formula-feeding
- Pacifier if your baby uses one
- Wallet, keys, and perhaps a cell phone for emergencies

What newborns see

Newborn babies usually keep their eyes closed for the first few days of life. Your baby has emerged from the dark womb into a world filled with light and color. For the first day or two, there is often some swelling of the eyelids created from the pressure of coming through the tight birth canal.

Newborns can see most clearly at a distance of 8 to 10 inches (20 to 25 cm); this is also the usual distance from baby to mother's face during feeding. Studies have shown that newborns are drawn to the contrasting shapes and colors of a human face. They also like to look at pictures of faces and contrasting black and white geometrical shapes. Even babies under 1 month will try to focus on objects.

Babies' eyes, however, do not work together at this age, and crossed eyes are often the result. Crossed eyes should start

to improve by 2 to 4 months of age as the baby's ability to use both eyes together (binocular vision) is established. Babies do not learn how to fixate and follow an object until 6 to 8 weeks of life.

When your baby is in a state of quiet alertness, hold him upright at 10 inches (25 cm) from your face and talk to him in a soft, high voice — he may respond and appear to be listening to and looking at you.

What babies hear

Babies' hearing is fully developed at birth. They often prefer high-pitched voices, and studies have shown that some babies are soothed by familiar sounds they were exposed to during your pregnancy. You don't need to tiptoe around your baby because he will likely block out loud noises, but babies do not like overstimulation. A safe rule of thumb is to play music at a level you can comfortably talk over.

HOW TO
Dress your baby for summer and winter

Dressing your newborn baby during the first months can be both fun and frustrating — fun because there is no better feeling than cuddling a newborn in a clean, cozy sleeper; frustrating because it sometimes seems as if you need a Ph.D. in engineering to fasten all those snaps properly as your baby squirms. Dressing is further complicated when you live in a climate where the seasons change, requiring a whole new set of clothes and approach to dressing your baby. Like us, babies don't like to be too hot or too cold, regardless of the weather.

Summer wear and care
Being outdoors is very important for babies and parents, but make sure your baby is appropriately dressed for the weather and protected from the sun.

1. Don't overdress the baby so that he appears flushed, sweaty, or uncomfortable. A good rule of thumb for summer dressing is to dress him as you are dressed, then add one extra light layer.

2. Cool hands and feet may suggest that another layer of light clothing is needed.

3. Dress your baby in clothing that covers the body, such as comfortable lightweight long pants, long-sleeved shirts, and hats with brims that shade the face and cover the ears.

4. Babies younger than 6 months should be kept out of direct sunlight, so be sure to shade your child from the sun with a hat, screening umbrella, or stroller canopy. UV screens are commercially available for strollers. When temperatures are very high (greater than 86°F/30°C) or there is a smog warning, limit your time outdoors. Sunscreen is not recommended at this young age because the risks and benefits of sunscreen use are not yet known. If your baby needs to be outdoors, discuss sunscreen use and other options with your health-care provider. If your baby gets a sunburn, it is advisable to see your doctor.

5. Do not leave your baby (or any child) alone in a car, even with the windows open. The inside of a car can heat up quickly to temperatures that could hurt or even kill a child.

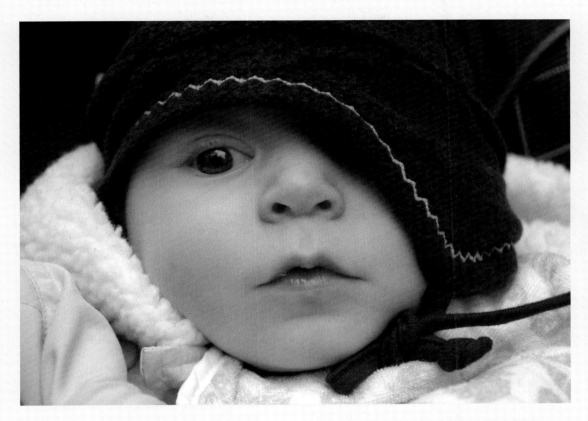

6. If your car has been parked outside on a hot day, make sure the car seat and seat belts are not hot before buckling your child into the car.

Winter wear and care

Infants are especially susceptible to fluctuations in external temperature because their bodies have a large surface area, allowing heat to be lost more easily through the head and skin, and because infants cannot produce sufficient heat through shivering.

1. When you're going out in the cold, dress your infant in a number of light layers. That way, articles of clothing can be easily removed or added as the weather dictates. A suitable outfit for an infant would include an undershirt, a sleeper, a snowsuit with coverings for hands and feet, and a blanket (not covering the face).

2. The extremities (hands and feet) and the lips, nose, and ears are the most susceptible to cold air and should be well protected with hats and scarves.

3. When temperatures are very low (below −13°F/−25°C), keep your infant indoors or limit your time outdoors as much as possible. Seek medical attention immediately if your baby's skin becomes pale or blistered (signs of frostbite), if your baby becomes very sleepy and difficult to arouse, or if he becomes cold to the touch (signs of hypothermia).

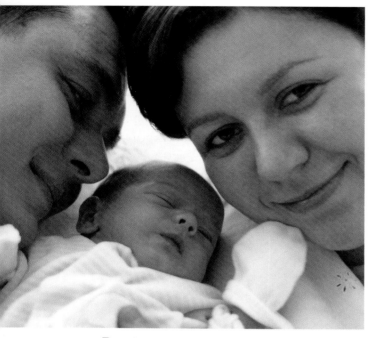

Receiving visitors

In the first month of your baby's life, you will be reeling from sleep deprivation, will feel constantly rushed, and will not always look your best. This is not a great time to entertain every relative, friend, neighbor, and casual acquaintance who wants to meet your baby. You may be excited to show off your beautiful newborn, but a constant stream of people into your home is likely not good for you or your baby.

Here are some tips on limiting your list of invitees, shortening the visits, and gaining some benefit from the intrusion:

- Discourage visitors with symptoms of a viral infection, such as a fever, runny nose, cough, rash, or diarrhea. Young children (unless they are your own) should probably avoid visiting or at least close contact with the new baby in the first month of life; they are often harboring a viral illness. Blame this rule on your doctor if people are offended.
- Let people know they should call before coming — this gives you some choice about what time is best for you and provides you with a bit of warning.
- When people ask what they can bring over, do not say "nothing." Tell them that dinner would be great!
- Ask all visitors to wash their hands as soon as they enter your house. You may want to place a container of antibacterial pump soap at your front door. Most viruses are transmitted from hand-to-hand contact.
- When your visitors arrive, put them to work! Once settled in, they can watch the baby while you have a quick shower, clean your dirty dishes in the sink, or get you something to drink. Real friends enjoy pitching in with the chores.
- Do not feel as if you have to entertain the entire world; if your visitors have children of their own, they will understand that the first few weeks are a period of adjustment and that eventually they will be able to meet your baby.
- Close family members who do not consider themselves to be visitors are often the worst offenders — set limits. You and your spouse may want some private time with your newborn away from parental advice. From the start, establish acceptable boundaries with your family members. Tell them what is really helpful and what is not so useful. They will usually get the message.

Treating common conditions

Most babies are happy and healthy most of the time, but for those times when your baby is not well, here is some advice and guidance for treating common conditions. For a quick reference to the symptoms and treatment of these conditions, see the final chapter in this book.

Crying

Crying is how your baby communicates with you. Crying could mean "I'm hungry"; "I'm wet"; "I'm cold"; "I'm frustrated"; or "I just want to be held." You may not believe it now, but there will come a time when you will be able to recognize some of your baby's needs by the type of cry. For now, responding to your baby's crying will likely be a process of trial and error.

All babies cry, but some babies cry more often and more vigorously than others. Some babies cry consistently for 5 to 10 minutes before they fall asleep, and other babies have crying episodes at times when there is extra stimulation in the home, such as when you have visitors or around mealtime.

Sometimes there seems to be no reason or explanation for a baby's crying episode. Episodes can last from 10 minutes to over an hour, and often occur at a particular time of day, such as the afternoon or evening. These episodes generally begin when your baby is 2 to 3 weeks old and end when he is 3 to 4 months old.

Colic

If you are wondering whether your baby has colic, he probably doesn't. Parents with colicky babies know who they are, and they are in good company. About one

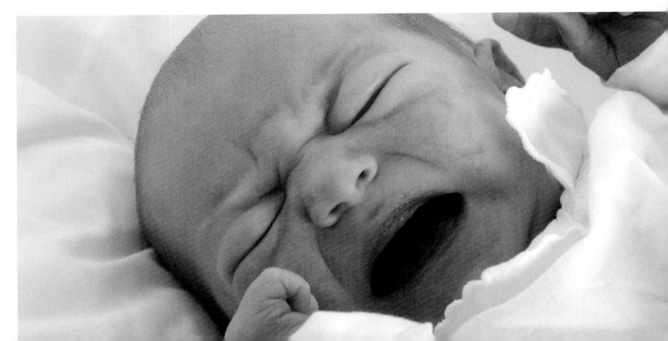

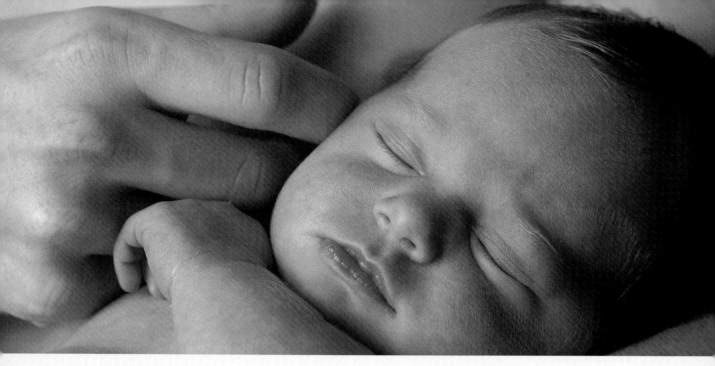

HOW TO
Calm your baby

Try these strategies for calming your baby when he is crying:

- **Reduce extra stimuli:** Keep lights low or off. Be as quiet as possible.
- **Respond:** Try to evaluate the cause of crying and take action. Change his diaper, try to feed him, ensure that he is dressed appropriately.
- **Rock:** Many babies like rhythmic movement; rock him in your arms or in an infant carrier.
- **Swaddle:** Some babies love to be wrapped up in a blanket. Make sure the blanket does not cover his face and he is not overheated.
- **Sing:** Babies like rhythmic sounds such as singing or the hum of an electric fan or vacuum cleaner.
- **Walk:** Most babies love to be taken for a walk outside. This is also a welcome excuse for parents to get out of the house!

- **Massage:** Infant massage includes gentle stroking of the skin over different parts of the head, limbs, and body using your fingertips. Massage is effective in decreasing crying in preterm infants and those whose mothers have depression.
- **Take a break:** The key to survival is good support, taking turns with other caregivers, and getting a break. Parents of babies with colic often feel frustrated, exhausted, and even inadequate.
- **Ask for help:** It is very common for parents of a colicky baby to feel anger and even violence toward the baby. This is the time to seek help: talk to your partner, a friend, or your doctor and find a way to take a break.

in five babies has crying episodes that are severe enough to be labeled as colic.

No one knows what causes colic. Various theories, such as milk allergy, bowel immaturity, parental anxiety, or difficult infant temperament, have been postulated but not proven. We *do* know that babies with colic do not have any long-term problems with their development or thinking skills.

An episode of colic is quite different from other crying. Without warning or cause, the baby screams, often turns red in the face, clenches his fists, furls his brow, and may pull up his legs. This episode can last 2 to 3 hours, and often occurs at a predictable time of day, such as the late afternoon or evening. During the episode, the baby is usually inconsolable. These episodes occur on most days.

Colic usually starts at week 2 or 3 of life, peaks in intensity at 6 to 8 weeks, and resolves by 4 to 5 months. Not all colic is alike; some babies have these episodes several times a day and seem to take longer to grow out of it (up to 6 months).

Soothing a colicky baby

Unfortunately, many popular treatments for colic are not effective. There are no safe, effective medications for colic; for example, studies using simethicone drops, which are supposed to counteract any gas, have not shown any benefit. Changing to soy or lactose-free formula has not been shown to reduce colic. Some babies may benefit from a hypoallergenic formula, but this should be discussed with your doctor. Crib vibrators (machines that can be attached to a crib and cause vibration) have not been shown to

be effective for colic and may cause overstimulation.

Fortunately, a few strategies, based on more than 200 studies of treating colic, have been shown to be effective for your baby and for yourself. The good news is that, whatever you do, colic will resolve by 4 to 5 months.

Diaper rash

The diaper area is a prime target for rashes because it is warm and moist. In addition, the delicate skin under the diaper is exposed to lots of irritating material. You can prevent diaper rashes by changing your baby's diaper frequently (at least every 2 hours) and avoiding the use of harsh soaps and detergents.

The most common form of diaper rash is diaper dermatitis (or inflammation of the skin in the diaper area). It begins as red, inflamed skin, does not involve the skin folds, and can lead to raw, open areas of skin.

Candida albicans yeast diaper rash is also common, and even more so if your baby has been treated with antibiotics. Antibiotics, in addition to getting rid of harmful bacteria, tend to kill off some of the good germs that usually compete with yeasts, thereby allowing the yeasts to flourish and giving rise to thrush and candida diaper rash. This rash looks bright red, with small red blotches beyond the margins of the rash ("satellite lesions"). Unlike diaper dermatitis, a yeast rash involves the folds between the chubby rolls of skin. Suspect a yeast rash if it does not respond to regular treatment and involves the folds.

HOW TO
Treat diaper rash

Diaper dermatitis
- Change diapers frequently and gently cleanse the area with a cloth soaked in warm water. Remember that this type of rash is caused by irritants on the skin, so removing them from the skin is at least as important as putting creams on it.
- Use a thick layer of barrier paste, which usually contains zinc oxide in varying strengths. The key to a good barrier cream is that it is difficult to wash off, which often means parents get covered themselves. The barrier keeps the urine and stool off the irritated skin and should be applied with every diaper change.
- See your doctor if the rash does not improve or involves skin breakdown. Sometimes a mild topical steroid ointment is needed.

Candida yeast rash
This rash is usually easily treated with antifungal ointments prescribed by your doctor.

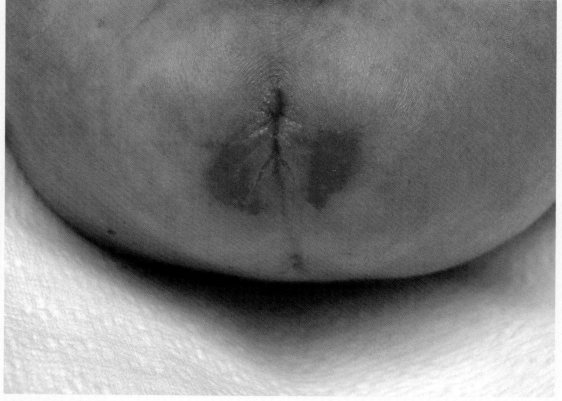

■ Diaper dermatitis.

Did You Know?

Thrush

Babies with *Candida albicans* yeast diaper rash sometimes also have oral thrush, a yeast infection in the mouth. It looks like a thick white plaque on the tongue, gums, or inside the mouth. Nearly one-third of all infants will develop oral thrush.

Oral thrush can cause pain with eating. The surface of the tongue or cheeks may be raw and may bleed slightly if you attempt to remove the thrush with a cotton swab. However, most infants are not bothered by it. Thrush does not usually interfere with feeding, nor does it cause a fever.

To prevent oral thrush, place bottle nipples and pacifiers in boiling water for 5 to 10 minutes. Make sure to cool them before your baby uses them. Putting them in the dishwasher is also effective. Handwashing is also important.

To treat oral thrush, your doctor can prescribe a medication called nystatin, which is painted onto the plaques in the baby's mouth three to four times daily for about 1 week. Another medical treatment, called gentian violet, is effective, but causes purple staining of the skin on which it is applied. This staining does go away, but be prepared for a week or two of a baby with a purple mouth!

If you are breast-feeding, be sure to be treated yourself. Breast-feeding mothers can develop itchy, crusty, burning nipples due to a thrush infection. Yeast infections can be passed back and forth from mother's nipples to baby's mouth, but rarely cause pain with breast-feeding.

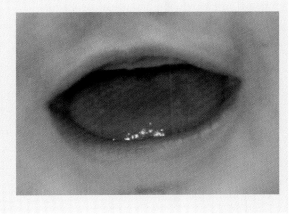

Heat rash

Heat rash (sometimes called prickly heat) is often seen in young infants when the pores of the sweat glands get plugged. Although most common in hot, humid environments, it may develop in cooler temperatures if the baby is over-bundled. Blockage of the pores causes tiny pink-red bumps to develop; they are most prevalent on covered parts of the skin, especially on the upper back and chest. As the name suggests, heat rash is worsened by heat and humidity. It does not cause fever. It usually settles on its own and can be prevented.

Preventing heat rash

To prevent heat rash, avoid over-bundling your baby, use cotton clothing that allows heat and moisture to escape, and reduce exposure to excessive heat and humidity. Ointments, creams, and powders are not useful in treating the rash because they can block pores and cause further heat rash.

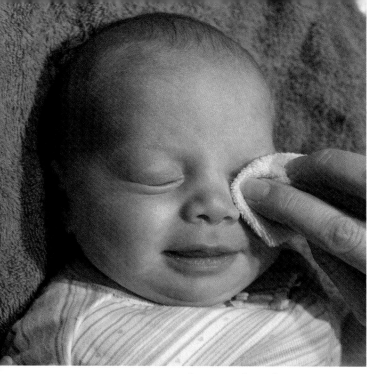

Tears and eye discharge

Tearless crying is common in newborn babies, but by the first few weeks of life, your baby's tear glands will produce enough fluid to bathe the eyes and create tears with crying. This fluid normally drains through a small duct called the lacrimal, or tear, duct in the inner corner of your baby's lower eyelid. These ducts drain into the top part of the nose, which explains why your nose often runs when you have a good cry!

Some babies, however, are born with blocked or narrowed tear ducts, on one or both sides. These babies may often look teary even if they are happy. Sometimes babies with blocked tear ducts have a collection of milky yellow discharge in the inner corner of their eyes. Occasionally, the baby will not be able to open his eye because the lids are a little stuck together with the yellowish crusty material.

Parents often mistake this as a sign of an eye infection. If the white parts of your baby's eyes are not red and there aren't copious amounts of thick pus, the problem is likely just a blocked tear duct or ducts. The eyes are not infected.

Treating eye discharge

Take a clean piece of cotton wool or gauze, wet it, and use it to wipe away the crusty material.

If still blocked, apply gentle pressure along the lacrimal duct beside the nose and underneath the eye several times a day. Ask your health-care provider how to do this.

Rarely, if the problem persists beyond the first birthday, the ducts need to be opened surgically by an ear, nose, and throat surgeon through a simple procedure that uses a probe to unblock the duct.

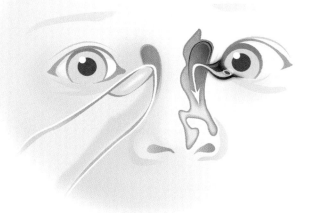

■ Apply gentle pressure downward against the nose over the lacrimal duct to help unblock it.

Irregular and noisy breathing patterns

If you watch your baby breathe, you will notice that he takes many short breaths of different lengths, the occasional deep breath and sigh, and even pauses of 8 to 10 seconds between breaths. This irregular breathing pattern, called periodic breathing, is normal; breathing usually becomes more regular around the end of the first month of life.

Many babies also breathe noisily, which many mistake for a cold or congestion. A newborn's nasal passages are very small, and even a slight amount of blockage can cause noisy breathing. Your baby may appear to be struggling to breath through his nose and may sneeze to clear his passages. This frequent sneezing is not a sign that he has a cold, but rather a protective reflex to clear his nose: a sneeze is a bit like nature's vacuum cleaner.

At the end of the first month, you may start to hear a gurgling sound in your baby's throat. This is caused by saliva pooled at the back of the throat. These sounds resolve once your baby learns how to swallow saliva effectively.

Clearing your baby's nose

Many approaches to clearing babies' noses have been tried. Here are a few strategies:

- To decrease irritation, lessen your baby's exposure to environmental irritants such as dust, lint, and tobacco smoke.
- If you are desperate for something to clear your baby's nose because the nasal congestion seems to be interfering with feeding or sleeping, try nasal drops or a suction bulb, but only continue with it if it seems to be helping. Theoretically, saline or salt water nose sprays or drops can loosen up the nasal mucus, allowing it to drain more freely or making it easier to suck out with a nasal aspirator. However, the use of nasal drops or aspirators has not been well studied for this purpose; they are generally felt to be ineffective.
- If your baby has a sudden onset of noisy breathing or changes in his breathing pattern, or if his breathing seems labored or difficult, it is best to see your doctor.

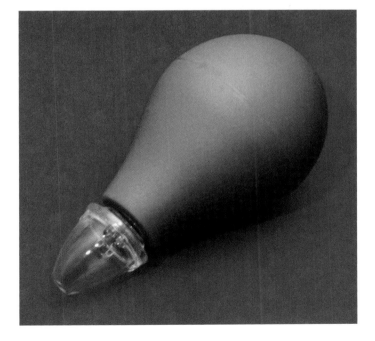

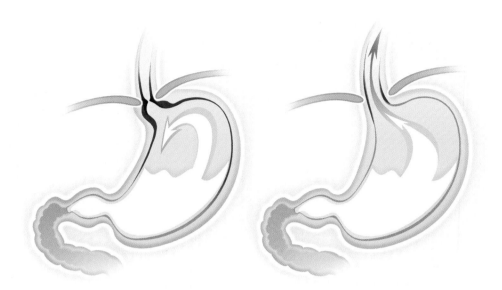

■ (Left) To prevent reflux, the sphincter between the esophagus and the stomach is closed; (Right) When reflux occurs, the sphincter is open, allowing milk to travel back up the esophagus.

Spitting up

Most infants regurgitate milk or formula from the stomach through the mouth or nose. In babies, the esophagus (the feeding tube that connects the mouth to the stomach) is relatively small, and the muscle at the end is not always fully developed. Reflux (spitting up) can result as food passes from the stomach back into the esophagus. This is a normal event.

For most babies, reflux is not bothersome — but parents can be alarmed by its impact on the laundry pile! It does not interfere with feeding or growth and should be considered a normal part of infancy. Spitting up is most common in the first few months; it improves spontaneously and becomes an infrequent occurrence (less than 5% of infants) by 1 year of age.

Did You Know?

Projectile vomiting

Projectile vomiting is the hallmark of pyloric stenosis, which differs from gastroesophageal reflux (when babies spit up food that dribbles out and soaks their sleepers). Vomiting from pyloric stenosis is forceful and can travel several feet in the air. The vomit does not contain bile (dark green fluid) and can sometimes have the appearance of curdled milk. Babies with pyloric stenosis usually appear very hungry and eager to feed, but with ongoing vomiting can develop signs of dehydration and inadequate nutrition, such as a reduction in wet diapers, constipation, and poor weight gain.

HOW TO
Manage problematic reflux

A minority of infants do have significant problems that can be related to reflux, including poor weight gain, discomfort during feeding, blood loss from the digestive tract due to the irritation of stomach acid, or recurrent respiratory problems (gagging, cough, or pneumonia) due to aspiration. For these infants, relatively simple measures may be helpful:

- Thicken formula with rice cereal.
- Avoid the sitting position (in car seats or swings, for example) after feeding.
- Place your baby on his stomach while he's awake. Almost all infants should still be placed on their backs for sleep, but keeping the head of the bed elevated by about 30 degrees may be beneficial. Holding him upright over your chest or shoulder for 20 to 30 minutes after feeding is also an option.
- For the occasional infant whose symptoms are significant, medications that reduce stomach acid or help in promoting more rapid emptying of the stomach may be considered in discussion with your physician.

If symptoms persist, consult your health-care provider, especially if your baby

- Is not gaining weight appropriately
- Seems to be in pain while feeding
- Coughs or gags with feeds/spit-ups or has frequent chest infections

You should also seek medical advice if the spit-up or vomit

- Contains blood (or "coffee grounds"), suggesting inflammation of the lower end of the gullet (although it is not unusual for breast-feeding babies to swallow some blood from the mother's cracked nipples)
- Is dark green (bilious) in color, suggesting a blockage in the small intestine below the level of the stomach
- Is "projectile" (can hit a wall a few feet away), suggesting a blockage at the outlet of the stomach (pyloric stenosis)

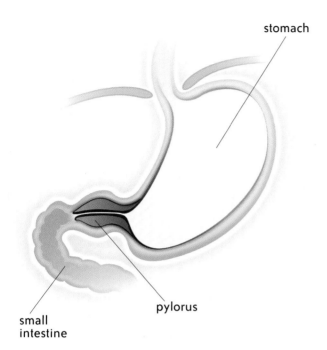

stomach

small intestine

pylorus

■ Thickening of the pylorus obstructs the emptying of the stomach into the intestine.

Pyloric stenosis

Pyloric stenosis is an obstruction in the upper bowel caused by a thickening of the pylorus, the muscular channel at the exit of the stomach. It is one of the most common surgical conditions of infancy, affecting one in every 300 to 400 babies. It is generally not present at birth, but develops over the first few weeks of life. Signs of pyloric stenosis typically become apparent at 2 to 4 weeks of age. The exact cause of pyloric stenosis is not known, but there is a strong genetic component. Boys are affected approximately four times as frequently as girls, and infants of mothers who themselves had pyloric stenosis as infants have a much greater chance of developing the condition.

Diagnosing pyloric stenosis

The diagnosis of pyloric stenosis is made by a combination of physical examination, blood tests, and imaging tests, usually an ultrasound of the stomach. Sometimes the thickened pylorus can be felt (it is said to feel like an olive) on palpating the stomach, but this requires a relaxed baby and an experienced examiner. If pyloric stenosis is suspected, blood tests are performed to look for signs of dehydration, and the vomited stomach fluid is examined for loss of acid and salts.

Treating pyloric stenosis

Pyloric stenosis is treated surgically with a relatively minor operation that usually requires only a 1- to 2-day stay in the hospital to ensure that feeding is well established after the procedure. Once it is fixed, there should be no recurrence or further problems.

Developmental dysplasia of the hip (DDH)

Disturbances in the hip joint in young infants are termed developmental dysplasia of the hip. DDH may be apparent at birth when the baby's hips are examined or may become evident during the first 6 months. Occasionally, DDH is noticed in older children when a limp is apparent.

DDH is actually a spectrum of conditions involving the way the thigh bone sits in relation to the hip joint. The top of the thigh bone (femoral head) is ball-shaped; this "ball" must fit in and be covered by part of the pelvic bones to allow proper growth and development of the hip joint.

Guide to

Infant birthmarks

Approximately 20% to 40% of infants have a form of birthmark. Most of these are normal and harmless, and often fade over time, but a small number of birthmarks are signs of an important medical condition.

SALMON PATCH

One of the most common birthmarks is the salmon patch — a flat, pink-red area apparent in the newborn period. These typically appear on the neck (stork bite) or eyelid (angel's kiss). The majority of eyelid marks disappear by themselves over the first year; those on the neck often persist longer.

MONGOLIAN SPOT

These marks are flat, blue-grey areas seen most often on the buttocks and back of darker-skinned babies. They may be mistaken for bruising because of their color. The markings disappear in 95% of children by the time they reach school age.

HEMANGIOMA

Hemangiomas are growths of immature blood vessels; they can appear as raised, firm, red areas (strawberries) or bluish lumps arising from the deeper skin and tissues. The growths, appearing most often on the face, scalp, and chest, are very common and are seen more frequently in girls and premature infants. They are typically very small or absent at birth but have a rapid growth phase (out of proportion to that of the infant) during the first 6 months, then shrink over a period of years. Approximately 60% disappear by age 6 and 90% by age 9. Hemangiomas do not require treatment unless they are in sensitive areas where they may obscure vision or are prone to bleeding.

PORT WINE STAIN

This flat, red-purple mark, made up of mature blood vessels, is evident at birth and grows in proportion to the child. Marks are treated with laser therapy if they are extensive or in cosmetically important areas.

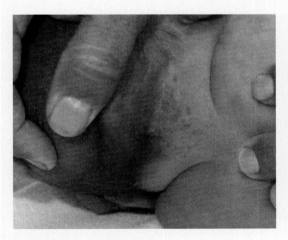
■ Salmon patch (stork bite).

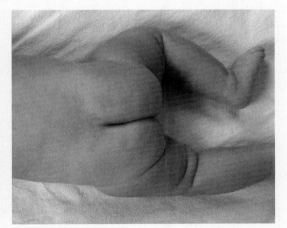
■ Mongolian spot.

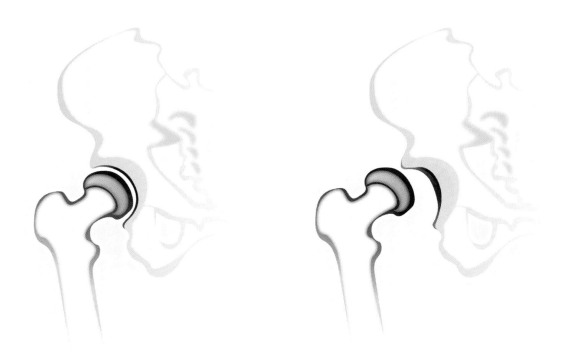

■ (Left) Normal hip joint; (Right) DDH: The hip tends to dislocate because the hip socket is too shallow.

Did You Know?

Hip dysplasia and club foot

Hip dysplasia occurs in approximately one in 1,000 infants. It is more common in girls and in babies who were in a breech position (legs or buttocks at the bottom of the womb, instead of the head). It affects the left hip more often than the right.

Hip dysplasia can be seen in isolation or along with other malformations caused by the positioning of the growing fetus or by lack of movement inside the womb. One such condition is termed clubfoot, a malformation characterized by a small, wide, and stiff foot with the heel and forefoot turned inward. A clubfoot is treated with casting, with or without surgery, for correction.

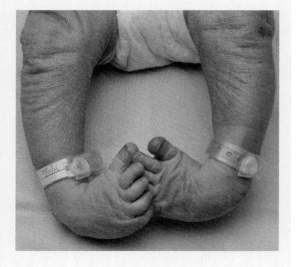

Dysplasia of the hip is not painful to infants, but untreated DDH can lead to a limp, a shortened leg, and arthritis in adulthood.

Detecting DDH

Regular hip examinations throughout infancy are an important part of routine health visits. The physician will check for problems by testing hip movement on both sides with the baby lying on his back. In DDH, the hip may be dislocated (where the head of the thigh bone lies outside the hip joint) or "unstable" (where the thigh bone can slip out of the proper covering of the joint). Dysplasia of the hip may be apparent to parents when the hips do not seem to have adequate movement during diaper changes or in older infants who have a discrepancy in the pattern of skin creases. An ultrasound is used to confirm the diagnosis in very young infants; an x-ray of the hips is used in older infants.

Treating DDH

Treatment requires the expertise of an orthopedic surgeon. In significant DDH, the young infant may need to wear a harness to encourage proper positioning and development of the hip joint. In more involved cases or in older children, surgery is often required to achieve better alignment of the joint.

Hypospadias and chordee

Hypospadias is a common malformation affecting almost 1% of boys. In this condition, the opening of the urethra is not located at the tip of the penis.

Hypospadias may be minor, when the opening is located very close to the tip, or severe, when the opening may be close to the base of the penis. Often associated with hypospadias is a condition called chordee, the bending of the penis on erection.

Hypospadias generally does not cause problems relating to the urinary tract, but it can make voiding with a direct stream while standing difficult to achieve. This difference can be awkward for a boy as he gets older. In addition, if chordee is present and significant, it can have an impact on sexual function and satisfaction. For these reasons, significant hypospadias and chordee are generally repaired, but for very minor degrees of hypospadias surgical correction may not be necessary.

Treating hypospadias and chordee

The type of surgical procedure depends on the degree of hypospadias. Infants with hypospadias should not be circumcised prior to any procedure by the urologist because the foreskin is often used for part of the repair. Mild hypospadias is often corrected during a short outpatient procedure. More extensive hypospadias and chordee repairs require more complex procedures and time in hospital. A catheter in the urethra may be used. Significant bleeding, even in extensive cases, is rare. Infection is uncommon. For extensive surgeries, fistula (a leak of urine from the newly constructed urethra), narrowing of the urethra, and recurrent chordee are the most important complications and may require further procedures.

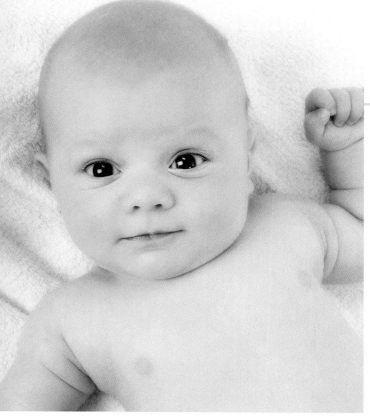

Hearing loss

Approximately two to three babies in 1,000 will have significant hearing impairment that can be detected during infancy. The known causes of this infant hearing loss include inherited genetic conditions, infections acquired during pregnancy, and problems related to premature birth. While hearing loss is detected in many infants at birth using screening tests, some infants will have a delayed onset of hearing loss or will develop conditions later in life that can lead to impaired hearing. Newborn screening programs, either hospital— or community-based, have been established in most communities, resulting in a reduction in the average age that hearing loss is detected from about 24 months to 2 to 3 months of age.

Hearing tests

In general, any concern about hearing or language development should lead to a hearing test. Early language development is often normal even in young infants with profound hearing loss, but if a baby does not engage in babbling or respond to his name being called by about 6 to 7 months of age, it could be an indication of a hearing problem. While being startled by loud noises does not rule out the possibility of hearing difficulties, infants who do not respond to loud noises should have their hearing assessed. Some of the risk factors for hearing loss that may require further testing include:

- Family history of childhood hearing loss
- Persistent fluid in the ear following ear infections
- Bacterial meningitis

Treating hearing loss

Early identification of hearing impairment is crucial to allow timely intervention that promotes normal language development. Infants who are found to have hearing loss on the newborn screening exam or after the newborn period are referred to an audiologist and an ear, nose, and throat doctor. The management of hearing loss depends on the underlying cause and the part of the hearing system that is affected.

For example, hearing loss caused by persistent fluid in the middle ear (the area behind the eardrum) is usually managed by the insertion of ear tubes. Many infants with profound hearing loss, who previously would have had significant difficulties with language, have been treated with cochlear implants (small electronic devices surgically implanted in the inner ear), which have allowed age-appropriate language development.

Urinary tract infection (UTI)

Infections involving the urinary tract are quite common in the first year of life. In older children and adults, UTIs can often be divided into bladder infections (cystitis) and kidney infections (pyelonephritis). In the first year of life, babies with a UTI are considered to have pyelonephritis.

The most common bacteria that causes UTIs is *E. coli*, which is found in the bowels and is often present on the skin in the diaper area. The infection is not caused by poor hygiene (inadequate cleaning or diaper changes), although baby girls should always be cleaned from front to back. UTIs generally occur in healthy babies.

Symptoms of UTI

Babies may have one or more of the following symptoms:

- Fever
- Irritability
- Vomiting
- Loss of appetite
- Crying with urination
- Discolored or foul-smelling urine

Diagnosing UTI

Diagnosis is made by taking a urine sample and testing it with a special stick, as well as sending it to the laboratory for culture. Unfortunately, to get a clean sample, the baby requires a very thin catheter to be placed into the bladder after a thorough cleaning of the genital area. The procedure is uncomfortable, but takes only a minute. Some doctors will use a bag stuck over the penis or vagina. This is more comfortable, but has a chance of picking up germs from the skin as well, which can make interpretation of the culture result very difficult. For that reason, this method is not recommended. Within 24 hours after the urine reaches the laboratory, your doctor will know whether a true infection is present.

About one-third of babies with UTIs have vesico-ureteric reflux, in which the urine refluxes from the bladder back up to the kidneys, exposing them to the germs present in the bladder. If your baby is diagnosed with a UTI, he will likely undergo an ultrasound of the kidney, as well as a VCUG (a special type of x-ray) to look for reflux. If reflux is present, you may be advised to give him a small dose of antibiotics on a daily basis until he grows out of the reflux, which usually occurs in the first few years of life.

Treating UTI

Treatment of a UTI consists of a 10- to 14-day course of antibiotics. If your baby is in the first few months of life, or is quite sick with a high fever and vomiting, then it is likely that, for the first few days, the antibiotics will be delivered intravenously, requiring a stay in the hospital. After that, the antibiotics can be given as a liquid by mouth. Most babies will make a quick and complete recovery from this infection.

More about fathering

You've listened attentively at prenatal classes, you've attended all the doctor's appointments, and you've even leafed through some of the baby books. You're eager to be an active part of your baby's life. The only problem is, you have little idea of what to do. Welcome to being a dad.

Inequality

When it comes to parenting, mothers and fathers should be equals, but the truth of the matter is that fathering a newborn is different from parenting a 10-year-old. You simply can't breast-feed your baby as your wife can. Still, you have a huge role to play, and the more involved you become, the more you will enjoy fathering.

Support and more support

Your partner needs your help now as much as at any other time in the parenting of your child. Provide her with the three S's — support, support, support. At the same time, you can bond with your baby.

For example, you can take responsibility for bathing your baby. All it requires is water, soap, and a pair of steady hands. You can also assign yourself designated time slots for caring for your baby, perhaps first thing in the morning, before work, and immediately after work when you come home.

Night shift

Even the most competent mother needs a break, especially in the middle of the night.

During the night, you can change the baby's diaper and prepare the bottle if he is formula-feeding. You can even volunteer to attend to your baby if he cannot fall back asleep. This is a win-win situation. The mother wins because she gets to go back to sleep, and you win because you get to hold your baby while reading or watching late-night television.

Social calendar

If you really want to help prevent your wife from becoming exhausted, take control of the social calendar. During the first month (and for as long as you can get away with it), be politely ruthless. Well-meaning friends and relatives can kill you with kindness and good advice. Send them packing.

It's worth it

Expect to be sleep deprived, exhausted, and irritable and to feel reduced in the family hierarchy. That's your current reality — but it's worth it. Your baby is beautiful, the best, more wonderful than you could have ever imagined.

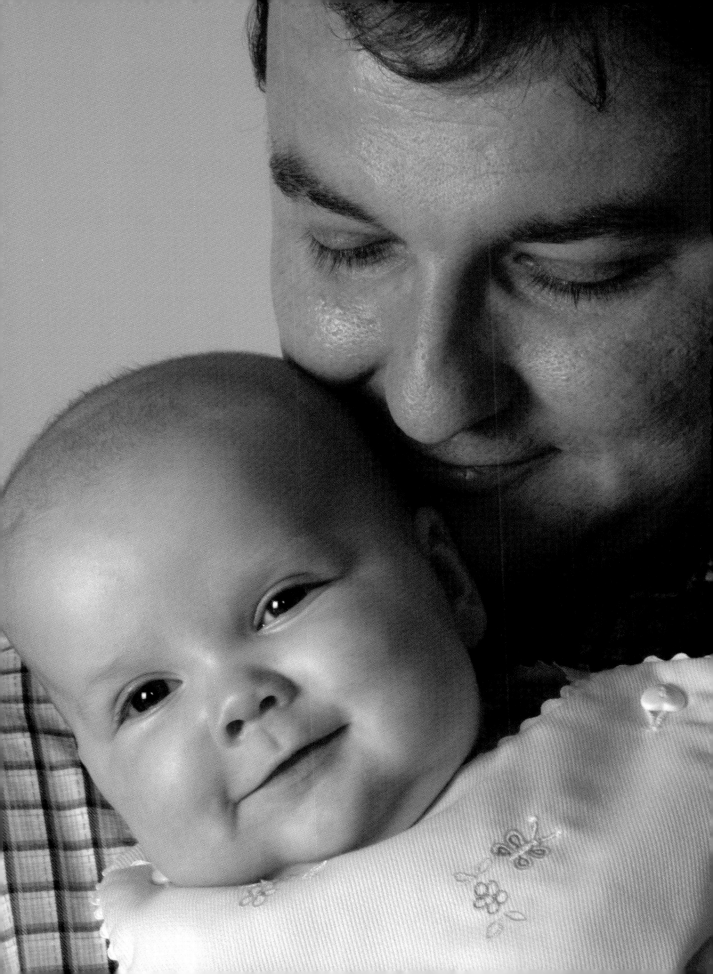

Frequently asked questions

As family doctors and pediatricians, we answer many questions from parents. Here are some of the most frequently asked questions. Be sure to ask your health-care providers any other questions that arise. If they don't have the answers, they will refer you to a colleague who does.

Q: I have a newborn and two other young children around the house. What is the best way to stop the spread of germs?

A: Frequent hand-washing with soap and water by all those who touch the newborn is still the most effective way to reduce the spread of germs. It is especially important if anyone has diarrhea, or is vomiting, coughing or sneezing. Remember to wash your hands and your children's hands after wiping noses and throwing away used tissues. Keep alcohol-based solutions and gels handy for those times when you aren't near a water source.

Q: I love our new baby, but there seem to be too many moments when I'm tearful. What should I do?

A: It's easy to blame your sadness on simple fatigue. But that would be wrong. Many women experience significant depression following childbirth. Although postpartum depression is often transient and relatively mild, it can sometimes pose a serious risk to both mother and baby. It's important to discuss your feelings with your partner and your health-care provider. You should have no feelings of shame or guilt if you're suffering from postpartum depression — it is a common problem that can be treated.

Q: I've heard a lot about the dangers of the flu. My baby boy is almost 1 month old now — should I be getting him vaccinated against it?

A: The current available vaccine for influenza can only be used from 6 months of age onward. If your baby will be over 6 months old in October or November, when it is time for the annual influenza vaccination, it is advisable to have him immunized.

Q: I am a first-time parent and have lots to learn about babies. However, everyone seems determined to offer me advice, even when I don't want it. How do I handle well-meaning but unsolicited advice?

A: It sometimes seems that everyone who has ever had a baby thinks she's an expert on parenting. The best advice is usually asked for, not imposed upon you. Try to listen politely and evaluate each suggestion objectively. But in the end, this is your baby. Trust your own instincts about what works best for you and your child. Repeat offenders, such as your mother and mother-in-law, may have to be diplomatically reminded that there are usually several correct ways to deal with a situation, not just theirs.

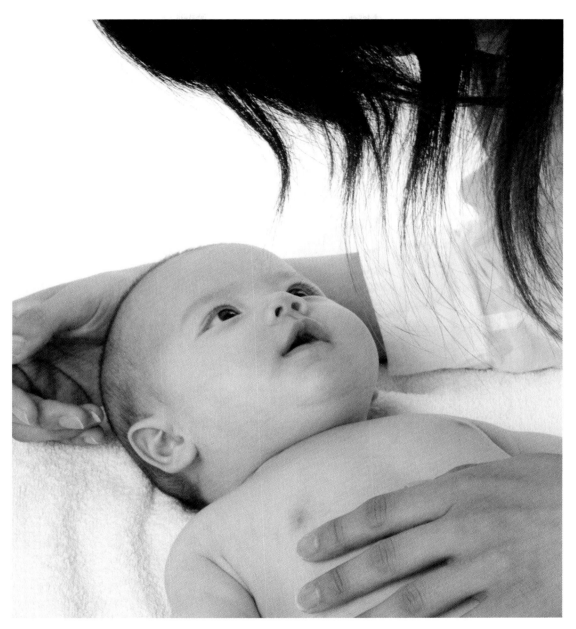

Q: I've heard that formula with iron can cause constipation. If my baby is constipated, should I find a formula without iron?

A: Actually, all types of formula have some iron. Those advertised as "with iron" just have a higher concentration of it. There isn't good evidence to suggest that formula "with iron" will cause constipation. If your baby is constipated, there are a number of potential solutions, depending on his age. Discuss this with your health-care provider.

Sam's Diary

February 22 (2 weeks old)

The last week has been quite hectic since we got home! It seems like you are feeding all the time, and when you aren't, Mom tries to catch up on some sleep. Dad has been off work and doing all the housework. He's doing a great job! Today your umbilical cord fell off, leaving a beautifully shaped belly button.

We saw Dr. Murphy a few days ago, and she was very happy with you — your jaundice is fading, and you have gained about 1 ounce (30 g) per day since you were born. It seems like you are enjoying feeding! We had so many questions, we had to write them all down so we wouldn't forget to ask.

Yesterday, we gave you your first bath at home — you weren't sure how you felt about this new experience, but we're sure you'll feel happier

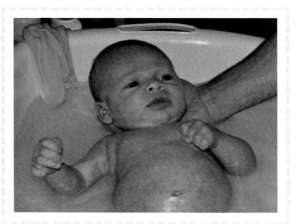

once you get used to it. Dad also cut your nails for the first time — what a delicate job.

March 17 (5 weeks old)

We think you've been smiling for a few days now, but it is still a little difficult to know what is gas and what is a smile. Today, though, you gave us a definite smile — what a joy!

Your grandparents are so excited about you — Granny loves to change you and bathe you at any chance she gets. Granddad has a big smile when he pushes you around in your stroller. You love going for drives in the car, as long as we don't stop too long at any lights!

Going out is not as simple as it used to be. We now have to pack a diaper bag and cover you from head to toe when we venture out into the cold.

April 3 (7 weeks old)

Every Tuesday we go to a mom and baby group. All the babies were born within 2 weeks of each other. You have been a little treasure. You are sleeping longer between feeds, and you'll allow Mom and Dad to put you down in your chair to play or sleep. You are smiling lots and lots, especially at your black and white mobile and when you are bathing. Sometimes you have a big cry, and we feel so bad because we don't really know what's

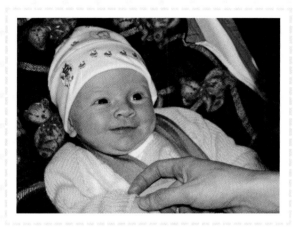

bothering you. Everybody has a suggestion, but when you're upset it is quite hard to get you settled again. Driving you around in the car sometimes seems to help. We even offered you a pacifier, but you weren't at all interested in it. Dad says that is a good sign of determination.

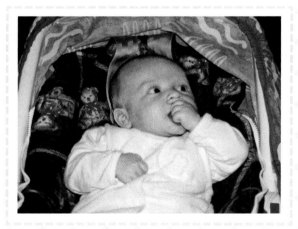

April 12 (2 months old)

You have just turned 2 months old, and today was a day of two "firsts." Last night you went for $5\frac{1}{2}$ hours between feeds, from 8:00 p.m. to 1:30 a.m. — that's the longest you've done so far. You also found your thumb, which you have been trying to suck. You seem to enjoy Mom's and Dad's facial expressions, and you try to imitate us by sticking out your tongue. You also love being sung to, especially "Twinkle, Twinkle, Little Star" and "Itsy-Bitsy Spider." You are always smiling. You have even started laughing and "talking" to us.

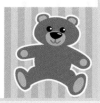

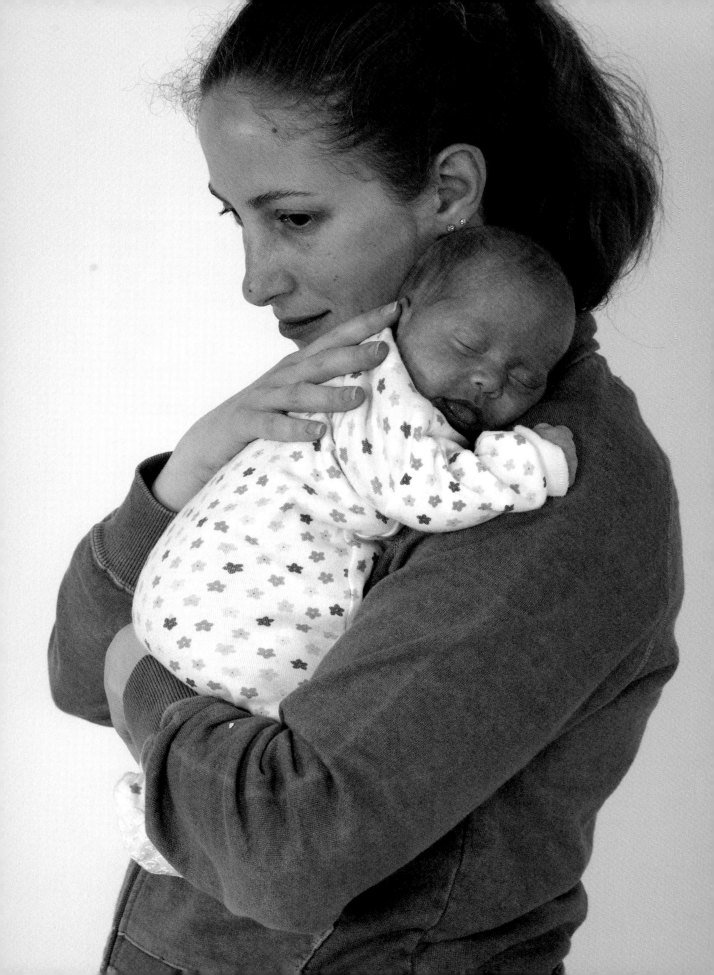

Helping
Your Baby Sleep

Understanding sleep

The birth of a new baby brings about many changes in a family's routine. One of the most distressing changes for parents is lack of sleep. Prior to the delivery of your baby, you probably received some "words of wisdom" on surviving with very little sleep, but only once you have your baby can you truly understand how precious a few hours of sleep can be.

There are many things you can do throughout your baby's first year of life to promote healthy sleep habits, starting as soon as your baby is born. The bad news is that your baby's sleep is very different from yours!

Good Sleepers

Are some children inherently good sleepers, while others aren't? Yes, but this is no different from many things in life. Does this mean that some children are destined to sleep poorly? Not necessarily, especially if you give your child the right cues to learn to sleep. Sleep is somewhat innate, but it is also learned. Providing

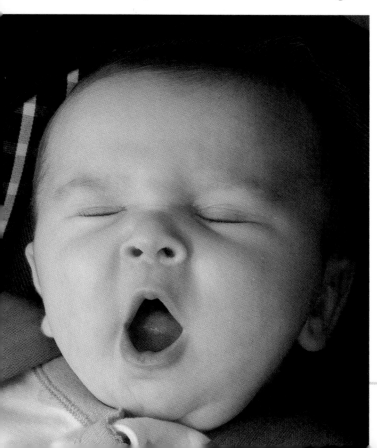

babies with a healthy sleep routine and teaching them how to put themselves to sleep without you will allow them to become "good sleepers."

Functions of sleep

Having a basic understanding of sleep is very helpful if you are going to teach your baby to be a good sleeper. Sleep is essential for the growth and development of your baby. Without sleep, our bodies cannot function properly. Sleep experts at the Hospital for Sick Children and elsewhere have identified several possible functions of sleep that promote good health:

- Restoration and regeneration of body systems
- Protection and recovery from infections
- Consolidation of memory
- Optimum daytime function of learning, memory, mood, attention, and concentration
- Growth and development of body and brain

Adapted by permission from Shelly Weiss, *Better Baby Sleep* (Toronto: Robert Rose, 2006).

Kinds of sleep

There are two main kinds of sleep: REM (rapid eye movement) and NREM (non–rapid eye movement) sleep.

REM sleep

REM sleep is commonly referred to as "dreaming sleep." In REM sleep, your brain is in an active state, even though you are asleep. Under your eyelids, your eyes move rapidly. Your heart rate and breathing rate may also fluctuate. While your brain is very active, your body is very still, apart from small muscle twitches — which is a good thing, depending on what you are dreaming about. In this state, it may be easier for someone to wake you up than if you were in NREM sleep.

In children, REM sleep is thought to help with the development of memory and contribute to learning.

NREM sleep

NREM sleep is a deeper, more restorative kind of sleep. There are different degrees of NREM sleep, from light to deep. If you are in deep NREM sleep, you may feel confused or disoriented if someone wakes you up. In fact, it may be very difficult to wake you if you are in deep NREM sleep.

This is the stage of sleep that allows a parent to carry a sleeping child from the car to the crib without the child waking. In this stage, your heart and breathing rate stay fairly consistent, and you do not dream as much as you do in REM sleep, because your brain is not as active.

In children, the purpose of this sleep is restoration of the body.

Sleep cycles

During an average night, your baby will go through several cycles of REM and NREM sleep:

- Infants typically fall asleep quickly, in less than 30 minutes, but may wake up soon after because this transitional sleep phase is easily reversed.
- Infants cycle from dreaming (REM) to restorative sleep (NREM) throughout the night. At 1 year of age, the cycle may last 45 to 50 minutes. The cycles lengthen with development.
- Infants typically have their first episode of deep sleep and continue to have their deepest sleep in the first third of the night. Your child may have a briefer episode of deep restorative sleep in the early morning hours, before waking.

Did You Know?

"Restless" sleep

Many parents are unaware of the different stages of sleep and often mistake normal sleep actions for discomfort or an unsettled baby. If your baby is in REM sleep (what we call active dreaming), she may smile, frown, suck, or twitch her limbs, and will be easily roused. She may appear to be restless, but she is actually just in a normal REM sleep phase. When your baby is in NREM sleep (restorative sleep), she will appear to be sleeping more deeply and will be more difficult to rouse.

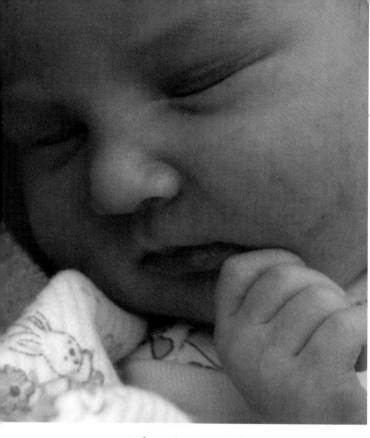

- Infants have their first episode of dreaming sleep about 90 minutes after falling asleep. The dreaming episodes become longer throughout the night, with most dreaming happening in the last third of the night.
- Infants may experience periods of brief arousal during the night. When your child ends one sleep cycle and starts the next, she may awaken briefly. This awakening is usually brief. These arousals occur out of REM or the lighter stages of NREM sleep.

- Infants typically wake up spontaneously in the morning.

Different cycles

Newborn babies spend half of their sleeping time in REM sleep, whereas adults spend only a quarter of their sleeping time in REM. By the time an infant is about 6 months old, her sleep cycles will have changed to resemble those of an adult. This is very important to know when you are trying to determine how to teach your baby to sleep. The sleep cycles of babies up to 6 months of age are not organized like those of an older infant or child; therefore, they may need more help from you to be able to sleep — you might comfort, hold, or rock them, for example. Once their sleep is more sophisticated, it is more reasonable to expect them to sleep on their own.

Circadian rhythms

Circadian (24-hour) rhythms also play a part in regulating our sleeping and waking. Light and dark, eating patterns, physical activities, and hormones all affect our biological sleep rhythms, regulating in a 24-hour period when we feel sleepy and when we feel awake.

Did You Know?

Partial arousals

Newborns cycle through REM and NREM sleep about every 60 minutes, whereas adults do so every 90 to 110 minutes. At the end of each cycle, we all have a partial arousal. When this happens in infants, they will commonly fall back into a deeper sleep. Unfortunately, many parents mistake this arousal for an awakening and pick up their baby, causing a true awakening (full arousal) and disrupting the baby's sleep. If you do not teach your baby how to fall asleep on her own, these partial arousals may develop into full arousals throughout the night.

How much sleep does my baby need?

Most parents wonder how much sleep their baby really needs. In their often tired state, they feel their baby does not sleep as much as other babies. Knowing how much sleep babies need on average can be reassuring during those nights when your baby stays awake.

Months 0 to 3

In the first months of life, don't expect your baby to sleep though the night. Newborn babies do not have the same ability as older infants to regulate sleep-wake cycles. In the newborn, sleep and wake states are usually driven by hunger. A newborn baby may feed every 2 to 3 hours during the day and at night. This is normal. In fact, if your newborn baby is sleeping through the night, this may not be normal. You should consult your health-care provider about this.

Average sleep

Newborn babies sleep an average of 17 hours per day, but "average" means just that, because some babies sleep 15 hours a day and others can sleep up to 20 hours a day. About 50% of sleep time for newborns occurs during the daytime. A normal newborn pattern is to sleep for 2 to 4 hours, then be awake for 1 to 2 hours, then sleep again. Some approaches have been shown to help babies sleep for longer stretches at night. There are, however, no guarantees.

Crying to sleep

Letting your newborn baby (0 to 3 months) cry herself to sleep is inappropriate. You should respond to the cries of a young infant during the first few months of life. For a newborn, crying is not manipulative behavior, but rather her only way of communicating a need, such as feeding, diaper changes, or soothing.

Did You Know?

Sleep regulation

Newborn babies do not have the ability to regulate their sleep as an older infant or child does and may want to be awake when most of us are asleep. As their bodies develop and they begin to learn from external cues, their sleep patterns evolve so that they are awake more during the day and asleep more at night. At 2 months of age, for example, your baby may be able to distinguish between day and night. As parents, providing infants with consistent cues is one way to help them begin to regulate this pattern.

Months 3 to 6

As your baby grows, she will start to sleep a little less during the day. By 3 to 6 months, she will begin to sleep through the night, with two to three naps during the day. The middle-of-the-night feeding is usually eliminated around this age, and by 6 months most healthy infants do not need to feed at night. Now is the time when helping your baby know what to expect in terms of daytime naps and nighttime sleep duration will make a difference in her sleep pattern — and yours.

Average sleep

The average total sleep decreases to 14 to 16 hours a day. For example, a 5-month-old may sleep from 7:30 p.m. until 6:00 a.m., have a morning nap from 9:00 to 11:00 a.m., and have an afternoon nap from 2:30 to 4:00 p.m. Some babies at this age continue to have three naps a day: a morning nap, an early afternoon nap, and a short nap before dinner.

Months 7 to 12

From months 7 to 12, babies sleep an average of 14 hours per day, sleeping through the night and having two naps during the day, each lasting from 30 minutes to 2 hours. This is a time of significant maturation in your baby's sleep patterns. She no longer needs to feed during the night, and should be able to soothe herself to sleep. By 7 or 8 months, a short period of crying prior to falling asleep is normal and not harmful. At this age, babies start to develop an increasing awareness of separation. They don't want to be left alone, and falling asleep by themselves may become an issue. When separation awareness develops, your infant might need a transitional object, such as a stuffed animal or blanket to cuddle.

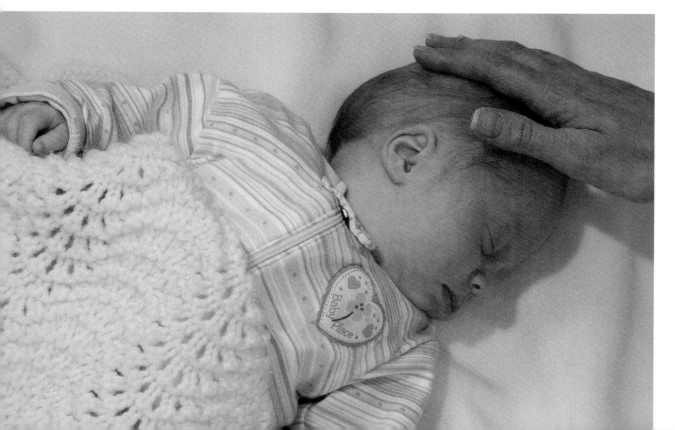

Developing healthy sleep habits

Parents can help their babies become good sleepers by teaching them healthy sleep hygiene. Good sleep hygiene involves establishing a consistent sleep routine. This consistency in sleeping habits is the key to preventing sleep problems.

Sleep hygiene

The first few months require the development of a secure, nurturing environment for your new baby to sleep. Your baby's room should be consistently quiet, dark at night, comfortable, and cool, to promote sleep onset and maintenance. Your child should also have a consistent space — bassinet, crib, or bed — to sleep in during the night and at naptime, whether in your room, in a room with a sibling, or in her own room. If your baby wakes soon after falling asleep or in the middle of the night, she should be in the same environment she was in when she fell asleep. That way, she can replicate the skills used initially to fall asleep to go back to sleep.

Despite having a healthy sleep environment, your baby may wake up soon after falling asleep and during the night. This is not uncommon. All people, but especially babies, have the potential to wake up as they cycle into the lighter stages of sleep (partial arousal). Babies under 6 months of age have an even greater chance of waking because they spend more time in REM sleep than in NREM sleep. The key to preventing this normal sleep pattern from becoming a problem is to teach your child the skills needed to put herself to sleep and to remain asleep at night. This involves establishing a consistent bedtime and naptime routine.

Healthy sleep routines

Months 0 to 3

Hunger often drives the sleep-wake cycle of the newborn baby, but even at this age, consistency helps. Regular feeding schedules that complement sleeping schedules are useful. Feeding should be

Did You Know?

Arousals

Until babies are 6 months old, it is not abnormal for them to wake up during the night or need some assistance falling asleep. Be prepared to soothe and feed your baby if necessary. Once they are over 6 months, babies should be able (for the most part) to fall asleep on their own and sleep through the night.

separate from sleeping, meaning that your baby should be awake when feeding (either by breast or bottle). Once she falls asleep, feeding should stop. If she is not finished a feeding, you may need to rouse her to complete the feeding. This will help her define distinct periods when she eats and when she sleeps, and she won't develop the habit of being able to fall asleep only when she is being fed.

Allowing your baby to fall asleep on her own at this age is just fine, but don't be surprised if she doesn't. You may need to hold her or rock her until she's sleepy. To establish a healthy sleep cycle, help your baby learn the difference between night and day. For example, during her awake period in the daytime, play with her in a bright, stimulating environment; at night, keep the light dim and just hold her.

Months 3 to 6

As your baby grows and matures, you will notice that she is awake more often and is more aware of daytime and nighttime. Consistent routines are being learned. Continue to follow her cues when it comes to feeding. By 3 months of age, some babies will be sleeping through the night and will no longer need to be fed during the night. Sleeping patterns vary from baby to baby, and the evidence on sleeping through the night shows no difference between breast-fed and bottle-fed babies as a group.

If possible, try to have your baby take naps in her crib. Stimulate and play with her during her daytime alert periods, but keep the lights low and your voice soft when she is awake at night. Her napping schedule and bedtime should start to take on some semblance of a routine. Try to determine when your little one is tired and put her into her crib while she is awake.

Months 7 to 12

By 6 months of age, your baby may sleep through the night (for a 5- to 6-hour stretch), but only if you have given her the tools to do so. Don't be disappointed if your 7-month-old still occasionally wakes up. Good sleeping takes practice.

A 6-month-old baby will usually nap two to three times a day and then sleep for 10 to 12 hours at night, though not always continuously. Once your baby is 9 months old, she will likely have only two naps and may sleep through the night for 10 to 12 hours. If possible, your baby should nap at the same time every day and go to bed at the same time every night. In the morning, a well-rested baby will wake by herself.

When your baby naps and goes to bed at night will be determined by your sleep-wake schedule. At 6 months, babies may have a morning nap, a noontime nap, and an afternoon nap. They may then go to bed between 7:00 and 8:00 p.m. Once they drop to two naps, the noon nap may disappear. Think about the scheduling of these naps. For example, naps that are late in the day (after 4:00 p.m.) are not recommended because they will prevent your child from falling asleep at the desired bedtime.

By this age, children of a normal weight do not need to be fed during the night; they can safely go without feeds for 6 to 10 hours overnight. If you are feeding your baby during the night, you will need to wean her from these feeds slowly so that she isn't waking because she is hungry.

HOW TO
Establish a healthy sleep routine

Although it is unreasonable to expect your 3-week-old baby to have a regular bedtime and naptime, there is evidence to show that instituting a consistent bedtime sleep routine from birth teaches your child the cues that sleep time is coming. Here are some tips to help you establish a healthy sleep routine from the start:

1. Before bedtime, create and maintain a quiet and relaxing atmosphere. Start by giving your baby a warm bath, feed her, change her into a fresh sleeper, read her a story, and sing your favorite songs.

2. After these comforting activities, place your awake or drowsy baby into her crib, giving her the opportunity to fall asleep on her own. Some children will be very good at this, while others will not, but practice makes perfect. Allowing your baby to try this over and over again will help her learn to fall asleep on her own, which will be particularly useful if she wakes up in the middle of the night.

3. For babies under 4 to 6 months, allow some fussing, but if your baby is crying consistently and hard, cuddle, hold, and soothe her before trying again to settle her in her crib.

4. After an hour or two, you may hear your baby move or fuss. Allow her the opportunity to put herself back to sleep before going in to check on her.

This awakening is likely to be a sleep arousal, an event that occurs every 60 minutes or so during sleep. Do not take it as a cue to awaken your child.

5. The same strategies for bedtime routines apply to naptime. Although a naptime routine does not generally include bathing, it should include placing your awake or drowsy baby in her crib to fall asleep. She will then learn that her crib is where she sleeps.

6. Some babies seem to need the warmth and comfort of their parents to sleep. Don't give up on consistent sleep routines and frequent attempts to place your awake baby in her crib — as she grows and develops, so will her sleep cycles and patterns. Sleep patterns become more organized in the second and third months of life.

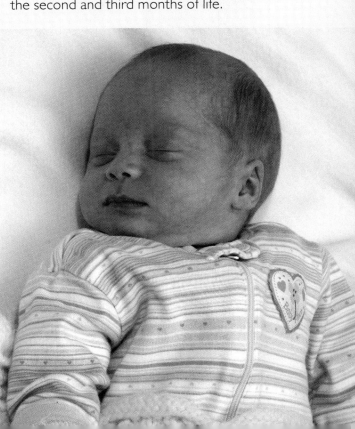

Did You Know?

Sleeping through the night

"Sleeping through the night" means sleeping for a period of 5 to 6 hours in a row, usually from midnight to 5:00 a.m. It doesn't mean sleeping from 7:00 p.m. to 7:00 a.m.! Also, infants have short sleep cycles (50 to 60 minutes), which means that during these 5 hours they may stir, but are able to soothe themselves and put themselves back to sleep. If your baby doesn't sleep through the night at 3 months, don't worry. This is still well within the limits of normal. No intervention is necessary — just continue with your routines.

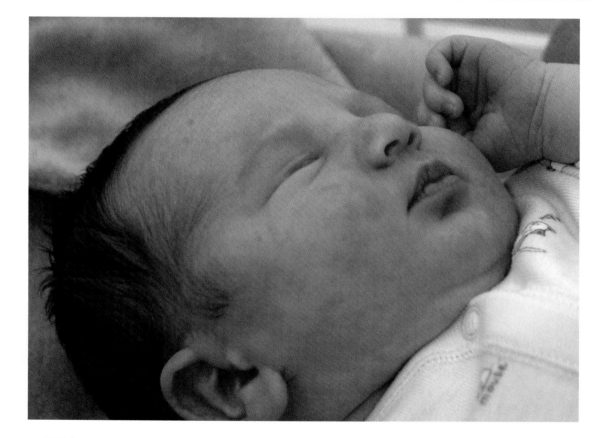

Did You Know?

Staying awake

Parents often believe that keeping a baby awake during the day will help her sleep at night. This is not true. At this age, it will just make her fussier and unhappy, potentially worsening her sleep.

Sleeping safely

Creating a safe sleep environment for your baby involves choosing a sleeping style that reduces the risk of sudden infant death syndrome (SIDS) and nurtures your child in a family setting. You need to ask yourself where your baby will sleep — in your room, in her crib or your bed, or in her own room, in her crib or her bed? Your answer to these questions should be informed by an understanding of the benefits and risks of various sleeping arrangements, especially bed-sharing and co-sleeping.

Bed-sharing and co-sleeping

Many parents choose to share their bed with their infant; in fact, this is the most common sleeping arrangement among many cultures in many parts of the world. Even if you don't actually share a bed with your child, you may choose to sleep in close proximity, with your child beside your bed in her bassinet or crib so you can easily bring her into your bed to feed or to be soothed when she wakes in the night. The American Academy of Pediatrics recommends a separate but close sleeping environment. Other medical experts feel that babies should be placed in their own rooms as soon as they come home from the hospital. This is a personal decision, and you may want to discuss it with your doctor.

Risks and benefits

Bed-sharing has been shown to encourage and sustain breast-feeding, likely because it is less disturbing to a mother's sleep to nurse her baby in bed. However, studies have shown that bed-sharing, as practiced in North America and other developed countries, is more hazardous to your baby than sleeping in a separate crib or bassinet because there's a chance that adults will roll over and suffocate their babies.

One solution recommended by the American Academy of Pediatrics is to have an approved crib or bassinet in the parents' room, beside the parents' bed, for the first

Did You Know?

Sudden infant death syndrome (SIDS)

SIDS is defined as the sudden and unexpected death of an apparently healthy baby in the first year of life. As you may surmise from the "sudden and unexpected" part of the definition, this tragedy is not well understood. We don't really know the true cause, or causes, of SIDS. However, we do know that the risk reaches a peak at 2 to 3 months of age, and that 95% of cases occur in the first 6 months. While we aren't sure about the cause, there are a number of things that parents can try to do to minimize the risk.

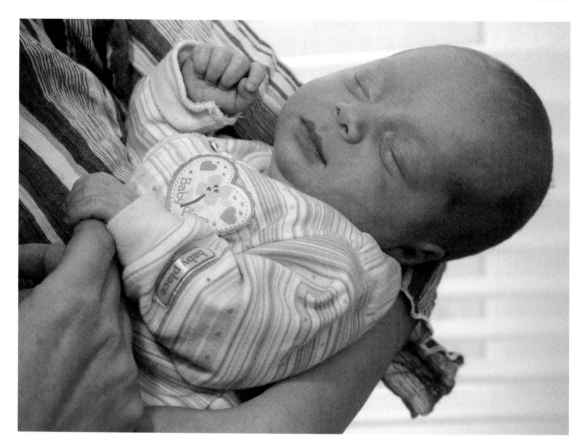

few months of life. This can facilitate breast-feeding and encourage close proximity to your baby while removing the potential risks of SIDS.

Other issues to consider include bed-sharing's effect on you and your partner, including the potential disruption of your sleep and your relationship.

Babies who co-sleep tend to breast-feed frequently during the night. When you decide to move your baby to her own crib, you may need to eliminate nighttime feeds and teach her new sleep associations. The transition from bed-sharing to sleeping in a crib is easiest on a relatively young baby (under 8 months).

Guide to

Bed-sharing safely with your baby
- Don't drink alcohol or use drugs or medications that increase fatigue.
- Don't smoke.
- Make sure your bedding (pillows and blankets) is not in the baby's sleep area.
- Never co-sleep in an unsafe environment, such as on a couch or waterbed or in an area where your baby could get trapped between the mattress and the wall.

HOW TO
Reduce the risk of SIDS

- **Place infants on their backs.** Babies should be placed to sleep on their backs until they are old enough to roll over from the back to the tummy. Avoid products developed to maintain sleep position, such as foam positioning rolls or wedges.

- **Place infants on a firm sleeping surface without pillows, quilts, comforters, loose bedding, stuffed animals, or toys.** Although they're not recommended, if bumper pads are used, they should be thin, firm, and well secured. If blankets are used, they should be thin, they should have holes, and they should be tucked into the mattress so that they cannot cover the baby's head. Instead of a blanket, you can use sleep clothing, such as a sack designed to keep the infant warm without covering her head.

- **Avoid bed-sharing.** The risks associated with bed-sharing are increased when a parent is a smoker, is under the influence of drugs or alcohol, or is extremely sleep deprived (which, unfortunately, may be the case for many new parents).

- **Prevent your baby from overheating.** Your infant should be clothed for sleep as you are, with one or two layers of light clothing.

- **Don't smoke.** Smoke in the baby's environment is a risk factor for SIDS, and is harmful for other reasons (including asthma). Even if you do not smoke in the home, smoke particles cling to your clothing and hair.

- **Consider using a pacifier.** Recent studies have shown that pacifiers may decrease the risk of SIDS, though it is not clear how (one potential explanation is increased arousal in babies accustomed to sucking while falling asleep). However, some experts believe that pacifier use may interfere with breast-feeding; they therefore suggest that pacifiers be used when putting the baby to sleep only after the first month of life. Pacifiers have also been shown to slightly increase the risk of ear infections in children, although these risks are low in babies under 1 year. The American Academy of Pediatrics suggests that a pacifier can be used when placing an infant to sleep for naps and at night, but should not be used if the infant does not want to take it and should not be replaced once the infant falls asleep. Pacifiers should not be coated with sweet solutions and should be cleaned and replaced regularly.

- **Avoid home monitors.** Electronic monitors that measure your baby's movement, breathing, or heart rate, or sounds in your baby's room, do not help reduce the risk of SIDS and may create a false sense of security.

- **Continue breast-feeding.** Babies who are breast-fed have a lower risk of SIDS. Again, this relationship is not well understood.

Positional plagiocephaly (flat head)

As a result of the successful campaign to encourage parents to put their babies to sleep on their backs to decrease the risk of SIDS, infants now have an increased incidence of positional plagiocephaly, or flat head (which sounds serious but generally isn't).

If a baby spends most of her time on her back and prefers to look toward the left (for example, at a toy), then after a while the pressure of the firm mattress will cause the left side of her fairly soft, malleable skull to become somewhat flattened. The flattening often becomes visible around 3 to 4 months of age.

No baby's head is perfectly round, but if you notice a big difference between one side and the other, see your doctor. There is no real danger of abnormal brain growth or development, but in some severe cases, your baby may need to wear a helmet that protects the skull and allows it to mold into a more rounded shape.

Tummy time

You can prevent positional plagiocephaly by encouraging your baby to spend time on her tummy while she is awake. Tummy time will also encourage good head control and upper body and shoulder strength. Many babies don't like tummy time at first because they are used to being on their back. Start by placing your baby on her tummy for 3 to 5 minutes at a time, several times a day, and gradually increase tummy time to at least 30 minutes a day. Try placing a brightly colored toy or a mirror in front of her to provide stimulation. Turn her head to face a different direction and rotate her body toward outside activity, such as the door.

Head Postion

Other ways to prevent flat head include holding your baby in an upright position as much as possible and limiting her time on her back when she's awake. Try changing her sleeping position each week.

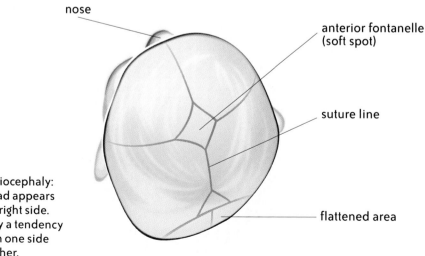

nose

anterior fontanelle
(soft spot)

suture line

flattened area

■ Positional plagiocephaly: Note that the head appears flattened on the right side. This is created by a tendency to prefer lying on one side more than the other.

Treating common sleep problems

There are two main types of sleep problems: those associated with difficulty getting to sleep (dyssomnias); and those that happen during sleep (parasomnias). Some examples of dyssomnias in young children are inappropriate sleep associations, frequent feeding through the night, and early wakenings. Parasomnias are defined as unusual behaviors while sleeping. In infants, these include rhythmic movements, such as head banging. As babies grow into toddlers, other common parasomnias include nightmares and night terrors.

Inappropriate sleep associations

Babies often develop sleep associations, or "props," to help them fall asleep. Parents are often the source of these associations. For example, if your baby always falls asleep while feeding, while listening to background music, or while her back is being rubbed, she might expect those conditions to be present each time she falls asleep. This may not be an issue at bedtime or naptime, but it becomes a *big* problem during the night, at the end of each sleep cycle, when she rouses and needs her prop to fall asleep again. Recall that babies can have arousals about every 60 minutes in the first few months of life. You won't be there to feed her, sing to her, or rub her back every 60 minutes.

Other sleep associations that may become problematic include excessive rocking, needing to be driven in a car to fall asleep, needing to be breast- or bottle-fed to fall asleep, and falling asleep with the television on. Your baby may fall asleep peacefully under these conditions, but each time she experiences a normal arousal during the night and these conditions are not present, she will likely awaken and be unable to fall back asleep.

A baby with inappropriate sleep associations can awaken seven to eight times a night, leading to disrupted sleep for both the baby and her parents. Ensuring continuous sleep for everyone is important.

Did You Know?

Appropriate sleep associations

Some appropriate sleep associations in infants include falling asleep in the same room and crib each night and falling asleep in a dark, quiet room. These conditions will be present while your baby is falling asleep and throughout the night when she experiences her normal arousals.

HOW TO
Improve sleep associations

Solving your baby's inappropriate sleep associations is not easy. She has likely developed these habits over a relatively long period of time, and it will take some time and effort to improve them.

Before embarking on a treatment plan, you and your partner need to agree that a sleep problem exists. Next, you will need to agree on the treatment approach. Making changes in your infant's behavior requires commitment, consistency, and fortitude. You and your partner, and all other caregivers, will need each other's support during the process.

You will need to choose a starting time. Some sleep experts suggest starting this process during a daytime nap (or on the weekend if you are not the caregiver during the daytime) because you may have more energy at this time of day. Other parents prefer to start this approach at the time they feel it is most important — during the night. This is a personal decision.

The goal is to have your infant fall asleep on her own by teaching her appropriate sleep associations and removing inappropriate associations. Once she knows how to fall asleep on her own, her awakenings during the night will not become full awakenings. She will learn to soothe herself back to sleep during the night.

Develop appropriate sleep associations

1. Establish a bedtime routine. This should include gently talking to, holding, and cuddling your baby, but she should not be asleep when she is placed in her crib.

2. Put your baby into her crib while she is drowsy but awake.

3. Ensure that your baby falls asleep in a consistently comfortable, quiet, and dark environment. Put her to sleep in the same room, in the same crib, and in the same manner each night.

Remove inappropriate sleep associations

1. If you have not already done so, wean your baby off her nighttime feeds (see page 250). She may be taking in a substantial amount of her daily fluid needs during the night. If she feeds before sleep, try to change her routine so that she feeds after she awakens. By slowly stopping her night feeds, she will learn to take in her feeds during the day and not awaken hungry at night.

2. If your baby has multiple sleep associations, remove these associations gradually, one at a time, day by day. For example, if your sleep routine is to walk your baby up and down the stairs, singing and rocking her to sleep, stop walking up and down the stairs for the first 2 to 3 nights. The next 2 to 3 nights, stop rocking her. Finally, for the last 2 to 3 nights, stop singing to her. It is perfectly appropriate to continue to rock and sing as part of your bedtime routine — just ensure that your baby is not falling asleep during these activities. Ultimately, you will put her into her bed while she is sleepy but awake.

Graduated extinction

After inappropriate sleep associations are successfully removed, some babies learn to fall asleep on their own, but others need further guidance in the form of a behavioral therapy called graduated extinction. Don't worry — it has nothing to do with dinosaurs or other threatened species. Extinction is a method of correcting sleep associations and encouraging self-soothing for sleep. Studies have shown this method to be effective in young infants, without any long-term negative side effects.

This approach is recommended for babies at least 4 to 6 months of age. The goal of this process is to slowly increase the amount of time you leave your baby in her crib to fall asleep, to teach her how to soothe herself to sleep.

1. First, decide on the amount of time you will initially leave your baby in her crib — that is, how long do you think you can stand to hear her cry? There is no magic number; some parents feel comfortable starting with 2 minutes, while others are happy to go 5 minutes. The important thing is to be consistent.

For example, on Day 1, after you place your baby in her crib while she is sleepy but awake, she may be upset and start to cry. If your starting time is 2 minutes, leave the room (out of sight of your baby) and wait for 2 minutes of significant crying before checking on her. If she is still crying after 2 minutes (likely she will be), spend 1 to 2 minutes in her room, speaking to her in a calm, gentle voice, place her lying down if she is standing up in her crib, and say a gentle and firm good night before leaving the room.

2. Now leave her for 4 minutes. If she is still crying after 4 minutes (which will feel like a lifetime), enter her room again and check on her.

3. Next, increase your waiting time to 6 minutes, and then to 8 minutes before checking on her. Repeat each 8-minute interval until she is asleep.

4. On Day 2, start by waiting for 4 minutes, then increase how long you wait by 2 minutes each time until a maximum time of 10 minutes is reached.

For the first several nights this process could go on for up to 2 hours!

Repeat the process for up to 7 days. By then, even the most strong-willed baby will get the message and fall asleep on her own.

When you check on your baby, do not inadvertently introduce new sleep associations; do not feed, hold, or rock her. The interaction should be short and reassuring. Speak to her in a soft voice, place her lying down if she is standing, and say a gentle good night. An example of what to say is, "Mommy and Daddy love you, and it is time to go to bed. Good night." Ensure that she does not hear or see you once you have left her room.

This routine should be repeated for all naps and bedtimes. Be consistent. All caregivers should use the same approach, both during the day and at night.

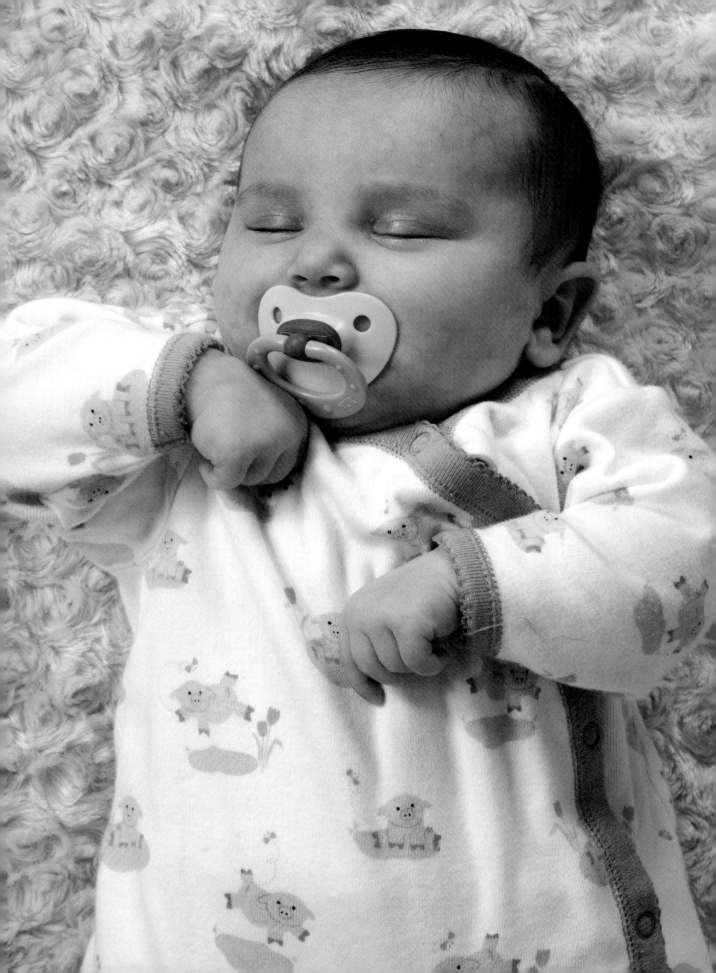

Consistent approach

Even after you have successfully taught your baby to soothe herself to sleep, she may still have nights when she needs you from time to time (for example, if she is not feeling well or is cutting a new tooth). Attend to her so she knows you are there, then resume the schedule.

Graduated extinction and removing sleep associations are very effective approaches to improving sleep problems; however, as with all other behaviors in children, the solutions require practice. It is common for babies to seemingly forget all their good sleep routines and practices as soon as their schedule is altered, such as when you are on vacation.

Try to stick to a consistent routine, even when you're traveling. If this is not possible, resume the steps to remove inappropriate sleep associations and institute graduated extinction when you return home. Once your baby has learned an approach, she is usually quick to pick it up again.

Frequent nighttime feeding

Babies with frequent feeding through the night often have sleep-onset associations; that is, they associate falling asleep with feeding and need to feed to put themselves back to sleep. For a variety of social or cultural reasons, parents themselves may differ in their expectations of their infant's sleep patterns. These expectations may also change as the infant gets older. For example, some parents may not mind that their 6-month-old continues to wake to feed two to three times per night; however, by 9 months of age, the parents and child

may be exhausted, and these frequent awakenings may be considered a problem.

This sleep problem usually occurs after 6 months of age and can affect babies who are bottle-fed or breast-fed. Some babies become accustomed to falling asleep while feeding, and then wake up frequently at night, requiring a feed to fall back asleep. They often fall asleep easily with feeds, but wake up during the night appearing hungry, and crying until they are fed. They may have excessively wet diapers during the night, leading to more wakenings and, subsequently, more feedings. Babies with this dyssomnia may feed three to nine times during the night.

By changing this pattern of frequent feeding early on, you can help your baby and yourself get a more restful, continuous sleep at night. The first step in solving this problem is to reduce the number of times the baby is feeding during the night. Once these feeds are decreased and the baby has learned to take in her nutritional needs during the day, she can learn how to fall asleep without feeding.

Sleep-stretching techniques

There are other techniques that can be used *from birth* to help your baby sleep for longer stretches at night. Their effectiveness will vary from baby to baby.

Focal feed

Introduce a "focal feed," offered to the newborn each night between 10:00 p.m. and 12:00 a.m. Babies offered such a feed may sleep for longer periods during the night.

HOW TO
Wean your baby from nighttime feedings

Slowly wean your child off wanting the breast or bottle during the night. It is not appropriate to allow her to feel hungry at night. Once your baby is accustomed to longer stretches without feeds at night, she will feed more during the day to make up for the caloric intake missed at night. This process can be challenging and may at first lead to more sleep disturbances. However, over a 2-week period, you should be able to change your baby's feeding habits and be well on your way to changing her sleep patterns as well.

This approach can be introduced at 6 months of age. Like any other behavioral treatment, make sure your partner knows and agrees with the plan; you will need to be consistent, and you will need to support each other for this to work. If your baby has difficulty with weight gain or growth, consult your doctor for advice before you change her feeding schedule.

Weaning your baby

1. Establish a bedtime routine.

2. Determine how much feeding your baby does during the night. For 2 to 3 nights, keep a diary of each night awakening and feeding. If you are breast-feeding, record how many minutes your baby feeds on each breast for each feed. If you are bottle-feeding, record how many ounces or milliliters of formula your baby drinks with each feed at night.

3. Determine the average or typical amount of food your baby takes in overnight. For breast-feeding, calculate the average amount of time your baby feeds per feed, in minutes. Add up all the minutes of breast-feeding and divide that total by the number of feeds for that night. For bottle-fed babies, calculate the average amount of formula or breast milk per feed in ounces or milliliters. Add up all the fluid your baby drinks, and divide that number by the number of feeds that night.

4. Decrease the breast or bottle feeds gradually over a 10-day period. If you are breast-feeding, decrease the length of time per feed by 1 minute each night. For example, if you were breast-feeding on average for 8 minutes per feed, then decrease this to 7 minutes per feed the first night, 6 minutes per feed the second night, and so on until you are not feeding at night. If you are bottle feeding, decrease the amount by $\frac{1}{2}$ ounce (15 mL) each feed per night. For example, if you are feeding 4 ounces (125 mL) each feed, decrease to $3\frac{1}{2}$ ounces (105 mL) each feed for the first night, 3 ounces (90 mL) each feed the second night, and so on until you are no longer feeding at night. Depending on the length of time or amount of feeds your baby is taking, this step should take 7 to 14 days to complete.

5. If you find that your baby is actually waking more often during this period, continue to feed her the same amount of food or for the same amount of time. For example, if she usually wakes four times to feed, but during this period wakes five times, give her the same amount of feed (or feed her for the same amount of time, if breast-feeding) that you have designated for the other four feeds. If you have determined that your baby will nurse for an average of 6 minutes each feed overnight, give her 6 minutes each feed.

6. It may be slightly more difficult for your baby to fall asleep during this process. Help her fall asleep by holding, rocking, or singing to her. Try not to feed her more than the predetermined amount for that night.

7. Be strong. This process may be more exhausting in the short term, but remember, you are providing the guidance your baby needs to have a more restful sleep and consume her required calories during the day.

8. Let your baby drink for longer periods of time or consume a larger amount of formula during the day and at bedtime. This ensures that she will receive the right amount of food, just at a better time.

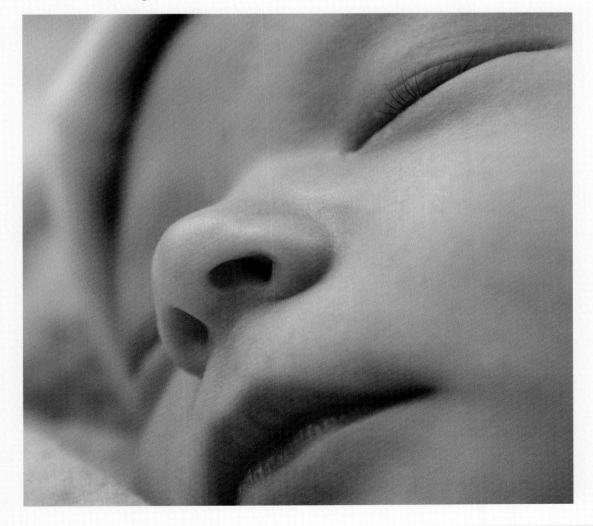

Nighttime cues

Help your baby understand the difference between day and night. A dark, quiet environment should cue a baby that it is night, while a bright, stimulating environment will let the baby know that it is daytime.

Non-feeding activities

Respond to your baby's awakening during the night with a non-feeding activity, such as a diaper change or short walk. This helps to lengthen the time between feeds during the middle of the night. Studies have shown that babies who are treated in this way feed the same amount as other babies, with a longer early morning feed. This approach should only be tried once feeding is established (usually after 4 to 6 weeks).

Scheduling

Before you establish a routine, you should be familiar with what time your baby usually goes to bed, wakes up, and naps. These times should remain consistent, even when your baby is up at night. For example, if she initially spends much of the night awake and crying, she should still be woken at her regular time and be kept awake until her regular naptime. This is sometimes very difficult — do the best you can. It is important to prevent your child from shifting her sleep schedule to sleep much longer during the day because she was awake all night.

Early awakening

Some babies develop very early awakening times, all of a sudden waking up at 5:00 a.m. on a daily basis, bright-eyed and ready to play. This may be your baby's normal sleep-wake pattern, and all efforts to ward off early morning awakenings may be futile. Your baby may have altered her biological clock and circadian rhythms. You may need to learn to cope with this sleep pattern, although in some cases it can be altered with behavioral therapy. Sleep patterns change frequently in the first year of life, and this pattern might too.

Managing early awakening

If early awakening is a problem for your family, you will likely have to go back to the basics on sleep patterns and sleeping environment.

- Ensure that your baby's room is dark and quiet by blocking out the sun and outside noise.
- Record your child's sleep patterns for a 2- to 3-day period. Think about how her sleep patterns might have changed recently. For example, is she going to sleep earlier or taking a late afternoon nap? She may be going to bed too early, or even too late. This may be her way of telling you that she doesn't need a late afternoon nap (if she is still napping twice in the afternoon) or that she doesn't need a morning nap (if she doesn't need both a morning and afternoon nap and her afternoon nap is starting later and later).
- Sometimes, her schedule hasn't changed; she is just waking up early, and then needing an earlier morning nap. For example, if your baby is

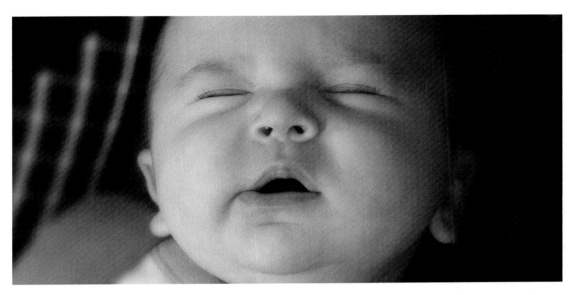

waking up at 5:00 a.m., she may also be napping from 8:00 to 9:00 a.m. In this situation, try to keep her awake until her regular morning nap at 10:00 a.m.

- If her naps seem appropriate, her bedtime may be too early; try moving it 10 minutes later each night for several nights until she begins to awaken later in the morning.
- If all else fails, keep a safe baby toy or book in her crib and encourage her to play alone for a while, to give you an extra few minutes in the morning.

Rhythmic movements

When babies fall asleep, they sometimes develop a soothing repetitive motion, such as rocking their bodies or banging their heads. These movements can be seen as the baby is first falling asleep at night and during the normal frequent arousals overnight. They usually last less than 10 minutes and cause no harm to the baby.

Although these movements may look strange or disturbing to parents, they are soothing and pleasurable to babies. They do not interfere with sleep or development, and they usually resolve during the toddler years.

Managing rhythmic motion disorders

- Make sure the baby is in a safe environment and is unlikely to harm herself during a rocking or head-banging event.
- Don't pay much attention to the problem. If your baby sees you react to the movements, she may increase them.
- If your baby has a chronic medical problem, such as seizures, autism, or developmental delay, seek the advice of your health-care provider.
- If your child displays rhythmic movements during the day while awake, and this is interfering with her ability to play, consult your health-care provider.

Frequently asked questions

As family doctors and pediatricians, we answer many questions from parents. Here are some of the most frequently asked questions. Be sure to ask your health-care providers any other questions that arise. If they don't have the answers, they will refer you to a colleague who does.

Q: I place my baby to sleep on her back, but over the last week I have noticed that she rolls onto her tummy. Should I be rolling her over onto her back again?

A: Placing a baby to sleep on her back has been shown to decrease the risk of sudden infant death syndrome (SIDS). However, once a baby has started to roll over from back to front, there is no advantage to turning her back over. The risk of SIDS is reduced significantly by 6 months of age, likely related in part to a baby's ability to roll herself over and lift her head effectively.

Q: I am worried that my baby may stop breathing overnight. Several friends have suggested that I buy a baby monitor to prevent SIDS.

A: It is normal to have worries about the health of your new baby. Sudden infant death syndrome is a very rare condition that is not fully understood. What we do know is that we can significantly reduce the risk of SIDS by placing babies to sleep on their backs on a firm mattress without pillows or heavy blankets, and by avoiding exposing them to smoke and overheating. Baby monitors that measure movement, sound, breathing, or heart rate have not been shown to reduce the risk of SIDS. They are not recommended because they

increase anxiety in families and usually result in less sleep for both babies and parents due to constant false alarms!

Q: My baby is almost 4 months old and is still waking up at 4:00 a.m. to feed. What can I do to get her to sleep through the night?

A: Don't be discouraged — many parents with a 4-month-old would be happy if they only had to get up once a night to feed him. Sleeping through the night at 4 months of age is considered to be a 5- to 6-hour stretch at one time. Consider trying a focal feed (see page 249) and see if it helps. Also ensure that you are giving your baby a chance to learn how to soothe himself to sleep by putting him to bed while he is drowsy but awake.

Q: My 9-month-old is still waking every 3 hours to feed at night. I think it is just a habit, but my husband feels she needs to be fed at night until she is a year old.

A: Your baby does not physiologically need to be fed at night if she is of a normal weight and height for her age. You can confirm this with your health-care provider. The majority of babies (unless they are underweight or have medical problems) do not need to feed at night

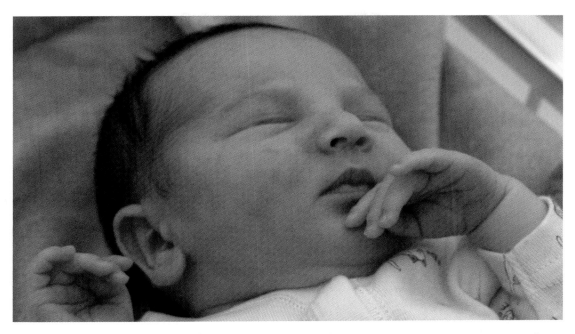

after 5 to 6 months of age. In fact, it is best for your daughter's growth and development if she sleeps through the night so she can benefit from the restorative functions of sleep. As you gradually start to wean her off nighttime feedings, she will start to eat more during the day.

Q: My 7-month-old son has difficulty falling asleep at night. My friend recently told me to play soft classical music to help him. Is this something tried and true?
A: Definitely not! While having your baby listen to Mozart during the day may be beneficial, listening while he falls asleep only creates an inappropriate sleep association that you will need to correct in the future. Your son's sleeping environment and sleep routines may give you clues as to why he is having trouble falling asleep.

Q: Every time we go away on vacation, I regret it. My 11-month-old daughter seems to sleep okay while we are away, but once we return home, she reverts to her old routine, needing me to cuddle her back to sleep four or five times per night. Is this normal?
A: This is very normal. Many parents end up reteaching their children how to fall asleep by themselves once they return from vacation. When families go on vacation, everyone's sleep environment changes, with new bedrooms and beds. Your baby may adjust to sleeping in the same room as you when she was previously used to being in her own room, or, if you are in a hotel, you may not be able to allow her to cry at night. These changes result in poor sleep behaviors once you return from vacation. Reinstitute her sleep routine. With consistency, your daughter will quickly revert back to her good sleep pattern.

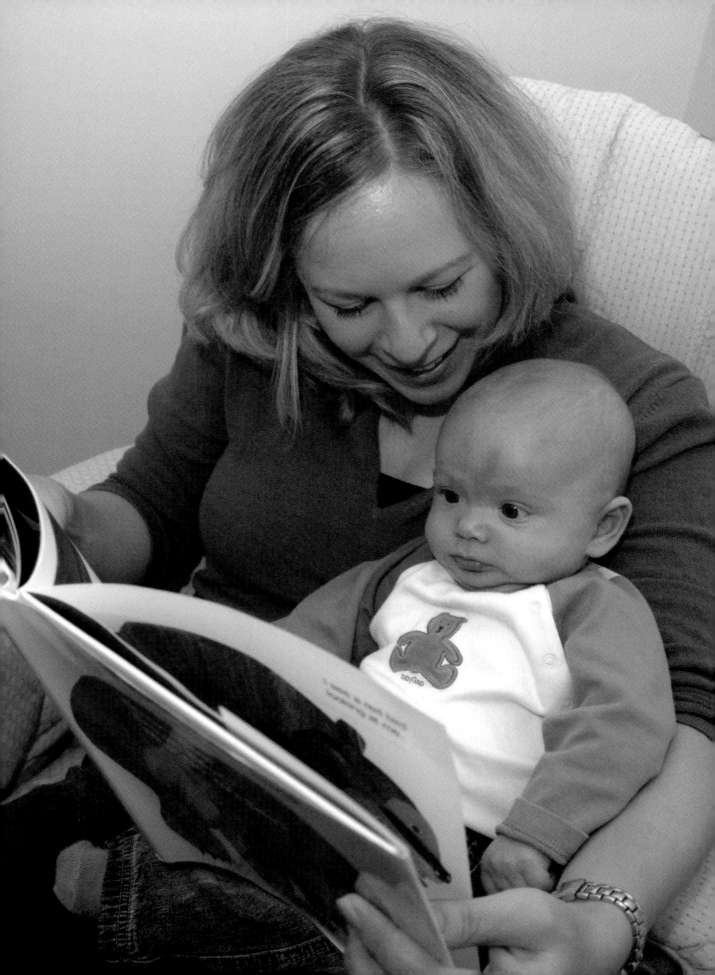

Your Baby's
Months 2 to 6

Establishing a routine

By your baby's second and third months, you are likely becoming more comfortable with your role as a parent and increasingly savvy at interpreting your baby's cues. Some infants of this age will naturally settle into a routine, around which you can begin to plan your day, even doing some things for yourself!

Over the next 3 or 4 months, your hard work in establishing a routine will pay off — not only will you get more sleep, but you'll also get more pleasure from your baby.

Striking a balance

The relative importance of routines largely depends on your own personality. Some parents thrive on structure and are anxious for their baby to have a schedule, while others are happy to live with unpredictable days for a while longer. If you crave structure, but your baby's days remain inconsistent, you can try to implement a consistent routine. If you enjoy a carefree lifestyle, appreciate it for as long as you like, but keep in mind that the older your baby is when you establish a routine, the more difficult it will be to implement.

When establishing a routine, it is best to base it on your baby's cues and natural rhythms. These will differ in each infant; there is no right or wrong schedule. By paying attention to your baby's cues, you will see what pattern he tends to follow. If you use this pattern as a basis for consistency in your care, you will likely find

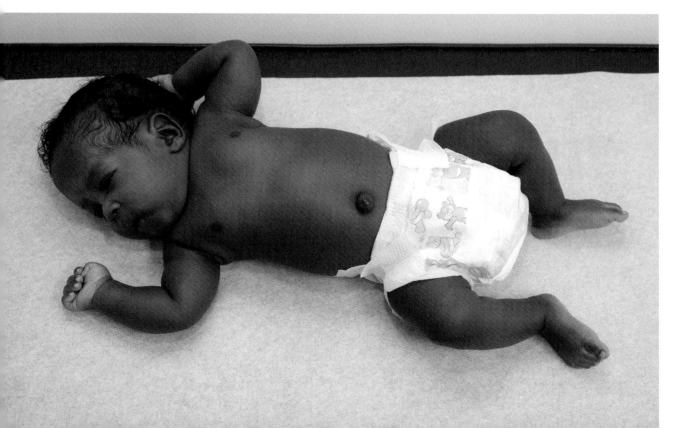

Did You Know?

Cyclical patterns

By necessity, any baby's routine will involve feeding, sleeping, and times when he is awake and alert. These activities will often fall into a cyclical pattern. For example, one desirable routine is sleeping and waking to feed, followed by an alert period before it is time to rest again. The length of such a cycle will initially be dictated by the interval between feedings; usually every 2 to 3 hours at first, and then gradually longer intervals. Your baby's periods of being awake and alert will gradually lengthen and, as he grows, will evolve into times when you can really enjoy interacting together.

Other babies prefer to be playful first, then feed before falling asleep. While this routine is perfectly acceptable, take care to avoid allowing your baby to fall asleep while feeding. It is natural for newborns to become sleepy during feeds, but if this routine becomes habit, your baby will associate the bottle or breast with falling asleep, which might contribute to sleep problems later on.

that, before long, a routine is established. If a routine is important to you, but your baby's activity does not even loosely follow a pattern, it is not unreasonable to create a schedule for him by feeding and allowing him to sleep at similar times each day.

Ultimately, though, his needs — adequate nutrition, rest, and alert time — must come first. Most importantly, continue responding to your baby's needs to aid him in establishing a sense of security and trust.

Bedtime routine

Between 2 and 3 months, many babies begin to sleep for longer stretches at night. You can encourage this desirable habit by initiating a bedtime routine. A consistent bath time and singing a lullaby at bedtime, for example, will help signal to your baby that it's time to say good night. Of course, at this age it is not unusual for babies to still require one or two nighttime feeds, but learning to differentiate night from day is a big step toward a good night's sleep for all.

Resuming your own routine

Once you understand your baby's rhythm, it will become easier for you to do things for yourself. For example, try showering while your baby has his first morning sleep, and time a daily outing to immediately follow a feed, thereby maximizing the time you have before he is hungry again. Most parents find that one activity outside the house a day is plenty; getting out the door with all of your belongings is no longer an easy task, though it's certainly a worthwhile one. Above all, don't forget the importance of getting adequate rest and nutrition!

Be flexible

Establishing a routine may be important, but keep in mind that flexibility is the key. Very few babies will follow a precise schedule at this early stage; instead, they will settle into a pattern. Even then, be prepared for the pattern to change frequently. He may seem sleepy earlier or later, stretch the length of time before he is hungry (or feed more frequently during a growth spurt), and vary his wakeful periods. Your baby is growing and changing quickly, and his needs evolve correspondingly. Follow his cues, allowing his pattern to change naturally. During the next few months, feedings will come to approximate your own meal and snack times, while sleepy periods will become regular naps as your baby naturally transitions to the later stages of infancy.

Medical checkups

By now, you have probably been to visit your baby's doctor a couple of times, likely in the first few days following your discharge from the hospital and again for a 1-month checkup. Your baby will continue to have regular checkups — usually at 2, 4, and 6 months of age. Some doctors schedule routine visits at 3 months as well. Although it may seem like you are at the doctor's office all the time, frequent checks are necessary during these early months because your baby is growing and changing so quickly.

While each health-care provider has a different style, the issues covered during these checkups are pretty much the same. You will be asked how your baby is feeding, sleeping, voiding, and stooling, as well as questions related to his developmental progress. Pediatricians learn very early on that a parent's instincts are usually extremely accurate, even in the case of a first child. So share your observations and any concerns you may have. The physician will see your baby for only a brief time and may not be able to observe that he is not focusing on an object or responding appropriately to noises, even if this is the case. Your answers alone will give your doctor a very good idea of how your baby is progressing.

Your health-care provider will likely ask how the family is coping with your new bundle of joy — and the cause of your sleep deprivation. Be honest about what you are feeling and how you are coping. Your doctor may be able to help you with some advice or practical tips, or, if necessary, refer you to someone who can help if you aren't coping as well as you'd like. In addition to answering your questions, your physician will likely also offer anticipatory guidance about what to expect in the coming months, sometimes including advice about safety or public health concerns. If your baby is due for an immunization, it is usually given at the end of the appointment.

Examining your baby

Your baby will have a full examination at each visit. Depending on his age and temperament, he may not mind being placed on the examining table, but your doctor can do much of the exam with your baby in your lap. Try to dress your baby in something that is easy to slip on and off — you don't want to be concentrating on closing all the snaps when you have important questions to be answered.

Measuring your baby again

Your baby's weight, without even a diaper on, will be taken on an infant scale, and his length and head circumference measured. All three measurements will be plotted on a growth chart, which is kept in your infant's medical record. While some babies are naturally big and

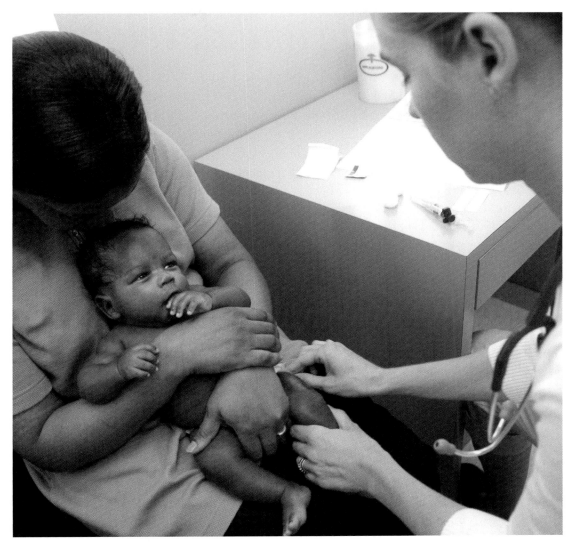

others small, this chart will allow your doctor to ensure that your baby is growing at an appropriate rate.

Booking appointments

To ensure that you keep up to date, ask your health-care provider at the end of each visit when she would like to see your baby next, and make an appointment on your way out. Some offices have specific times set aside in which to see "well babies." Take advantage of this to minimize the likelihood of exposing your young baby to illnesses while you're sitting in the waiting room. If possible, schedule the visit for early in the day; your waiting time will usually be shorter. Bring a list of questions with you to make the most of your time with the doctor. Make sure you know whom to call after hours and what you should do if you have questions before your next scheduled appointment.

Still growing and developing

Your baby's growth will be measured and plotted on a growth curve by your health-care provider at least three times during the first 6 months (2 months, 4 months, and 6 months are the most common times), and more frequently if there have been concerns.

Growth curves, 2 to 6 months

Your doctor will continue to watch to ensure that your baby is growing at the expected rate and following one of the curves in the growth charts. Remember that growth can and does occur in spurts, so weight gain measured on a day-to-day basis is not as helpful as the progression over weeks and months.

Weight

By 2 months of age, an average North American baby weighs between 8.5 and 14 pounds (4 and 6.5 kg) and measures 21 to 25 inches (54 to 63 cm). Gains in weight continue at an average of 0.5 to 1 ounce (15 to 30 g) per day, slowing slightly toward the end of the first 6 months. By 6 months, your baby has likely doubled in weight since he was born!

Height

Gains in height also continue, though at a slightly slower rate. By 6 months, an average baby measures between 24.5 and 28.5 inches (62 and 72 cm).

Head circumference

Rapid brain growth continues, as demonstrated by your baby's head growth, which increases on average 0.5 inch (1 cm) every 2 weeks for the first 3 months and 0.5 inch (1 cm) every month between 3 and 6 months.

Development milestones, 2 to 3 months

As the second and third months progress, your baby gradually becomes stronger.

Head control

You will notice that he is gaining some control of his head. When you hold him against your shoulder or place him on his tummy, he will start to raise his head on his own and move it from side to side. However, if you pull him up to a sitting position, his back will remain rounded and his head will lag behind — he is not yet strong enough to support it completely.

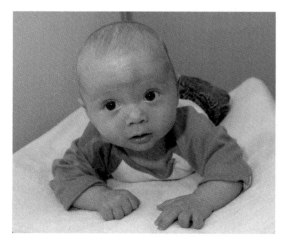

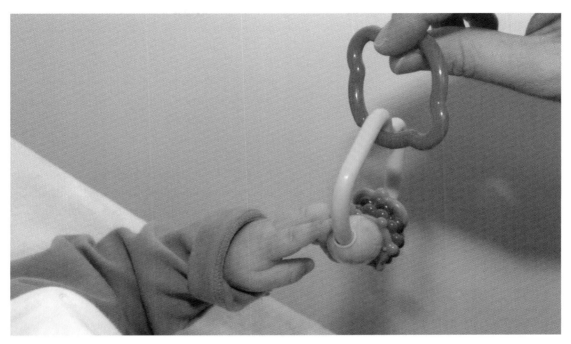

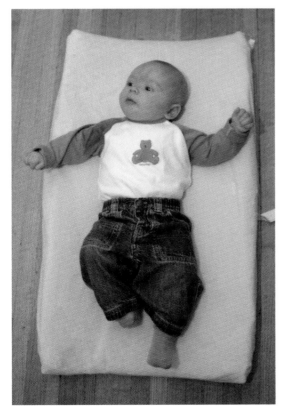

Leg kicking

As your baby gains strength and control, he will kick his legs more. Be careful not to leave him unattended where he could fall.

Holding objects

Although your baby's hands are held open more frequently now, he is not yet ready to hold objects. A block or rattle placed in his hand will fall right out again. He is also not quite ready to reach out for objects — don't worry, these skills will be coming soon.

Alertness

Throughout these months, your baby is becoming more alert. He will turn his head to follow your face or an interesting object, will quiet briefly when you speak softly to him, and will turn to look toward a noise. When picked up or stimulated, he will respond with smiles and excited movements.

Development milestones, 4 to 6 months

This is a period of rapid motor development. Your baby may now start to become more mobile! Most babies of this age are able to roll over independently; near the end of this period, a few may even start to crawl.

Head control

By 4 months, head control has usually become established. When pulled up to a sitting position from lying on his back, your baby will support his own head. An infant is now able to lift his shoulders and head when lying on his tummy. As he gets stronger, he will be able to support his weight on his outstretched arms and, eventually, on his hands and knees. By 5 months, many infants are able to sit briefly if supported, and by 6 to 7 months most babies are able to sit up alone for short periods.

Reaching and holding

By 4 months of age, babies start to reach for and hold interesting objects. You can help your baby's development in this area by placing him on his back with interesting toys for him to reach toward. You can also

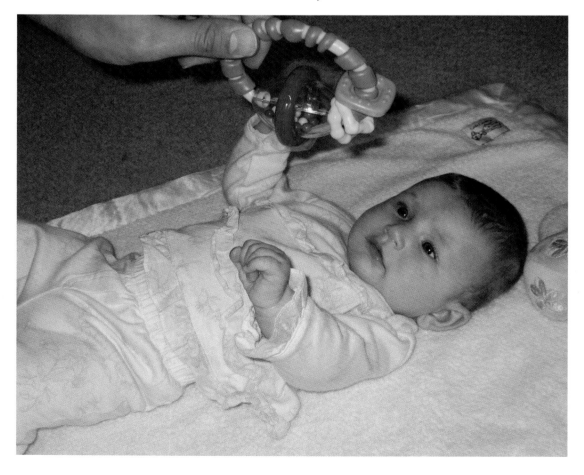

try using an infant chair or "exersaucer" with a variety of different-shaped and -colored objects for him to reach for, touch, and manipulate.

As your baby gains practice and dexterity, typically by 6 months, he will be able to transfer objects from one hand to the other. All objects seem to find their way eventually into his mouth, so beware of small ones he could choke on or swallow, or anything that has small appendages that are not tightly fastened, such as the noses and eyes on teddy bears.

Conversation

Just as his motor skills are taking off, you will also notice a change in your baby's sounds. By 4 months, your baby will probably have a "conversation" with you; that is, if you imitate his sounds, he will answer back with another sound. He is learning that sounds have meaning!

By 6 months, these sounds will change from cooing vowel-based sounds to babbling sounds that include vowels and consonants, such as "dadadada" or "lalalala." Your delighted response and imitation of these sounds will encourage his language development.

Object permanence

At this age, your baby will enjoy looking at and manipulating toys — and putting them in his mouth! — but he probably has not yet developed "object permanence," the recognition that an object no longer directly in view still exists. So, if he drops a toy, he won't yet look to see where it went.

Stranger anxiety

Infants of this age begin to discriminate between parents and strangers and may seem wary of adults they don't know well. This is known as stranger anxiety. Don't worry, it's normal — though Grandpa may get upset when your baby cries at the sight of him.

Did You Know?

Percentile concerns

Some parents become concerned if their baby is slimmer or smaller than average — if, for example, his weight plots on the 10th percentile, while his height is on the 25th percentile. No parent wants to hear that anything about their child is average (50th percentile), and especially not below average (less than the 50th percentile).

If your child is feeding well and seems healthy, you likely have nothing to worry about. Some babies are born small and take a bit of time to catch up. If both you and your partner are small or slim, your child will likely continue to grow along this course.

What is important is that the progress of his height and weight are routinely recorded at every visit to your health-care provider. If he appears to be falling below his expected growth curve, a review of his nutritional intake and general health can be performed.

Temper, temper

Generally speaking, parenting just doesn't get much better than when your baby is 4 to 6 months old. Earlier in infancy, most of a baby's activities are somewhat reflexive, governed by the more primitive parts of the brain. Babies at this early stage tend to behave in a generic fashion: they sleep, they cry, they feed, and, occasionally, they smile. At this earlier stage, most new parents are just beginning to hone their child-rearing techniques. Parenting may feel a little overwhelming, and at times they may find it almost surreal.

At 4 months of age, however, individual personality and temperament start to rapidly emerge. Babies at this stage become very interested in the world around them, and particularly in the people who hold and feed and smile at them. Parents, with their improving skills and growing confidence, find this period easier, and even fun.

Temperament

When it comes to having babies, parents generally must take what they are given. It's not like buying a new car — you can't choose the make and model that best suits you. An individual's temperament is largely determined very early in life; temperament may even be innate. "Temperament" refers to how individuals naturally respond to people and situations. By 4 to 6 months of age, a baby's behavioral patterns have definitely begun to emerge. How parents react to their baby's temperament is critical, not just for this period but for a lifetime of parenting.

Easy and difficult children
The elements of temperament often occur in recognizable patterns. Some infants can be labeled "easy children." Their temperament allows them to adapt easily to most situations; they quickly fall into recognizable routines that simplify their care; and they usually seem happy. Such infants are a joy to parent.

Not every father and mother is so lucky. At the other end of the spectrum lies the "difficult child." These babies are intense; they dislike change; they have trouble establishing routines; they cry easily and are hard to settle; and they often seem negative about everything.

A third pattern is the "slow to warm up child," who is initially apprehensive and tense in new situations but, when given a chance to adapt, usually does so.

Elements of temperament
The landmark research of Thomas and Chess described nine elements that constitute a child's temperament:

- **Activity level.** Some babies seem to lie placidly most of the time. Others seem to be constantly in motion, their arms and legs usually moving one way or another.

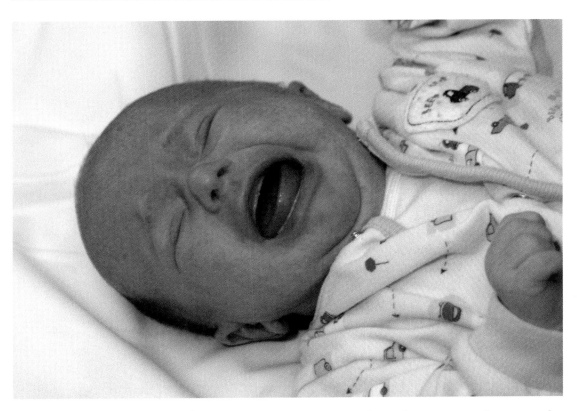

- **Distractibility.** Some infants can tune in to the task at hand and more or less ignore distractions. Others are easily distracted by a different activity.
- **Intensity.** Some babies react much more strongly to a stimulus. For example, if they are upset or frightened, their cries seem louder and more shrill, and they persist for an unduly long period of time. It can be real work to settle these babies.
- **Regularity.** Some babies establish routines for sleeping and feeding quite readily. You can tell without too much effort when they are likely to nap, nurse, and even fill their diapers. Others seem to have no predictable schedule at all.
- **Sensory threshold.** Some babies respond much more strongly to sound, sight, and taste than others.
- **Reaction to new situations.** Some babies appear apprehensive in the presence of strangers or when placed in a new situation. Others seem relaxed in a strange environment, behaving like born politicians.
- **Adaptability.** Some children readily adjust to change and transitions; others don't.
- **Persistence.** Some children are able to stay focused and persevere with the task at hand more than others.
- **Mood.** Some infants seem serious, very negative, and dour. Others are constantly smiling and babbling contentedly. Most babies are somewhere in between these extremes.

HOW TO
Parent the difficult child

Clearly, parenting an "easy baby" is less exhausting and less frustrating than caring for a "difficult child." You did not choose your baby's temperament, but you must learn to deal with it. Here are some helpful tips:

- **Remember, it's not your fault.** Temperament is innate: you did nothing wrong. You are not a worse or better parent than the mother of that smiling baby sitting next to you in your parenting group.

- **Be consistent.** Try to identify his behavior patterns and routines, to the extent that they exist, then try to solidify these routines with consistency.

- **Take a break.** No executive in human resources would ever design a job that went on 24 hours a day, 7 days a week. Parenting is also a job, so make sure you recharge your batteries. Schedule time for yourself each day. A fitness class, a coffee date with a friend — anything will do.

- **Get out.** Taking the baby for a walk with another new mother is a lot more enjoyable than going alone. Enroll in parenting groups or infant gym classes for your sake as well as the baby's.

- **Share the load.** Chances are that Grandma would love to get a little more involved with the baby. Let her! And once your spouse unwinds from a busy day at work, he will probably relish a little one-on-one time with his baby.

- **Cherish the good moments.** Somewhere in your memory bank, store the fact that the intense, determined infant often grows up to be the most successful adult.

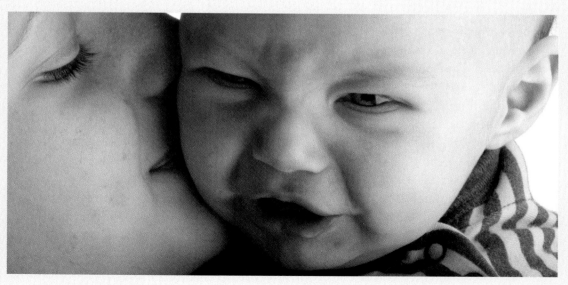

All about vaccinations

An important part of well-baby visits in the first year is immunizations. With the advent of vaccines over the past 50 years, infectious diseases that previously caused sickness and death in many children are now rarely seen. Unfortunately, these illnesses have not been eradicated entirely, so unprotected children and adults remain vulnerable to them. Ensuring that your baby receives his vaccinations is one of the best preventive health measures you can provide.

Administration

Immunizations are usually reserved for the end of your doctor's visit, and may be given by either the physician or the nurse. Until babies are walking, the shots are administered in the big muscle of their upper leg. Following his physical exam, get your baby partially dressed, with his leg exposed, and hold him in a sitting position on your lap. Your doctor or nurse will hold his leg, clean the site with an alcohol swab, quickly administer the injection, and cover it with a Band-Aid.

Many schedules require that two or more shots be given at the same visit. They are administered at different sites (one in each leg, for example), and this is a perfectly safe practice. If your child has a cold, it is usually okay to go ahead with the immunization, though vaccines are usually deferred if a child has a fever or is very unwell.

Immunization cards

The specific immunization schedule varies between countries and provinces or states, but in developed nations, the same coverage and protection is achieved. Your physician or nurse will give you an immunization card that records your baby's vaccinations. Bring it with you to subsequent doctor's visits so you can keep track of your baby's shots. In the future, you will likely need to show it to child-care facilities such as daycares, schools, and camps. It is also important to take it with you if you are seeking health care from anyone other than your regular doctor, for example, the emergency room of your local hospital.

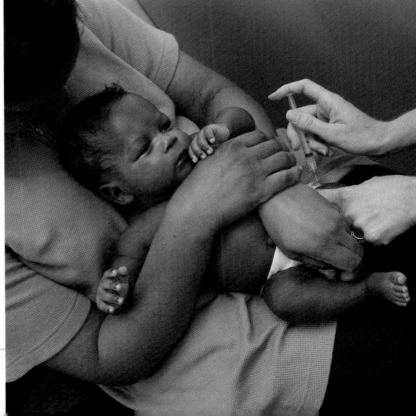

Vaccinations

Because immunization schedules vary among jurisdictions and can be difficult to interpret, be sure to discuss your baby's vaccination program with your health-care provider soon after your baby is born. If you plan to travel with your baby, particularly to developing countries, other vaccinations may be required in addition to the routine series.

DTaP vaccine

DTaP is the abbreviation used for a vaccine that immunizes your baby against diphtheria, tetanus, and acellular pertussis.

- **Diphtheria** is caused by bacteria, resulting primarily in difficulty breathing, in addition to heart and nerve problems. Babies who get diphtheria have a significant chance of dying from it.
- **Tetanus (lockjaw)** occurs when the tetanus bacterium, found in soil, gets into an open cut in the skin. Painful muscular spasms occur, the muscles that affect breathing may be affected, and long-term neurologic problems may result. Thankfully, immunization and proper hygiene practices have made tetanus very uncommon in developed nations.
- **Pertussis (whooping cough)** is caused by bacteria that enter the lungs and cause a severe cough. Pertussis remains relatively common. Many adults lose their immunity to it over time and can develop pertussis in the subtle form of a persistent cough; they can then pass the germ on to their

baby. Young babies with pertussis may become critically ill and can even die from the disease when their cough becomes so severe that they have trouble breathing. In older children, the cough can last up to 3 months.

IPV vaccine

The inactivated polio virus (IPV) vaccine will protect your baby from the polio virus. Many people infected with polio have very few symptoms, while others experience fever, headache, vomiting, muscle pain, and weakness. Some children even develop permanent paralysis. In years gone by, entire hospital wards were filled with children afflicted with polio who needed an "iron lung" respirator in order to breathe.

Hib (Haemophilus influenzae type B) vaccine

This vaccine immunizes against *Haemophilus influenzae* type B, a bacterium associated with many childhood infections. Most importantly, Hib was previously one of the most common causes of meningitis, a potentially devastating infection of the brain and spinal cord. Since the vaccine was developed in the early 1990s, Hib is very rarely seen as a cause of such serious infections.

5-in-1 vaccine

In Canadian jurisdictions, a "5-in-1" vaccine is available to protect your baby from five diseases: diphtheria, tetanus, pertussis, polio, and Hib. It is given at approximately 2, 4, and 6 months of age, and again at 18 months. In the United States, DTaP, IPV, and Hib are given at similar intervals, but in separate injections.

Pneumococcal conjugate vaccine

This vaccine will protect your baby from *Streptococcus pneumoniae*, a common bacterium that causes meningitis, blood infections, pneumonia, and ear infections. These illnesses affect an enormous number of children, and, despite antibiotics, infections such as meningitis can still cause permanent brain damage or death. While this immunization is recommended for all children under 2 years of age and is increasingly considered routine in developed countries, it is relatively new and may not be covered by all jurisdictions and health plans. Be sure to ask your health-care provider for more information.

Meningococcal C conjugate vaccine

Meningitis gets a lot of press when outbreaks occur in college residences, but babies less than a year old may also be at risk. This vaccine protects against one strain (type C) of meningococcus, a bacterium that causes meningitis and life-threatening blood infections.

However, babies less than a year old are very rarely affected by type C; rather, they contract another strain of the bacterium for which no vaccine is currently available. Many public health agencies thus view multiple immunizations with meningococcal C conjugate vaccine in the first year as not cost-effective.

The Canadian Paediatric Society recommends that babies be immunized with three doses while under 1 year of age. In the United States, this vaccine is

---

Did You Know?

Vaccine safety

Many parents are concerned about the safety of the vaccines themselves. In fact, immunizing your child is extremely safe.

Your baby may experience some redness or soreness at the site where the needle was given, and, depending on the vaccine, a fever or rash is possible, but more serious side effects are exceedingly rare. Once the immediate discomfort of the needle has passed, most babies are not bothered at all. You may give your baby a pain medication, such as acetaminophen, to minimize side effects. If you are breast-feeding your baby, he may be comforted

by nursing soon afterwards.

Children who have had an allergic reaction to a vaccine, involving trouble breathing or severe swelling on the skin or in the mouth, should not be immunized with that vaccine. If your child has immune problems or HIV infection, speak to your health-care provider about specific recommendations.

At one time, there was great concern that the MMR (measles, mumps, and rubella) vaccine was associated with and, in fact, caused autism. However, large studies have proved that such concern is completely unfounded: the MMR vaccine does not cause autism.

not recommended in infancy, but is given at 11 to 12 years of age. Speak to your health-care provider about what is recommended in your area.

MMR vaccine

MMR stands for measles, mumps, and rubella. These three diseases, all caused by viruses, are covered by one vaccine. Two doses are needed — the first at 12 months, and the second at least 1 month later, but usually at the age of 4 to 6 years.

- **Measles (red measles)** causes fever, runny nose, cough, red eyes, and a rash. In some children with measles, the virus affects their brain, leading to serious consequences.
- **Mumps** results in fever, headache, and painful swelling of the mouth's salivary glands. It can also cause meningitis and deafness. In adult men, it may result in sterility.
- **Rubella (German measles)** causes fever, rash, and swollen glands. Pregnant women who contract rubella have a high chance of passing it on to their babies, which can be very serious. Depending on the stage of pregnancy when the fetus is infected with rubella, it can result in blindness, deafness, or heart problems. One out of 10 babies born with rubella will die during their first year of life. When you vaccinate your baby, his immunity against rubella will last for the rest of his life.

   If you are thinking about getting pregnant and did not have the vaccine or the disease when you were a child, speak to your health-care provider about getting it now. This immunization cannot be given once you are pregnant.

Chicken pox (varicella) vaccine

Chicken pox is a common illness caused by the varicella-zoster virus. You might think that chicken pox is no big deal, causing just a fever and an itchy rash. While this is often the case, complications of the infection include scarring, skin and blood infections, pneumonia, and inflammation of the brain. Chicken pox can be severe and even life-threatening in young babies, adults, and those with immune problems. An effective vaccine against chicken pox is now available; one dose is recommended for children older than 1 year. In the United States, a second dose is given at 4 to 6 years of age.

Hepatitis B vaccine

Hepatitis B is a virus that leads to infection of the liver. If a mother carries the virus, it can be transmitted to her baby at birth. Other routes of transmission are from infected blood products, sexual contact with an infected individual, and injection drug use. The hepatitis B vaccine is given in a series of three shots, usually over a 6-month period. Depending on where you live, the vaccine is given beginning either at birth or in early adolescence.

Hepatitis A vaccine

This virus causes an acute, self-limited illness usually associated with fever, nausea, malaise, jaundice, and loss of appetite. Infection is spread from person to person through the fecal-oral route. In the

United States, the hepatitis A vaccine is recommended for all children at 1 year of age (two doses, at least 2 months apart).

Influenza vaccine

Influenza is the virus that causes "the flu," common in the late fall and winter months. The flu can cause serious lung disease, particularly in those at high risk — young children, the elderly, and people with chronic medical conditions such as asthma or diabetes. The flu vaccine is given annually in the fall to those over 6 months of age, but is not mandatory. Speak to your health-care provider about a flu shot for your baby.

Rotavirus vaccine

Rotavirus is the most common cause of gastroenteritis. Approved in the United States by the Food and Drug Administration (FDA) in 2006, this vaccine is recommended by the Advisory Committee on Immunization Practices (ACIP) for universal immunization in infancy, with three doses administered at 2, 4, and 6 months of age.

Recommended immunization schedule for infants

Age at vaccination	DTaP	IPV	Hib	MMR	Var	Hep B	Hep A	Pneu-C	Men-C	Flu	Rota
Birth	●	●	●					●	●		❖
2 months	❖	❖	❖			● 3 doses during infancy or in schools ❖		● ❖	●		❖
4 months	● ❖	● ❖	● ❖					● ❖	●		❖
6 months	● ❖	●	● ❖			❖		● ❖	●	● ❖ 6–59 months, given yearly	❖
12 months	● 18 months ❖ 6–18 months	● 18 months ❖ 12–18 months	● 18 months ❖ 12–15 months	● ❖ 12–18 months	● ❖ 12–18 months	3 doses: birth, 1–2 months, 6–18 months	❖ 12–23 months: 2 doses, 6 months apart	● ❖ 12–15 months	● 12–15 months	6–59 months, given yearly	

DTaP:	Diphtheria, tetanus, acellular pertussis	Hep B:	Hepatitis B vaccine
IPV:	Inactivated polio virus vaccine	Hep A:	Hepatitis A vaccine
Hib:	*Haemophilus influenzae* type B conjugate vaccine	Pneu-C:	Pneumococcal conjugate vaccine
		Men-C:	Meningococcal C conjugate vaccine
MMR:	Measles, mumps, and rubella vaccine	Flu:	Influenza vaccine
Var:	Varicella-zoster virus (chicken pox) vaccine	Rota:	Rotavirus vaccine

❖ Recommended in the United States, as adapted from the Department of Health and Human Services, Centers for Disease Control and Prevention.

● Recommended in Canada, as adapted from the National Advisory Committee on Immunization, Public Health Agency of Canada.

Treating common conditions

Other health conditions that are not exclusive to your baby at this age may arise during these months. For a quick reference to the symptoms and treatment of these conditions, see Part 11, "Caring for Your Sick Baby."

Baby's first cold

Healthy children may have eight to 10 colds a year in the first years of life, and infants who have older siblings or are in daycare may seem to have a permanent cold. Colds are caused by a variety of viruses that are present throughout the year but are more common during the fall and winter months. Nasal congestion, clear

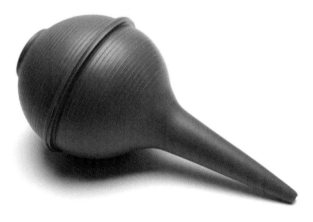

to yellow/green nasal discharge, cough, fever, and mild sore throat are common symptoms. Because infants are nasal breathers and need to breathe through the nose when feeding, those under 3 months may have particular difficulty feeding if dealing with a blocked nose.

Treating colds

Most colds last from a few days to a week and resolve on their own. Salt-water sprays or drops and a bulb-style suction syringe can benefit some young infants if nasal congestion is prominent and is interfering with feeding. Acetaminophen (Tylenol, Tempra) or ibuprofen (Advil, Motrin) can be helpful to treat discomfort and fever, but are not recommended in the first 3 months of life because they might mask a fever, which could be a clue to something more serious. Over-the-counter decongestants, cough suppressants, and antihistamines should not be used — they

Did You Know?

Cold complications

If your infant has any of the following complications from a cold, he should be seen by a health-care provider:

- Rapid or labored breathing

- Listlessness and lack of interest in his surroundings
- Persistent fever lasting more than 48 hours
- Fever (in infants under 3 months)
- Inability to feed or keep fluids down

are ineffective in young children and have the potential for serious side effects. Antibiotics, which treat bacterial infections, have no role in treating a cold.

Diarrhea and vomiting

A self-limited episode of vomiting and diarrhea (that is, an episode that resolves on its own) is common in young children, usually due to viral intestinal infections (gastroenteritis), most prevalent in the winter months. These viruses are hardy (living on tabletops and objects for several days) and very contagious, spreading easily among children in daycare and among family members. Wash your hands carefully after changing your baby's diaper.

Viral intestinal infections can cause fever, vomiting, cramping, loss of appetite, and frequent, watery stools. These symptoms may last several days to a week in most children, although the vomiting and fever usually resolve within 48 hours. While most episodes can be managed simply at home, these infections can be distressing for families (particularly when several individuals are sick at once) and lead to significant time away from school and work, with frequent visits to medical centers and emergency departments.

Treating gastroenteritis

- **Feeding:** Mild episodes of gastroenteritis require no change in diet. Breast-fed infants should continue breast-feeding without restrictions in their diet. The majority of formula-fed infants can continue their usual formula. Temporary use of lactose-free formulas may benefit some infants who have had profuse diarrhea and have significant cramping and rapid diarrhea immediately after drinking their regular formula.

- **Rehydration:** Children who have persistent vomiting or are dehydrated should be offered a commercially prepared oral rehydration solution (Pedialyte or Enfalyte, for example). These are available at most drugstores, and no prescription is required. They do tend to have a slightly salty taste, so picking a flavored variety is a good idea. Other fluids, such as flat pop, juice,

Did You Know?

Diarrhea and vomiting complications

The major risk to children with intestinal infections is dehydration — the loss of water and salts from excessive vomiting or diarrhea. While mild dehydration can be managed at home, more significant dehydration can be dangerous and needs to be treated in a hospital.

Watch for these signs:

- Listlessness and lack of interest in his surroundings
- Failure to wet diapers (urine may be difficult to differentiate from watery diarrhea)
- Dry mouth, without saliva
- Sunken eyes or soft spot (fontanelle)
- Inability to keep fluids down

tea, rice water, and soup, do not have the appropriate mix of water and salt and should not be used to manage dehydration. Rehydration solution should be offered in frequent but small amounts (1 to 3 ounces/30 to 90 mL per hour in infants under 6 months, 3 to 4 ounces/90 to 125 mL per hour in babies 6 to 18 months) if vomiting is present.

- **Medical care:** Children who exhibit signs of complications should be seen by a health-care provider. While small amounts of blood in the stool can infrequently occur, large amounts of blood suggest a bacterial infection; your physician will ask for samples of the stool, and antibiotics may be prescribed.

Undescended testicle

The testes develop inside the abdomen while your baby is inside the womb and normally descend into the scrotum during the last trimester of pregnancy. When a testicle fails to descend into the scrotum, it is called an undescended testicle.

The potential problems with an undescended testicle can include reduced sperm production and infertility; increased risk of testicular cancer; twisting of the testis, causing loss of its blood supply; and the adverse psychological effects of having a half-empty scrotum.

Changes inside the testicle and their adverse effects on sperm development can be seen as early as 6 months of age. The risk of developing a tumor of the testicle is up to 10 times greater in males who have an undescended testis. This risk does not change with bringing the testis down into the scrotum, but it makes examination and detection of any mass easier.

Treating undescended testicles

If an undescended testicle has not come down into the scrotum by about 6 months of age, it is unlikely to spontaneously descend. The testis can usually be brought down into the scrotum with a simple outpatient surgical

---

Did You Know?

Undescended testicle facts

Approximately 30% of premature male infants have a testicle that has not descended into the scrotum, while about 3% of boys born after a full-term pregnancy have an undescended testicle. Most undescended testicles come down into the scrotum over the first several months of life, but about one in 150 boys has a testicle that remains undescended.

This condition must be differentiated from a retractile testicle, which can appear undescended because a reflex causes the testis to pull up from the scrotum, but the testis can be easily manipulated down into the scrotum. This is completely normal.

Most undescended testicles are felt higher up in the groin area. In 10% to 20% of cases, both sides are affected. Rarely, neither testicle can be felt; in this case an ultrasound is done to check for the presence of the testicles in the abdomen.

procedure called orchiopexy, usually performed when the child is between 9 and 15 months of age. Hormonal treatment has been used, but is not generally successful.

Hernias

An inguinal (groin) hernia is seen in about 2% of children, more commonly in boys. About 50% of groin hernias are found before a child's first birthday. Some infants may have a hernia under the belly button area (umbilical hernia).

A groin hernia usually results from a persisting connection between the abdominal cavity and groin area, which usually closes as the baby is developing in the womb. If the connection remains open, contents of the bowel can move into the groin area and cause a lump, which is how a hernia is noticed and brought to a doctor's attention. In male infants, a hernia must be differentiated from a hydrocele, a fluid collection around the testicle that is apparent in the scrotum but does not extend up into the groin. A hernia is usually painless unless the bowel extends into the groin area and becomes stuck.

Treating hernias

Because there is a risk that, over time, the bowel will become stuck in a groin hernia, these types of hernias are repaired by a general surgeon on a non-urgent basis. Most infants and children are operated on and go home from the hospital on the same day. If a hernia seems to be painful, or the area is red or hot, your baby should be seen immediately — the bowel may have become stuck in the groin area.

Umbilical hernias generally close by themselves before your child reaches school age and no treatment is necessary.

umbilical hernia

inguinal hernia

testicle

fluid (hydrocele)

■ (Left) A hernia can present as a swelling in the groin area (inguinal hernia) or at the belly button (umbilical hernia); (Right) Hydrocele: A fluid collection surrounding the testicle.

Eczema (atopic dermatitis)

One of the most common rashes, affecting up to 10% of people, is eczema, which is characterized by patches of red, raised, dry, scaly, and itchy skin. Approximately 60% of people who have eczema develop signs in the first year of life. While eczema resolves by school age in about 50% of infants, 25% of individuals continue to be affected into adulthood. It is more prevalent in individuals with a personal or family history of allergic conditions (asthma, food allergies, and hay fever). In infants, the areas most commonly affected are the face (particularly the cheeks), knees, and outer areas of the arms. The diaper area is typically not involved.

Managing eczema

There are no available treatments that prevent or cure eczema, but there are effective measures to manage the symptoms. Irritants to the skin (harsh soaps, fabric softener, bubble baths) should be avoided, while gentle soaps for infants (such as Baby Dove) and bath moisturizers (such as Aveeno) are helpful. The skin can be kept lubricated with petroleum jelly, which helps to trap moisture in the skin. Your physician will advise you on the use of topical steroid creams or ointments if there are inflamed areas.

Seborrheic dermatitis (cradle cap)

Seborrheic dermatitis is another common rash that usually develops during the first 3 months of age. When the scalp is involved, it is termed cradle cap. Other areas typically affected include the folds in the diaper area and the skin behind the ears.

This rash appears as a scaly yellow eruption with reddened, greasy skin often appearing around or under the scales. The rash is not usually itchy.

Treating seborrheic dermatitis

Cradle cap is usually self-limited and does not require treatment. In fact, baby oils often exacerbate the condition. Anti-sebborheic shampoos can be used for more extensive, cosmetically bothersome, or inflamed scalp eruptions. Used three to four times a week, the shampoo is left on for approximately 5 minutes, followed by gentle combing of the scales. Vigorous removal of the scales should not be attempted. A mild topical steroid medication may also be advised by your physician for areas that are inflamed.

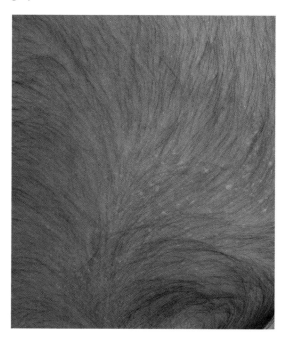

Pertussis (whooping cough)

Whooping cough is a potentially serious infection that can affect people of all ages but is most dangerous to young infants. Whooping cough is usually a dramatic illness that, once seen, is never forgotten. The term "whooping cough" comes from the characteristic "whoop" sound made by a forceful inhalation after a spasm of coughing. Coughing spells from whooping cough characteristically come in fits lasting up to several minutes at a time, often followed by vomiting, whooping, breath-holding, and blue spells. The illness usually starts as a nondescript cold with runny nose and briefer coughing episodes before progressing over several days into the typical whooping pattern. Young babies who become infected with pertussis, however, may not develop a "whooping" pattern but may only exhibit breath-holding and blue spells.

Treating and preventing pertussis

Once whooping cough has developed, there is no effective treatment that shortens the duration or severity of the illness. In some parts of the world, the name for whooping cough is "the 100-day cough," indicating the length of time it takes for the signs of the infection to resolve. The disease must run its course.

Young infants under 6 months are usually hospitalized initially for supportive care, which consists of oxygen, management of mucus and secretions, and help with feeding. Antibiotics are given mainly to prevent the spread of infection to others, not to cure the symptoms.

The most effective treatment for whooping cough is immunization in infancy. Immunization is now also available for adolescents and adults (combined with a tetanus booster) to further reduce the incidence of infections.

Meningitis

There are few words that strike fear in parents more than "meningitis." The term refers to an inflammation of the brain and its lining caused by bacterial or viral infection. Bacterial meningitis, the life-threatening form of this condition, is treated with intravenous antibiotics. Even with timely antibiotic therapy for bacterial meningitis, brain injury can occur, leading to hearing loss, seizures, and visual

Did You Know?

Whooping cough immunization

Prior to immunization, pertussis infections caused many deaths in infancy and can still lead to outbreaks and deaths, even in developed countries with well-established immunization programs. Infants are routinely immunized against pertussis beginning at 2 months of age, but infections still occur because vaccination, while effective, does not provide complete immunity, and a person's immunity diminishes over time. Adolescents and adults who have not had a booster immunization are often sources of pertussis infection.

impairment, as well as physical and mental handicaps. Prevention is the most effective treatment against bacterial meningitis. The recently introduced vaccines are more than 90% effective against several of the most common forms of bacterial meningitis.

Meningitis caused by viral infection is generally much less serious and does not usually lead to significant long-term health problems. Most forms of viral meningitis resolve on their own without any specific therapy, but antibiotic treatment for bacterial infections is often given initially until the results of the spinal fluid analysis are complete.

Heart murmurs

Heart murmurs are sometimes worrisome for parents, but a heart murmur does not mean heart disease. Up to 50% of children may have a heart murmur during childhood, but only a small fraction of these children have heart disease.

The sound of a heart murmur is produced by blood flowing through the chambers and valves of the heart and can be heard using a stethoscope. In newborn infants, whose circulatory system has changed significantly since they were in the womb, a murmur can be heard transiently in the first few days after birth. Other types of murmurs can commonly be heard throughout infancy or childhood. These are called "innocent" or "functional" heart murmurs.

The most common signs that suggest a possible heart problem during infancy are rapid breathing and increased work at breathing, particularly during feeding; excessive sweatiness during feeding; and blueness, noticed best around the mouth. A health-care provider may sometimes be concerned about a heart murmur or other signs that may indicate a heart problem, and will arrange for an electrocardiogram, an x-ray of the chest, or an echocardiogram (an ultrasound picture of the heart). If there is concern about heart disease, an opinion from a cardiologist will be sought.

Did You Know?

Diagnosing meningitis in infants

One reason that meningitis is so frightening is the difficulty, in the early stages, in differentiating it from a self-limited viral infection in young infants. Signs seen in older children and adults, such as a stiff neck, are usually absent in young infants. In babies, the signs and symptoms of meningitis can include fever, poor feeding, lethargy, a mottled skin color, bulging fontanelle (soft spot), and seizures. Some of these signs, however, may be absent or apparent only late in the course of the illness. That is why tests to screen for meningitis are often suggested for infants under 3 months of age with fever. Meningitis is diagnosed by performing a lumbar puncture (spinal tap) and testing the spinal fluid for infection.

Frequently asked questions

As family doctors and pediatricians, we answer many questions from parents. Here are some of the most frequently asked questions. Be sure to ask your health-care providers any other questions that arise. If they don't have the answers, they will refer you to a colleague who does.

Q: Nearly every morning, we discover our 6-month-old baby lying on his tummy. We know he should be sleeping on his back to prevent SIDS. Must we keep getting up during the night to rotate his sleeping position?

A: No, for two reasons. First, getting up night after night will exhaust you, which would probably constitute the greater risk for your baby. Second, a baby who is old enough to roll over by himself is already past the peak age for incidence of SIDS, probably because he is neurologically more mature, and having the ability to roll over appears to be protective against SIDS.

Q: Should we be worried that our baby's weight percentile is less than the percentile for his length?

A: Actual weight loss, when it occurs, is worrisome. But don't be too concerned if your baby is growing steadily along a certain weight percentile, even if it is less than his percentile for length. There's nothing wrong with long and lean; in fact, most adults would probably choose that body build for themselves if they could.

Q: Our breast-fed 5-month-old seems a little chubby. What should we do about it?

A: Nothing. Even though obese children often become fat adults, obese infants — especially those who are breast-fed — don't necessarily become fat children. These infants tend to slim down once they become mobile. Breast-feeding on demand is the preferred form of infant nutrition. Restricting nursing time is seldom a good idea.

Q: Our baby drools all the time. Is this a sign of teething?

A: Teeth get the blame for pretty much everything. Drooling does not equate with teething. Many babies drool a lot. If yours is one, use a bib and, if a rash develops, put some petroleum jelly on the affected area after first cleaning and drying it.

Q: Can I safely fly with a 2- to 6-month-old baby?

A: Yes, but use some common sense:
- Book a non-stop flight when possible.
- Give yourself lots of extra time to get to the airport. You'll need it.
- Change the baby shortly before boarding, then take advantage of early boarding opportunities, if offered.
- To reduce earache, encourage your baby to suck on something during ascent and descent.
- Book an extra seat for the baby: the cost may be worth it by journey's end.

Q: My baby still gets up at night. Will feeding him cereal at bedtime help him sleep through the night?

A: No. Cereals aren't sedatives. Babies sleep through the night when they are ready to do so.

Q: My 6-month-old baby loves to stand and bounce when I support him, but I worry that it will cause bowed legs. Will it?

A: No need for worry. Standing supported at this age is good exercise, not a cause for bowed legs.

Q: Is something wrong if my 5-month-old still isn't rolling over?

A: A baby's developmental milestones are individualized. Some skills will come earlier than usual, while others might appear later. It's the overall developmental pattern to which you should pay attention. Now that babies are placed on their backs to sleep, many seem in no rush to roll over by 4 or 5 months.

Q: Why does my son put everything in his mouth?

A: Infants love to explore the world around them. Often, they use more than sight and sound to do so: they also use the mouth and tongue to explore shape and texture. The real trick lies in ensuring that what goes in his mouth is safe.

Q: Can I "spoil" my baby at this age?

A: Being responsive to your baby is just meeting his needs. At some point, children must learn that the world doesn't revolve around them, but this is not that time.

Q: When my 5-month-old daughter sees her grandfather, she often cries. It is very upsetting for everyone. What can we do?

A: By this age, infants have developed the ability to differentiate caregivers from strangers. They prefer caregivers. Some babies are quite cautious and react poorly even to people who love them. Allow your baby time to warm up to new situations and individuals who don't care for them on a daily basis. Frequent exposure and shared pleasurable moments will ultimately forge positive bonds.

Q: My baby and I love to spend time outside. But sunscreens are not recommended until 6 months, so what can I do to protect him?

A: Keep going out, if that is what you both enjoy; just avoid the peak hours of sun exposure, between 10:00 a.m. and 2:00 p.m. Use clothes and umbrellas that block ultraviolet rays. And if it comes down to a choice between sunburn and sunblock, choose sunblock. Products that contain microparticles of titanium dioxide are unlikely to cause problems, even in young babies.

Q: When should a cup be introduced?

A: There is no rush; wait until your baby can sit supported. Drinking from a cup in the sitting position reduces the risk of choking, compared to drinking while supine (on the back). Babies at 4 to 6 months of age are quite "oral": they love to explore with their mouths. If you are interested in supplementing breast-feedings, it is quite reasonable to introduce a cup at this age.

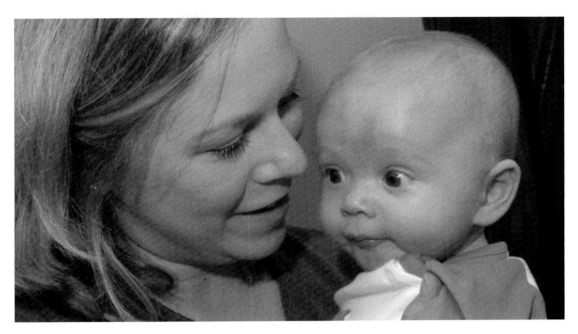

Q: My baby will soon be starting to eat solids. Do I need a high chair?

A: By now, your baby can sit supported, and feeding him in a high chair is appropriate. Of course, high chairs must be safe. The restraint system must fit between the legs to prevent the baby from sliding out, and must fasten securely across the hips. There should be no sharp corners or edges. The high chair should be stable — look for a wide base. Cleaning the chair properly should be easy to do. Comfort should also be a priority. Look for a well-padded seat for the baby and an easily removable feeding tray to make it easy on you. Finally, it is a good idea to purchase a chair that adjusts to a growing baby and folds easily. Once these criteria have been met, it is a matter of taste and budget.

Q: At what age can we use a framed backpack-style baby carrier?

A: Most backpack-style carriers can be used once a baby turns 6 months of age. The baby should have good head control and trunk strength.

Q: My baby's eyes still seem crossed. Is that normal for a 4-month-old?

A: In the first month or two, an infant's gaze may not be coordinated, or "conjugate." By 4 months, though, the eyes should not be turning in. Have your doctor look into the problem.

Q: My 5-month-old still spits up. Will it ever stop?

A: Spitting up, or gastroesophageal reflux, is still normal at this age. You don't need to worry unless your baby repeatedly chokes or wheezes at feeds, is gaining weight very poorly, or seems irritable when swallowing (which suggests that the esophagus is inflamed). In over 90% of infants, gastroesophageal reflux resolves before the first birthday.

Sam's Diary

April 22 (2½ months old)

For 2 nights in a row, you have gone for 7 hours between feeds — what a milestone! You are able to entertain yourself for short periods by looking at your mobile or sucking your thumb. Thanks for being such an amazing little man.

May 9 (3 months old)

Today is your 3-month birthday and Mom's first Mother's Day, and she felt very spoiled! Dad gave Mom a photo frame with a picture of you in it, and you bought Mom a ticket to the ballet. You are taking a bottle beautifully now, so Mom pumps her breast milk, and we give you one bottle-feed a day. Mom even went to the gym for the first time since you were born. You have some routine to your day now — one sleep sometime in the morning and another around 3:00 p.m. At night you are sleeping from about 8:30 p.m. until about 3:00 or 4:00 a.m. Mom feels like a different person now that she has been getting 4 to 5 hours of sleep at one stretch at night. People are always commenting on how alert, aware, and friendly you are — you are a happy, smiley, chatty bundle of joy.

June 16 (4 months old)

Since your cold in May — about the same time you started feeding frequently — we've all had a tricky time with lack of sleep. You have been waking up every 1 to 2 hours. We are all a bit sleep deprived.

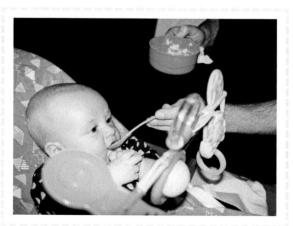

Although we knew that babies should start eating solid foods at 6 months, we decided to try you on rice cereal mixed with breast milk — and you loved it! We noticed that you were paying a lot of attention to watching Mom and Dad eating, and you want to put everything in your mouth, so we thought, why not see if you'd like to try something yourself? After only a few meals, you were insisting on holding your own spoon and feeding yourself. It's a messy business, but you manage really well. We hoped you might sleep better with some solids in your tummy, but no luck so far!

At your 4-month checkup you weighed 16.3 pounds (7.4 kg) and were 25 inches (64 cm) long. You had your second set of needles, which caused you to have a bit of a cry, but you were fine a few seconds later.

August 8 (6 months old)

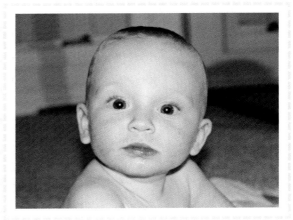

We have finally solved your sleep problems, and you have learned to go to bed without being rocked to sleep. You've become a great sleeper. We can now put you down awake in the crib. You talk to your mobile and crib toy, then roll over onto your tummy and fall fast asleep. This has made life so much easier for everyone! Your nighttime routine goes like this: you have your supper around 6:00 or 7:00 p.m., then you have a bath (which you absolutely love), then you play a little, feed around 7:30 or 8:00, and by 8:00 or 8:30 you're off to sleep.

A few weeks ago, you went swimming for the first time and had the most amazing time with Dad. When he held you on your tummy, you knew exactly how to kick. You just loved splashing the water with your hands. We decided to buy you your own little plastic pool so that you can splash around whenever you want to.

These days, your favorite form of transportation is the "Sam-Mobile," which is what we call the backpack we got as a present. You are happy riding around on Dad's back and checking out all the action. The car is a different story! You cry desperately for quite a while, until you either fall asleep or we reach our destination and take you out of your car seat.

You have just started to babble, saying "da-da-da" and other sounds. You're now able to hold your bottle by yourself.

You went for your 6-month checkup and weighed 17.9 pounds (8.1 kg). Mom fed you while you got your shot — you were so brave. The good news is, no more shots for the next 6 months!

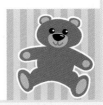

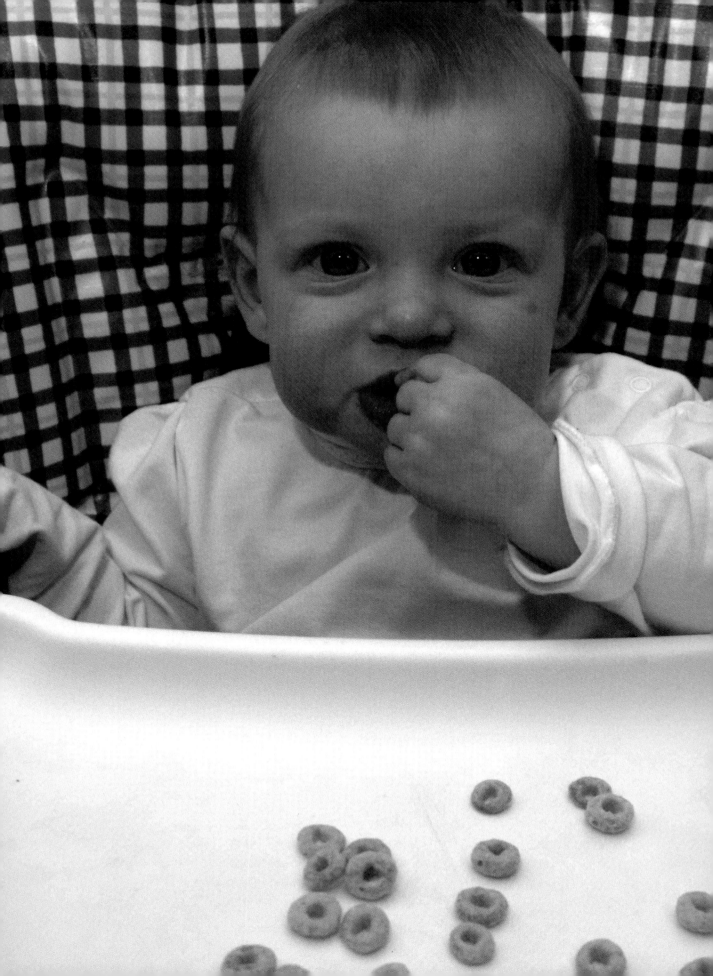

Introducing
Solid Food

Another milestone

Remarkable changes occur in a baby's diet during the first year of life. The tiny newborn who once fed exclusively on breast milk or formula has, by the age of 1 year, become a regular member of the family, sitting in a high chair, joining in mealtime activities, and eating more or less the same meal as everyone else.

Parents view the introduction of solid food to their baby's diet as a significant milestone, marking a new stage of infancy. This is understandable — your baby is growing up. But introducing solids to your baby can be confusing. When should solid foods be offered, what foods should be offered, how much food should be offered, and in what sequence — these are questions you will need to answer in consultation with your health-care providers, but there are some general guidelines you can follow.

When to start

No healthy, thriving baby, whether breast- or formula-fed, requires solid food during the first 6 months of life. In fact, the World Health Organization, the American Academy of Pediatrics, and the Canadian Paediatric Society recommend that babies be breast-fed exclusively for the first 6 months.

Solid foods are sometimes started as early as 4 or 5 months by parents who simply can't wait to begin. Introducing solid food long before 6 months or long after 6 months is not recommended.

Not before 4 months

There are several good reasons not to start solids earlier than 4 months of age. First, solid foods simply aren't needed until then. Breast milk or infant formula provides ample nutrition. Second, your baby may be neurologically too immature to be fed solids safely. An infant may still have her primitive extrusion reflex, which helps with nursing but interferes with solid foods moving easily from the front of the mouth to the back of the throat. Even supported, it is difficult for a very young baby to be placed properly in a sitting position. Third, a baby's gut is still quite immature before 4 months of age; as a result, digestion of some of the protein in solid foods may be incomplete, which

Did You Know?

Iron needs

Increasingly, medical science is recognizing how essential iron is for learning and development in infants. Up until about 6 months of age, your baby benefits from iron stores acquired in the womb. At 6 months, however, those stores are running out, and your baby needs supplementation from solid foods in her diet — over and above what breast milk or formula provide.

Did You Know?

Feeding principles

Though common sense and parenting instincts should always prevail when you're feeding your child, here are a few general principles to follow:

- Decide what your child eats and let her determine how much she eats.
- Choose healthy foods. Save chocolates and deep-fried foods for special treats. Select natural products, free of excessive preservatives or sugar substitutes.
- Allow your baby to feel in control of her mealtime. Let her open her mouth by herself before you try to place food in it. Let her explore the food, touch the spoon, or use her fingers to put food in her mouth. Let her decide on the pace of things and, when she seems to have had enough, stop feeding her, even if some food is left on her plate.
- Introduce your baby to a wide variety of foods, but hold off on peanut products, egg whites, and honey until she is at least 1 year of age because of possible food allergies or toxicity associated with these foods.
- Avoid adding extra salt or sugar to your baby's food. (The same advice should probably apply to everyone in the family.) However, it's okay to season food gently with common herbs and spices such as rosemary, thyme, sage, or even mild curry, allowing your baby to become accustomed to your family's tastes.

can lead to a food allergy in some cases. Finally, although you may have heard that giving your baby cereal at night will help her sleep, there is no scientific evidence to suggest that this is true.

Not long after 6 months

There are equally good reasons not to wait longer than 6 months before starting solids. Though breast milk or infant formula will continue to be your baby's primary source of nutrition between 6 months and 1 year, neither provides the amount of iron your baby requires. In addition, if solids are not introduced before your child reaches 9 months, she might decide that drinking fluids is much easier than eating solids and resist being introduced to textured foods.

When she's ready to eat

In addition to these medical considerations, your baby will be ready to eat solid foods when specific physical and developmental milestones are achieved:

- She can sit with support and hold her head up nicely.
- She shows an interest in your food and may even begin to try to feed herself.
- After breast-feeding or bottle-feeding, she seems to want more.
- She wants to feed more often.
- She opens her mouth to put toys in, and if you put a small spoon in, she can keep her tongue low, as opposed to pushing the spoon out.
- She uses her tongue to help move food into the mouth and shows signs of a chewing motion.

Feeding equipment

Feeding is no exception to all of the other milestones your baby reaches — it is accompanied by a deluge of information from marketing companies about the equipment you must buy. In truth, there are only a few items you need to get started.

High chairs

Initially, you may choose to feed your baby in any infant seat in which she is upright and secure. Ultimately, you will need a

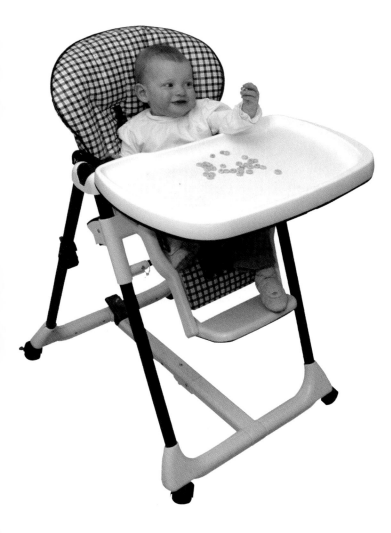

proper high chair for your baby's comfort and safety.

Features of a good high chair include a comfortable seat, strong straps with a proper buckled harness, and a footrest.

Other features to consider are wheels, if you plan to move the high chair around your kitchen, height adjustments to allow for your baby's growth, and a removable tray that can be easily cleaned. It is useful if the tray has a lip so that food remains on the tray rather than gravitating toward the floor. To prepare for this eventuality, it is a good idea to lay some plastic underneath the high chair to collect flying food.

Depending on your lifestyle, you may wish to invest in a portable high chair. Made of plastic, with straps that allow them to fasten to a regular chair and a tray that snaps on and off, these are relatively inexpensive. Although many restaurants have high chairs, some aren't suited for smaller babies in terms of the support they offer. You may find a portable chair useful not only for restaurants, but also when visiting friends or grandparents.

Bowls

When your baby begins solids, no special bowls are required because you are feeding her. As she develops and begins to feed herself — either with her fingers or a spoon — your need for plastic bowls will depend on your tolerance for broken dishes! Inexpensive plastic bowls or plates are a practical option. There's no real need to spend money on compartmentalized dishes, bowls with suction-cup bases to stick to the tray, or dishes with special sections (even heat sensors) for the spoon.

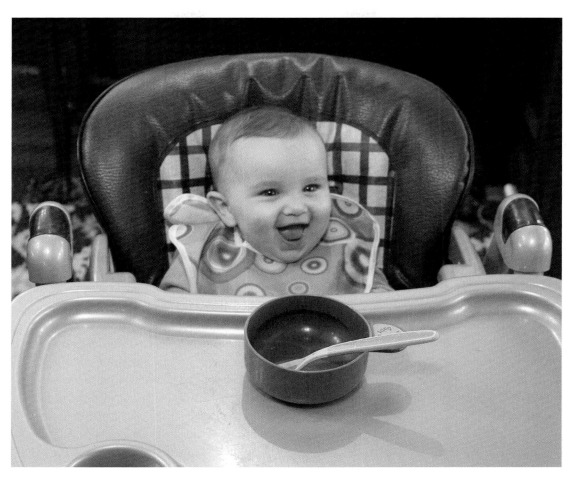

Spoons

Plastic infant spoons are a nice way to start, and several can be purchased in one package. Their flexible handles and shallow heads make them ideal for little mouths. Older babies or toddlers can graduate to slightly deeper spoons or little forks, but make sure the handle is small enough for their hands to grasp.

Bibs

Starting solids will be — and should be — a messy experience. Your baby will explore each new texture with her hands and her mouth as she determines her likes and dislikes while learning to eat with increasing independence.

Needless to say, bibs are a must! Either cloth or plastic is acceptable, though you will probably find the plastic ones more convenient for wiping off with soapy water between meals. Most fasten around the neck with either a snap or Velcro, and bigger ones will cover most of your baby's front. Some are sold with plastic sleeves, but this is certainly not a necessity. A nice feature as your baby begins finger foods is a pocket along the bottom of the bib to catch at least some of the food that doesn't quite make it into her mouth.

Portable containers

You will want to be prepared to carry food for your baby with you, whether you're traveling far away or just to a friend's house for lunch. Food is easily carried about in plastic containers with tops. Some bowls for babies come with accompanying lids, but any resealable container will do. If your baby is eating infant cereal, just pour the desired amount of powder into the bowl and add the liquid when it's time to eat. Baby food in jars is easily portable; if you're making your own, simply place an appropriate portion in a container. There are lots of portable healthy snacking options for children who are exploring finger foods.

Finally, it's a good idea to keep some basic accessories in your diaper bag so that you're not constantly packing up. A plastic bib, spoon, and washcloth will fit easily into a small container, and you'll be glad to have them on hand.

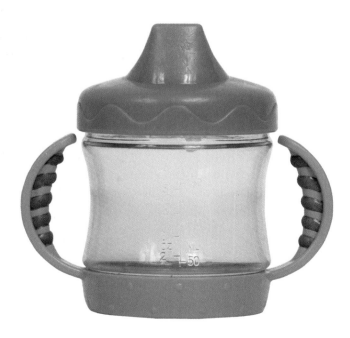

Bottles and "sippy" cups

Unless babies are nursed exclusively, most will use a bottle at some point. Most babies love their bottles — and so they should, given how much good nutrition the contents provide. Unfortunately, babies quickly learn to love the bottle itself, and not just what's inside! If you're able to curb your baby's intake to an appropriate volume, continuing with the bottle for all or some of her fluid intake is fine, but remember not to let her take milk or juice to bed.

An alternative option is to introduce a "sippy" cup, a plastic cup with a lid and a valve system in place to prevent liquids from spilling out when the cup is turned upside down. Though you may associate their use with toddlers, there is no reason they can't be introduced to a baby. The valve dictates that a certain degree of "suck" be generated for your baby to get the fluid out, but babies as young as 6 months can begin to get the hang of it. Though babies learn to love sippy cups, they don't tend to be as "addictive" as the bottle, which makes volume control and transitions easier.

There are lots of ways to introduce sippy cups. Try offering water from the cup early on, then gradually offer milk or formula from the cup one feed at a time. If you've nursed your baby exclusively for several months, you could even go directly to the cup (in addition to continued nursing) for water and eventually milk, skipping the bottle stage altogether. Even if your baby doesn't understand right away that the cup is for drinking, let her play with it and watch you drink from a cup. She will certainly work it out in time!

What to eat

Your baby's transition to solid foods should be gradual. Introduce one new food at a time and wait a few days before introducing the next. That way, you can easily identify the cause of any reactions or allergies, if they occur.

Food groups

Aim to feed your infant from the four basic food groups — cereals and grain products, vegetables and fruit, meat and alternatives, and milk and dairy products — to create a well-balanced diet of carbohydrates, protein, and fats, rich in vitamins and minerals.

Cereals

Serving single-grain, iron-fortified baby cereals is the best way to start solid foods. Iron is the most important nutrient your baby needs from solid foods at this stage, and infant cereals provide an excellent source of iron.

Infant cereals are bought as a powder, which can be mixed with expressed breast milk, formula, or even water to the desired consistency. If your baby is thriving, there is no reason you can't simply mix the cereal with water. At this stage, breast milk or formula is still your infant's primary source of calories.

Many commercial brands are available, and there is no best one to choose. They are all iron-fortified, but be sure to read the labels because some come pre-mixed with powdered formula.

Most people begin with a rice cereal, as rice is the grain least likely to produce an allergic reaction. Once your baby has adjusted to eating rice cereal by spoon, she can try other single-grain cereals such as oatmeal or barley. Wait about 3 days after introducing a new food before you try another, so you can observe how well each is tolerated.

After your baby has tried each of the single-grain cereals, you may introduce her to mixed cereals, most of which contain wheat. In the past, it was believed that foods containing wheat were difficult for a baby's immature gut to handle and could potentially produce allergies. While wheat allergies do occur, they are rare. There is no evidence that the introduction of wheat-based cereals should be delayed.

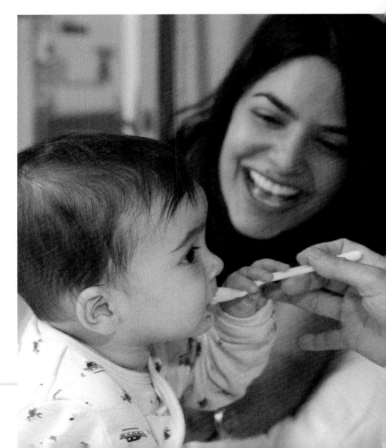

HOW TO
Prepare infant cereal

1. Initially, mix cereal to the consistency of thin porridge, then gradually thicken it to whatever density your baby seems to prefer, which in most cases is a soft mush.

2. Serve cereal at body temperature, as with milk feeds, and feed your baby from a bowl, using an infant spoon.

3. Never feed your baby cereal from a bottle; the texture will be diluted, and this method can interfere with the development of her feeding skills.

4. Start with approximately 2 to 3 teaspoons (10 to 15 mL) of cereal, given once daily; as your baby catches on, gradually progress to whatever amount seems to interest and satisfy her, usually 2 to 4 tablespoons (25 to 50 mL) twice a day. These volumes are just a guide.

5. Feed your infant as much or as little as she wants to eat. Some babies take longer than others to adjust to textures. Your baby may take very little one day and surprise you with higher volumes the next. The most important marker — not just with cereals, but with your infant's nutrition in general — is that she is growing and developing normally, not the number of teaspoons she takes at each feed.

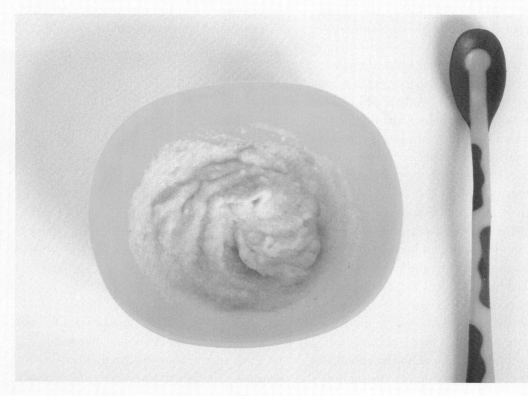

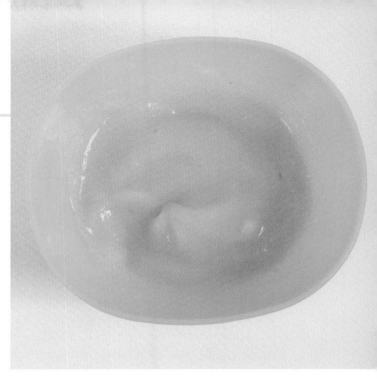

Vegetables and fruits

Once your baby is accustomed to infant cereals, usually between 6 and 7 months of age, it is time to add cooked and puréed vegetables and fruits. Yellow, green, and orange vegetables, as well as all varieties of fruit, are appropriate. Common choices include carrots, squash, green peas, pears, applesauce, and bananas, but anything goes.

There is no "right" order in which to introduce these foods, though many people suggest serving vegetables before fruits so that your baby doesn't become accustomed to sweet flavors and reject her veggies. There is no science, however, behind this largely theoretical suggestion. In fact, your baby may love sweet potatoes and dislike applesauce or pears. Offer a variety of vegetables and fruits and enjoy watching your baby experiment with new tastes and textures.

Begin by offering vegetables or fruit twice a day, in addition to infant cereal. At the beginning, the consistency should be a smooth purée because your baby is just learning about different textures and doesn't yet have the ability to chew. Introduce each new flavor with a positive attitude. Your baby will pick up on your feelings about what you're providing, so try not to influence her with your own likes and dislikes. Eventually, your baby will determine her own favorites and express dislike for some foods. When this happens, wait a few days or longer, then try the food again — you may be pleasantly surprised as your baby adjusts to the new flavor or texture.

As you introduce solid foods, don't be concerned if the color and consistency of your baby's stools change. What you see in the diaper will vary depending on her diet each day, and it is not unusual for small undigested pieces of fruit or vegetables to appear in the stool. This is normal, as long as your baby is growing well. What goes in is generally more important than what comes out.

Meat and alternatives

By the time a baby is between 7 and 9 months old, cereals, vegetables, and fruits have usually been successfully incorporated into her diet, and you can try giving her a source of protein, such as red meat, poultry, fish, egg yolks, beans, or tofu.

At this stage, your baby's food should be puréed. Meats can be puréed in a food processor, while egg yolks and soft tofu are easily mashed. Commercially prepared protein foods for this age group are all in purée form.

Now that your baby has increasing variety in her diet, these new foods can be given at the same feed as cereal or offered separately as a third or even fourth feed.

Did You Know?

Food allergies

Food allergies occur when a person's immune system reacts to a food protein that the body identifies as "foreign." Symptoms range from severe anaphylaxis (facial swelling, hives, and difficulty breathing, requiring immediate medical attention) to non-specific symptoms such as abdominal pain and diarrhea, wheezing, or skin rash. True allergies are different from food intolerance, in which symptoms occur in response to a particular food but are not due to an immune or allergic reaction.

While people of any age can develop allergies, children's immature digestive systems make them more susceptible. Some common allergies, such as those to cow's milk protein or egg whites, are outgrown by the majority of children. If you are worried that your baby may be at increased risk of allergies, discuss this with your health-care provider.

Milk and dairy products

Dairy products can also be introduced around this time to provide an important source of fat, protein, and calcium. Be sure to give your baby full-fat options until she is at least 2 years old — fat is vital for proper brain development.

Plain yogurt, grated cheese, and cottage cheese are excellent choices. Homogenized cow's milk can be introduced at 9 months, but it is better to wait until your baby is a year old. Before then, her gut may be too immature to handle cow's milk protein. Continue to feed with breast milk or infant formula until that time. Of course, breast milk may be continued even longer, if desired.

Mealtimes

Initially, it's better to respond to your baby's signals than to a clock. Begin by offering cereal just once a day, and progress to twice daily as your baby gets the hang of things. This affords her twice the opportunity to learn that the pasty stuff on the spoon is actually satisfying. Remember that your baby's primary source of nutrition remains breast milk or formula, so these cereal feedings should not interfere with nursing or the bottle.

Hunger response

The earliest morning feed should be breast milk or formula; if you're nursing, this will also help relieve any overnight engorgement. Cereal can be offered when your baby expects her second feed of the day. Generally, it's best to offer cereal at the beginning of the meal and then "top it up" with breast milk or formula. That way, the baby is a little hungrier and thus more motivated to experiment with new tastes and textures.

However, when she's first starting solids, if your hungry infant cries persistently because she hasn't yet learned to appreciate cereal, you can settle her and her "hunger pangs" by offering the breast or bottle for a brief initial period. When she has settled, retry the cereal. The second feeding of cereal can be offered any time later in the day, usually in the late afternoon.

A regular schedule

As your baby is introduced to more food groups, her feedings will begin to resemble meals in terms of the variety offered and satisfaction achieved. As your schedule allows and your baby demands, two feedings a day will gradually become three meals. When your baby is older still, morning and afternoon snacks will be incorporated.

Though a strict schedule is not necessary, it is never too early to introduce positive eating habits by establishing a routine. Offer the first meal, for example, when the rest of the family is up and ready for their breakfast; enjoying breakfast together is a wonderful start to any day. Provide your baby with supper when everybody is gathered again at the end of the day. In that way, mealtime can be a family event.

Food cautions

Before you know it, your baby will be enjoying a balanced and varied diet. Although variety is the spice of life, some foods are better introduced a little later in your baby's life. Wait until your baby is at least a year old before introducing egg whites and honey. Peanut butter is best deferred to even later.

Egg whites

Though yolks may be introduced earlier, egg whites contain many different proteins that can contribute to the development of allergies. Once your baby is over a year old, it will be easier to identify a potential allergy, and it may be handled better by your baby.

Honey

The bacterium *Clostridium botulinum* may contaminate unpasteurized honey, posing a theoretical risk of contracting botulism. Botulism is a very serious disease that results in severe swallowing difficulties, muscle weakness, and constipation. Honey is not recommended until after your baby's first birthday.

Peanut butter

Peanut allergy is common. In some cases, it can be life-threatening. Do not give peanut products in the first year of life. The American Academy of Pediatrics recommends introducing peanut butter no earlier than the age of 3 years.

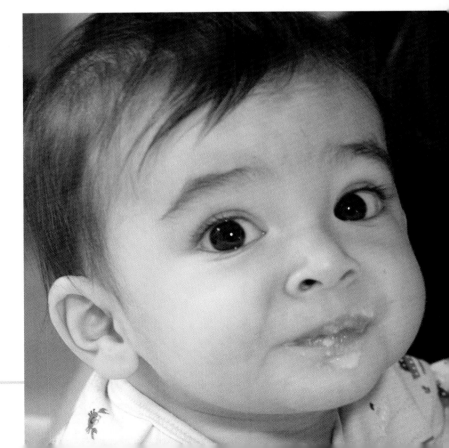

From purées to finger food

Preparing food for your baby at this stage is an exciting experimental process of introducing new textures, colors, and flavors. Your baby will quickly let you know her likes and dislikes. Have fun preparing her favorite foods.

Homemade vs. store-bought purées

Whether you make your own baby food or buy commercially prepared puréed food is up to you. Homemade foods are simple to prepare and allow for more variety at a lower cost; however, they can be time-consuming to make. Store-bought foods are manufactured under stringent hygiene conditions and are equally nutritious. Organically grown brands of infant food are also widely available (at a premium) if you have concerns about added chemicals. Alternatively, you may choose to buy organic produce with which to prepare your own food.

Sugar is often unnecessarily added to commercially prepared baby food, while homemade foods are more apt to have unnecessary salt. Give your baby the opportunity to appreciate the natural flavors of fruits and vegetables, without added sugar or salt. In a few months, when she is eating a broader range of foods, feel free to experiment with mild seasonings and spices, allowing your baby to adapt to your family's tastes.

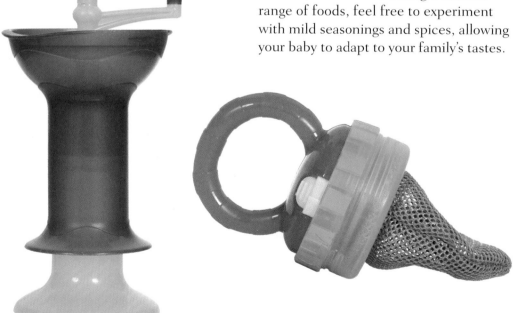

■ (Left) An inexpensive food mill purées fresh fruits, giving them a texture babies enjoy; (Right) Food nets allow babies to suck the juice from larger pieces of fruit without the risk of choking.

HOW TO
Prepare homemade baby food

- Wash fruits and vegetables carefully. Peel and remove stems and ends.

- Cook, bake, or grill meats; do not fry them. Be sure to remove any skin, bone or gristle.

- Mash or purée most food to the consistency of applesauce.

  - Food mills work well for fruits such as apples and pears. Wash the fruit, cut it into chunks, and soften it in the microwave. When you add it to the food mill, the juice and pulp will nicely squeeze out into your bowl, leaving the skins, cores, and pits behind.

  - A food processor or blender makes puréeing all varieties of fruits and vegetables easy and is also ideal for beans and meats. Fresh vegetables can be boiled or steamed until soft. Thaw frozen varieties and cook according to package directions. Place the cooked produce in the food processor or blender and purée for 30 to 60 seconds. You'll need to add a little water — usually between 1 and 3 tablespoons (15 and 45 mL), depending on the vegetable — to reach the desired consistency. Meat and poultry require more water and a longer processing time.

  - Some foods don't require any special preparation. Examples include bananas, avocados, and soft tofu, all of which are naturally soft and can be mashed as required with the back of a spoon.

- Prepare batches of food for several meals, cooking a whole bunch of carrots or asparagus, for example, at one time.

- Store freshly prepared purées in the refrigerator or freezer. Refrigerated food can be safely stored for up to 2 days, while frozen food can last for months. To freeze purées, first pour them into ice cube trays. (Some specialty baby stores sell trays with lids specifically for this purpose.) Once the cubes are frozen, transfer them to freezer bags. Be sure to write the contents and date on each of the freezer bags — sweet potatoes and squash can look very similar! Thaw the cubes as needed. Cubes are an easy way to measure out portions.

- Try using food "nets." Some babies enjoy sucking on larger pieces of fruit using nets designed for this purpose. Pieces of melon, for example, are placed inside the net so that your baby can suck the juice from the fruit without the risk of choking on larger pieces. Both washable and disposable nets are available.

Guide to

Appropriate finger foods

As with purées, continue to offer your baby a variety of foods, both to satisfy her tastes and interest and for their diverse nutritional value. Ensure that food is soft enough to be easily mashed by your baby's gums and that it is cut into small pieces — generally no larger than ¼ to ½ inch (0.5 to 1 cm) in size.

Following are some common examples of foods to try initially, but the options are endless, so feel free to be creative!

- Peeled soft fruit, such as bananas, ripe cantaloupe, pears, or peaches, cut into bite-sized pieces
- Soft cheese, or hard cheese that is grated or thinly sliced

- Cooked tender meat, ground or cut into small chunks
- Fish, soft tofu, mashed beans, or cooked egg yolk (all are good sources of protein)
- Mashed or diced cooked vegetables (favorites include green beans, spinach, carrots, potatoes, and tomatoes)
- Soft bread, oat rings, or crackers that easily dissolve (try them out in your own mouth)
- Cooked short pasta

Meat is often the most difficult food for infants to adjust to because it can be difficult to chew. Many recipes can be made with ground meat, including meatloaf or lasagna, which can then be cut into small pieces. Try softening meat with gravy or tomato sauce.

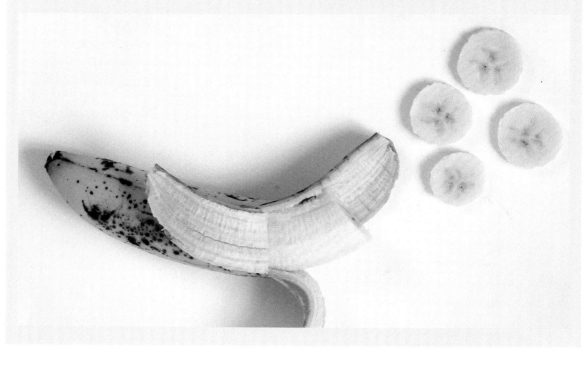

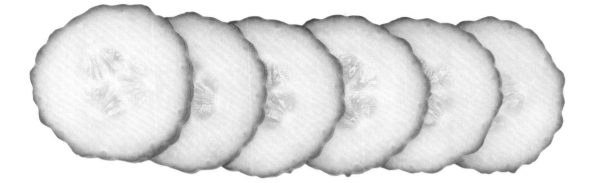

Finger foods

While every baby is different, by the age of 8 or 9 months, most infants are ready to try more textured finger foods (foods that can be held in their hands). Children who are ready for finger foods have probably been introduced to all of the major food groups and have developed the skills to sit alone, pick up food with their fingers, bring it to their mouth, and chew with some degree of success. These newly acquired skills represent quite an accomplishment, but don't expect this process to be neat — just enjoy the feeding experience, however messy.

If you're not sure whether your child is ready for finger foods, offer a trial of soft food, such as grated cheese or small pieces of very soft fruit, and watch to make sure she doesn't gag or choke. Take note of whether she enjoys this new experience. If she is not yet ready, continue with purées for another few weeks, then try again.

When you do make the transition from purées to finger food, be sure to do so gradually. It will take your baby time to adjust to new textures and the work involved in eating finger foods, so her diet is best supplemented with ongoing offerings of a well-balanced diet of purées.

Continue to feed your child cereal as a source of iron, though you may decrease cereal feeding from twice to once a day as her diet expands to include other iron-rich foods such as red meat and leafy green vegetables. Breast milk or formula feedings should also continue, though their quantity will naturally decrease.

Snacks

Along with finger foods, you can now introduce nutritious snacks to your child's diet between meals. Try giving her

- bite-sized fruit
- soft veggies and dip
- crackers with cream cheese or small pieces of hard cheese
- oat rings or infant cereal
- yogurt (3.25% milk fat or higher)
- muffins

How much to eat

Your baby's energy needs are unpredictable. Trust that she will know what she requires. The amount of food consumed day to day, feed to feed, and baby to baby will vary. That's normal. After all, you probably don't know exactly how much food you will eat for lunch two Wednesdays from now!

Offer your baby the amount of food she seems to crave, but don't force her to take more than she wants. Conversely, don't withhold food if she appears hungry. Long before she has words, your baby will communicate very clearly when she's hungry or full!

Specific guidelines

The typical 6- to 9-month-old infant will thrive on 4 to 6 tablespoons (60 to 90 mL) of vegetables and 6 to 7 tablespoons (90 to 105 mL) of fruit daily, in addition to 2 to 4 tablespoons (30 to 60 mL) of cereal twice daily, as well as meats or alternatives and dairy, when they're introduced. Most infants this age will begin eating two meals a day and work up to between three and five.

If you are concerned about the overall adequacy of your infant's diet, focus on recording her weight, plotted serially on the growth chart in your doctor's office, rather than on measuring her day-to-day intake. In most cases, her growth curve will confirm that she is doing just fine.

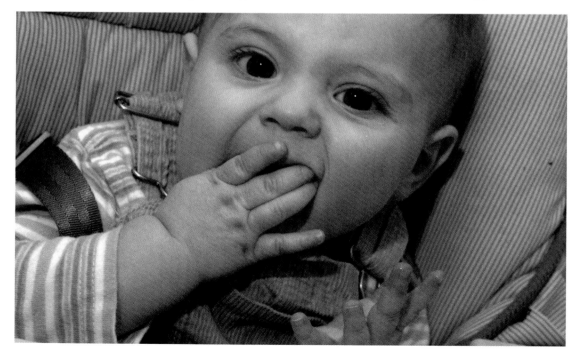

Diet plan for introducing solid foods

Foods	From 6 to 9 months	From 9 to 12 months
Breast milk	Nursing on demand	Nursing on demand
Iron-fortified infant formula	On demand, about 3 to 5 feedings every 24 hours	On demand, about 3 to 4 feedings every 24 hours
Iron-fortified infant cereal	Offer 2 to 3 tbsp (30 to 45 mL) twice daily	Offer 2 to 3 tbsp (30 to 45 mL) twice daily
Other grain products	Introduce other grain products, such as dry toast or unsalted crackers	Introduce other plain cereals, such as bread, rice, and pasta, 8 to 10 tbsp (120 to 150 mL) daily
Vegetables	Offer puréed cooked vegetables (yellow, green, and orange), progressing to soft mashed vegetables, 4 to 6 tbsp (60 to 90 mL) daily	Offer mashed or diced cooked vegetables, 6 to 10 tbsp (90 to 150 mL) daily
Fruit	Offer puréed cooked fruits or very ripe mashed fruit (such as bananas), 6 to 7 tbsp (90 to 105 mL) daily; fruit juice may be offered from a cup	Offer soft fresh fruit, peeled, seeded and diced, or diced canned fruit packed in water or juice, 7 to 10 tbsp (105 to 150 mL) daily
Meat & alternatives	After vegetables and fruit, offer puréed cooked meat, fish, chicken, tofu, beans or egg yolk, 1 to 3 tbsp (15 to 45 mL) daily	Offer minced or diced cooked meat, fish, chicken, tofu, beans, or egg yolk, 3 to 4 tbsp (45 to 60 mL) daily
Milk & dairy products	Offer plain yogurt (3.25% MF or higher), cottage cheese, or grated hard cheese, 1 to 2 tbsp (15 to 30 mL) daily	Introduce whole cow's milk, moving from a bottle to a cup. Continue with plain yogurt (3.25% MF or higher), cottage cheese, or grated hard cheese, 1 to 2 tbsp (15 to 30 mL) daily

Adapted by permission from Daina Kalnins and Joanne Saab, *Better Baby Food* (Toronto: Robert Rose, 2001).

Safety first and last

Choking is a significant hazard when solid foods are introduced. Babies like to explore with their hands and mouth and may inadvertently swallow food before you have mashed it for them. Signs of choking include coughing, gagging, wheezing, and sputtering. Consider taking an infant CPR course so you'll be confident should this situation arise.

Reducing the risk of choking on solid foods

- Never leave a feeding baby unattended.
- Don't allow your baby to crawl or walk with food in her mouth.
- Feed her in a high chair.
- Carefully examine fish for bones, even tiny ones.
- Cut all foods into small pieces. Foods such as hot dog slices or whole grapes can completely plug the throat or windpipe. Cut them lengthways into quarters to be safe.
- Avoid foods that can crumble or shred and be aspirated into the lungs, such as whole nuts and whole raw carrots. Serve carrots cooked or grate raw carrots to prevent choking.
- Avoid hard candies, cough drops, popcorn, nuts, sunflower seeds, gum, and any other food you're not sure your baby can handle.

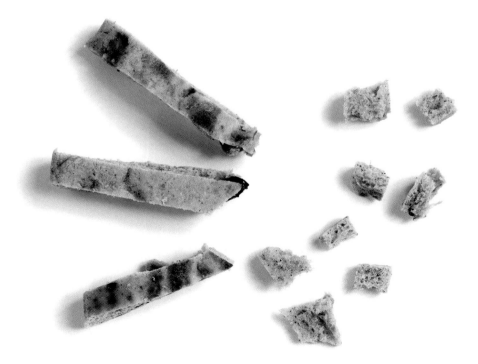

Frequently asked questions

As family doctors and pediatricians, we answer many questions from parents. Here are some of the most frequently asked questions. Be sure to ask your health-care providers any other questions that arise. If they don't have the answers, they will refer you to a colleague who does.

Q: Should I feed my baby or allow her to try feeding herself?

A: When you first introduce your baby to solids, she will not have the developmental capability or the desire to feed herself. At this stage and for the first few months, she will rely on you to feed her with a spoon. Between 8 and 12 months, she will begin to use her fingers to feed herself, initially by grasping soft cookies or crackers. Give her the opportunity to feed herself at least some of the time. One tactic is to feed her for the first part of the meal, ensuring that a good portion of the food winds up in her mouth, and allow her some independence as she finishes off.

Your baby will also learn from you as you use utensils to eat. By all means, offer her a soft spoon to explore. She'll initially play with it, but by 11 months of age or so, she may impress you by picking it up by the handle. Though she likely won't feed herself exclusively until several months down the road, these early opportunities to explore and learn are invaluable. Ignore the mess — and be sure to offer praise and encouragement as success is achieved!

Q: My 9-month-old son insists on feeding himself. He's not very good at it, and I worry that he won't get enough to eat. What should I do?

A: Don't worry — his desire for independence will not result in starvation. Hunger inevitably trumps autonomy. By this age, your son has probably developed a pincer grasp and finds picking up food by himself quite enjoyable. It's okay for him to experiment with textured foods, such as pieces of cooked macaroni, well-cooked ground meats, and mashed bananas or potatoes. He won't be able to use a spoon yet, but will probably let you feed him his favorite purées or, at least, let you help him use the spoon.

Q: How much should I feed my baby?

A: Most people's food intake varies from day to day and often from meal to meal. Babies are no exception. Some infants also seem to eat more than others. Don't worry if your nephew gulps down everything in sight, while your own child seems quite picky. Rather than sticking to a strict feeding regimen, it's best to let your baby's appetite determine how much she should consume.

Q: How often should I feed my baby?

A: Because mealtime is a great family time, try to make breakfast, lunch, and dinner an important part of your baby's routine between 9 and 12 months. Around this time, morning and afternoon snacks are also introduced to satisfy your baby's hunger between meals. Snacks add an important nutritional component to your baby's diet, provided that healthy snacks are offered. Depending on your baby's nursing or bottle routine, her snack may be finished off with some breast milk or formula.

Q: When can I introduce milk?

A: As your baby's nutritional requirements are increasingly met by her solid food intake, the quantity of breast milk or formula she drinks will gradually decrease. While you may choose to nurse your baby for longer than a year, formula may be replaced with homogenized cow's milk by 1 year of age. This transition is not recommended prior to 9 months of age, and closer to 12 months is preferred to ensure that your baby's gut is mature enough to tolerate the cow's milk protein.

When you do introduce your baby to cow's milk, remember that, while it is an excellent source of calcium, it does not contain the same quantity of iron or other nutrients found in infant formula. You may choose to transition your baby gradually, continuing to offer some formula, as well as infant cereal and meat.

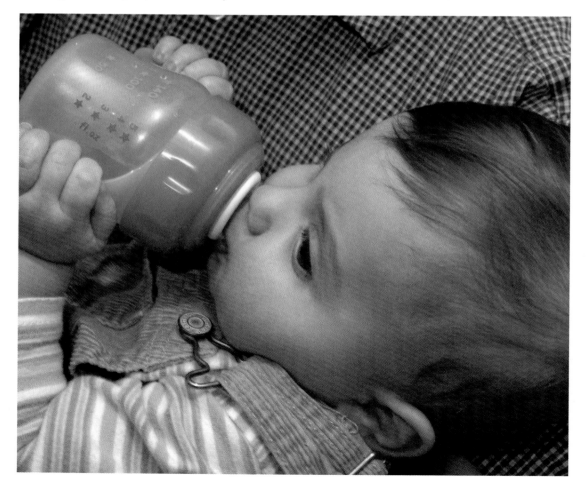

It is also important to limit your baby's milk intake to 16 to 20 ounces (475 to 600 mL) per day. More than that will place her at risk for iron deficiency, due to possible microscopic blood loss from the gut. Babies also have a tendency to "fill up" on milk in place of nutritious solid food; decrease the chance of this happening by offering milk during or after mealtime, not before.

Q: Should I give my baby water?

A: While newborns do not need water, by 6 months of age it is appropriate to offer your baby water to quench her thirst. Of course, water has no nutritional value, so your baby shouldn't fill up on water prior to mealtimes. Offering it with meals, however, or on a hot day, is a good idea. In terms of quantity, there is no guideline as to how much water your baby needs. Just as you drink until your thirst is quenched, so too will your baby. Let her be the judge.

Q: What about juices?

A: Many parents view fruit juices as a "natural" food that can be harmlessly consumed by babies without concern or limit. Wrong. Fruit juices are loaded with sugar and can cause many problems. A bottle of juice in the crib at bedtime may soothe your baby — but it can also produce serious tooth decay. Undiluted juice may cause cramps or even diarrhea. Fruit juices can also kill a baby's appetite for more nutritious foods, including milk. Of course, this doesn't mean an infant should never be offered apple or grape juice. Just remember that moderation is the key. Here are some helpful guidelines to consider:

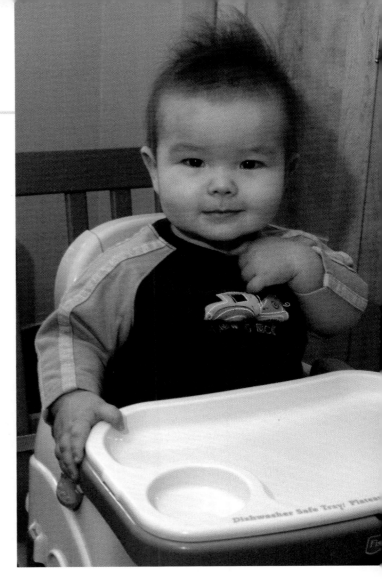

- Encourage your baby to drink water instead of juice to quench her thirst.
- Introduce fruit juice no earlier than 6 months of age (some say to wait until 1 year).
- Dilute fruit juices with equal amounts of water to reduce unnecessary calorie intake. Unsweetened apple juice, for example, contains 124 calories in every 8-ounce (250 mL) bottle.
- Limit the amount of juice a baby receives daily in the first year to 4 to 6 ounces (125 to 175 mL).
- Don't let a baby take a bottle of juice or milk to bed — the sugar in these drinks can cause tooth decay.

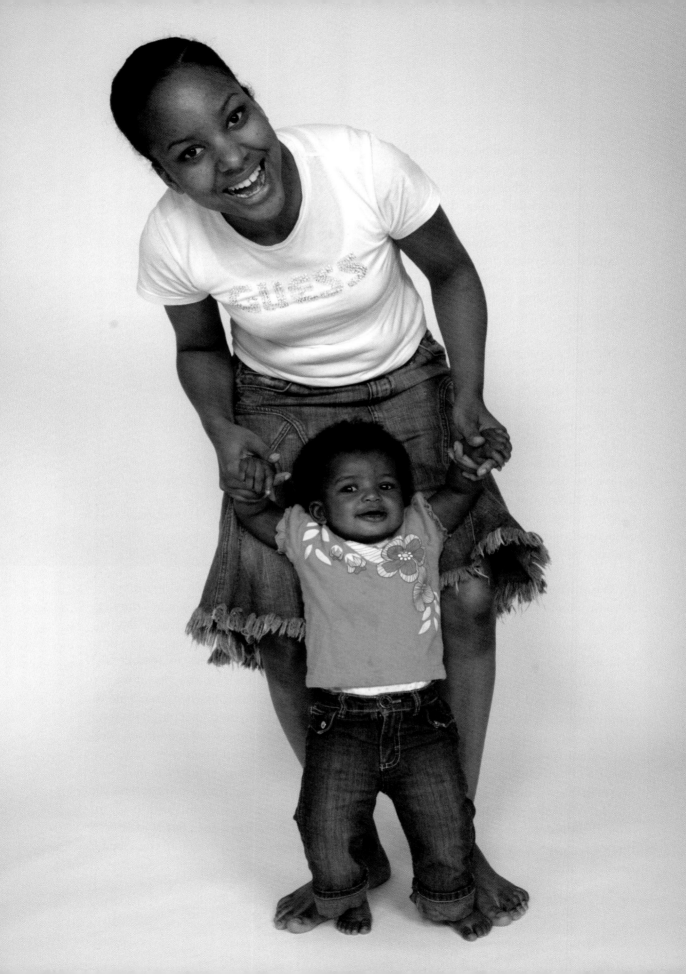

Your Baby's
Months 7 to 12

Disciplining your child

It may seem premature to start thinking about disciplining your baby at this age. After all, he is not even a year old! However, by introducing your values and expectations early on, you can lay a solid foundation for your child's behavior for many years to come.

There are no absolute rules of discipline. Individual children have different temperaments, and parents have varying approaches, priorities, and expectations. So methods of discipline should be individualized. Caregivers should be consistent, so that it is clear to your baby what the limits are. Children, even the very young, quickly figure out who can be easily manipulated and who will allow them to break the rules. Discipline is most effective in an environment where a child feels comfortable and secure. In older children, negative consequences are sometimes necessary to reduce undesirable behavior, but, at this age, positive reinforcement and encouragement are the most effective forms of discipline.

Discipline defined

Many people equate the term "discipline" with punishment. But discipline is not punishment. The word is derived from the Latin word for "teaching." According to the American Academy of Pediatrics, "discipline is a whole system of teaching based on a good relationship, praise and instruction for the child on how to control his behavior. Punishment is negative; an unpleasant consequence for not doing something. Punishment should only be a very small part of discipline." The goals of discipline are to teach your child how to conduct himself in a manner that will ensure his safety and allow him to become a socially acceptable member of society. This involves teaching your child self-control.

Did You Know?

Appropriate strategies

Time out, spanking, and punishment are not appropriate strategies in the first year of life, but distraction, removal, and ignoring unwanted behaviors are useful techniques. For example, if your baby keeps pulling your hair, give him something else to play with or pull on. Alternatively, tie your hair up so that he cannot reach it. He will probably become bored with the game and move on to something more entertaining. Sometimes a firm "no," coupled with a negative facial expression, gets the message across very clearly. But remember, although we are all human, acting out of anger is not good parenting, no matter how tired or frustrated we feel. If anger, not teaching, drives our discipline, then it's time to get some help.

Safe behavior

In this age group, safety is a major focus for discipline. Infants 7 to 12 months of age are very curious about the world around them. They reach and grab objects. When they become mobile, they seek to explore their environment. This curiosity is not matched with judgment and experience.

Children must be taught their limits and appropriate boundaries. Not only should you ensure that their environment is safe and provide close supervision, you must teach children safe behavior. If your child tries to grab something that is hot or fragile, firmly say "no," remove him from the object, and distract him by giving him something else to play with. If you are consistent, he will learn that some objects are not appropriate for him to play with.

Consideration for others

It is not too early to begin teaching your baby to be considerate of others. If you are attending to the needs of an older brother or sister, it's okay to deal with the older child first. It's not necessary to drop everything and immediately respond to the baby. A gentle voice should reassure your infant that you will get to him as soon as you can. The world revolves around no one individual; after all, your baby is just one part of your family.

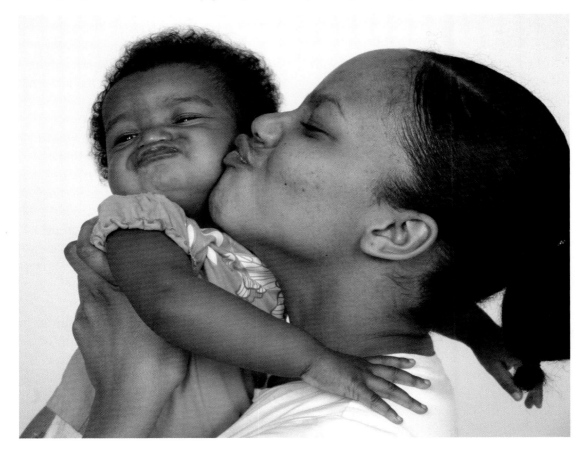

Still growing and developing

As your baby progresses through this period, his growth continues in weight, height, and head size, but at about half the rate of the first 6 months. Infants at this age continue to develop motor skills rapidly. As a result, they become much more interactive and playful.

Growth curves, 7 to 12 months

Growth measurements will typically be taken two to three times during this period, usually at around 9 months and again at the 1-year visit.

By 1 year of age, an average infant has tripled his birth weight, has grown by one-quarter of his initial length, and has gained about 4 inches (10 cm) in head circumference.

Your child's growth should be followed carefully as he transitions to eating solid foods to ensure that he continues to meet his nutritional requirements. It is

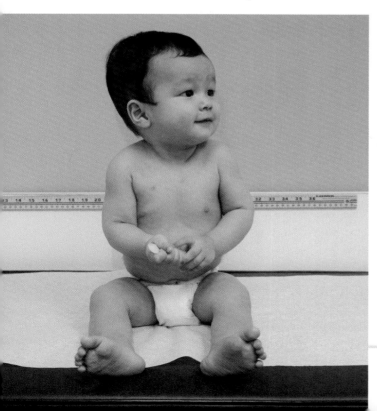

expected that he will continue to follow along the curves on his growth chart.

Development milestones, 7 to 9 months

Suddenly, it seems, your baby is able to sit, crawl, stand, and even say "Mama" or "Dada."

Sitting and holding

By 7 months, most babies are able to sit securely and hold objects in their hands at the same time — quite an accomplishment!

Crawling

Most infants of this age are able to crawl, with varying degrees of dexterity. Some begin with "commando crawling," as soldiers do in war movies, dragging their body by pulling ahead of them with alternating arms. Others progress straight to their hands and knees. Some babies never crawl.

Standing

Many infants are able to pull themselves up to a standing position by 9 months of age. Once they are up, they may have a hard time getting back down. If you haven't already done so, this is definitely the time to move things from coffee tables and night tables up higher! Make sure there are no sharp edges to bump into. At this stage, when mobility far exceeds agility, many little falls are likely to occur.

Picking up small objects

Growing control of hands and fingers leads to attempts to pick up smaller objects, initially by trapping them between the baby finger and palm, and gradually moving toward a thumb and index finger pincer grasp. These hands are inquisitive, and whatever they pick up will inevitably make its way into the mouth, so make sure that little objects are not left lying around, especially by older brothers and sisters whose playthings are likely full of choking hazards. At this stage, your baby may start to hand a toy to an adult, but has trouble letting go.

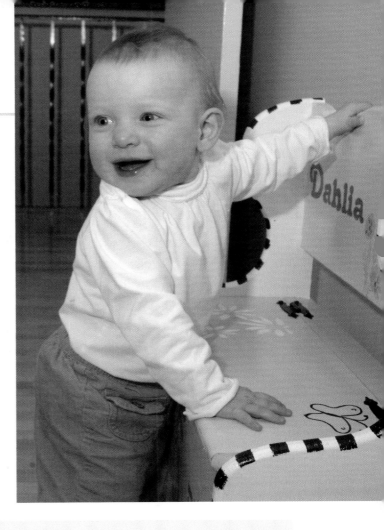

Did You Know?

Reaching his potential

Some parents become overly concerned about the short stature and chubbiness of their children at this age. Remember that a big part of your child's ultimate height was decided when you chose your partner. You don't see too many short parents watching their sons play basketball in the NBA! The best predictor of ultimate height is probably the midpoint between the mother's and father's height. The vast majority of children in the developed world will reach this potential, even those with rather odd eating habits in the early years.

Some parents fear they are over-feeding their babies. Excessive chubbiness usually becomes less of an issue when the baby starts to become more active and increases in height. It is not appropriate to make dietary adjustments in the first year of life — for example, cutting down on fats or carbohydrates — because your baby needs these to fuel his growth and development. As he gets older, there will be ways that you can encourage the development of healthy eating habits. The most important thing you can do now is to ensure that he is being weighed and measured on a regular basis and is following his growth curves appropriately — that is, he is not dropping off his expected course of growth.

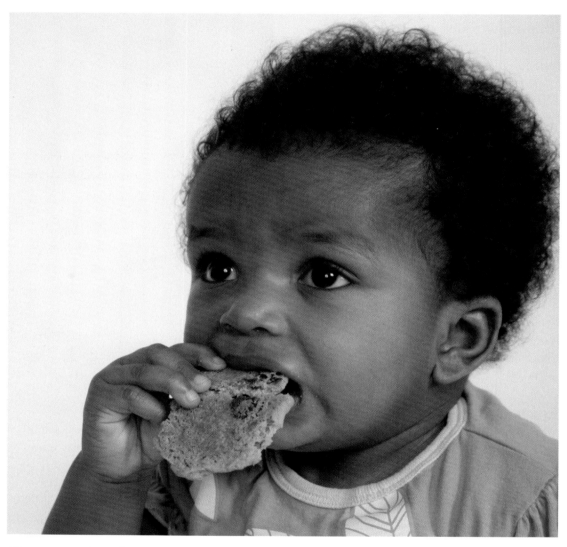

Communicating

At this age, your child will continue babbling and should be using a number of different sounds. He will imitate funny sounds you make and laugh at them. He is capable of shouting and is not afraid to practice this new ability.

Throwing objects

Your baby is now aware that objects out of view are still there and will look for a toy that has fallen or rolled away. In fact, he is likely to practice this newfound wisdom by repeatedly throwing objects, such as food, spoons, and dishes, from his high chair and expecting you to pick them up. This is not done with the intent of driving you crazy — it is a normal stage of development!

Playing games

At this stage, your child will become interested in games, such as peekaboo.

Development milestones, 10 to 12 months

By now, your baby is on the move!

Cruising

At 10 months, many infants start to cruise: walking along while holding onto furniture with both hands. Soon this will progress to walking with his hands held by an adult, and just when you think your back can't take it any more, he will take those exciting first steps. Don't worry if he's not quite there yet — most babies generally start walking between 12 and 15 months.

Picking, pointing, and marking

By this time, your baby will be able to pick up small objects, such as Cheerios, fluff, and dust specks, with his precise thumb and index finger pincer grasp. He is starting to point to objects and is able to hold a bottle or cup. Around 1 year of age, infants can hold a crayon in one fist and make marks on paper with it.

Speaking

Your baby's babbling is becoming more purposeful. By 1 year of age, many babies are able to use "Dada" and "Mama" with meaning — sweet music to the ears of parents who have been waiting for this moment for some time! By 12 months, your child will generally know and respond to his own name. Your continued positive reaction to these gains and imitation of these sounds will help encourage your child's language development.

Interactivities

As your baby gains more understanding of the world around him, he will become increasingly interactive. Peekaboo and tickle games engage his attention. He will start to clap his hands and wave goodbye, new skills that bring with them a host of new clapping and bye-bye games.

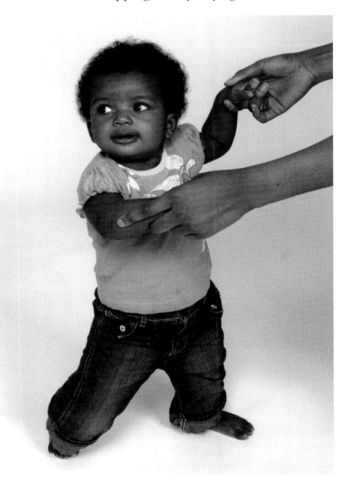

What's normal, after all

As babies grow older, they love to explore the world that surrounds them and continue to develop their unique personalities. In so doing, they may exhibit several behaviors that appear unusual to you. The majority are normal and usually transient.

Separation anxiety

Separation anxiety is a normal stage of development during which infants develop emotional discomfort and seem anxious when separated from familiar caregivers. The degree and duration of separation anxiety can vary tremendously between infants depending on their individual temperaments. Some babies develop separation anxiety at a few months of age, while others are always happy to be picked up and entertained by strangers. These are the extremes. Most infants develop some degree of separation anxiety around the age of 9 months, not only when you leave your baby with someone else but also when you try to put him down for the night.

Typically, separation anxiety lasts until about 2 years of age, although new experiences, such as starting school or going to camp, can precipitate separation anxiety in older children.

Coping with separation anxiety

Having your baby cry every time you leave him can be very upsetting for a parent. Most infants settle quite easily once their parents are out of earshot, so check in with the babysitter to see if this is indeed the case. In addition, here are some strategies for alleviating separation anxiety for your child and helping you with your emotional response:

- When possible, try to leave your baby with a consistent caregiver, with whom he will become accustomed to spending time.
- Having the babysitter come over a while before you need to leave is sometimes helpful — it gives her a chance to engage the baby in a fun activity while you are still there.
- Some parents think it is easier to sneak out and avoid a scene. This is probably

Did You Know?

Object permanence

Separation anxiety should be seen as part of normal development as your baby develops a sense of object permanence and memory. Object permanence means that he knows you are still around even when he can't see you. For younger babies, out of sight is usually out of mind! The development of memory means that, when he sees the babysitter or sees you getting ready to go out, he remembers that this means you will not be there for him for a while. This is distressing to him.

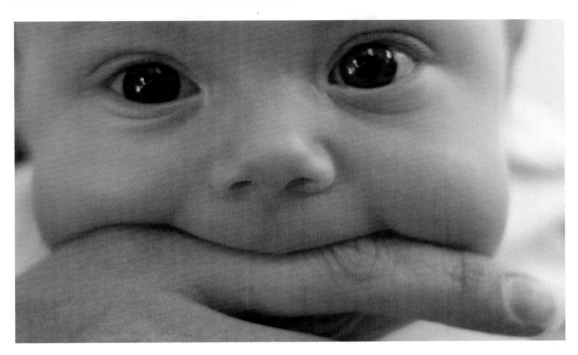

not a good idea because it can be confusing and anxiety-provoking for the baby if he hasn't seen you leave. He may start to cling to you to make sure you don't disappear again. A better plan is to give him a little advance warning that you are going out and a big hug and kiss as you are leaving, reassuring him that you will be back and will see him later.

Biting

The primary teeth usually start to erupt during the second 6 months of life, and your baby will subsequently learn to bite and chew. Many infants will take the opportunity to bite down on anything that comes close to their mouths, including Mom's breast and other people's fingers, cheeks, noses, and ears. As the teeth get bigger and more numerous, this can be very painful for the victim.

Despite your misgivings about this behavior, your baby is not being angry or hostile. Biting is a normal part of experimental behavior, and is usually a transient phenomenon. However, if biting behaviour persists into the toddler years, it will make your child very unpopular.

Preventing excessive biting

Your baby needs to learn that biting is not acceptable. Biting is sometimes reinforced by the reaction it provokes: it is natural to startle and react with facial and verbal expressions when you are bitten. Try not to respond dramatically.

The most effective response is to calmly remove your baby from the body part he has bitten, firmly say "no," then move on to another activity to distract him. If you do this repeatedly and consistently, your baby will learn not to bite.

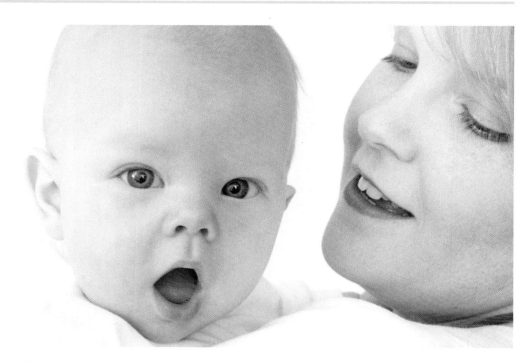

Do not bite the baby back — that will teach him that it is okay to bite because Mom and Dad do it too!

Pulling hair

Pulling people's hair is another common behavior in infants. Some babies enjoy the reaction it provokes. To discourage this behavior, gently pull back your baby's fingers from your hair, say "no," and distract him by engaging his attention in something else. It may also be helpful to tie your hair back.

Some babies like to stroke, twirl, and play with their own hair, especially when they are tired. This is usually a comforting, soothing habit, and is not of concern. However, if he is pulling out chunks of his hair, this should obviously be discouraged. Cutting his hair very short may help. You can also provide a toy or blanket for him to hold as a replacement

for playing with his hair. Again, distraction may be a useful technique.

Tooth grinding (bruxism)

Tooth grinding occurs in up to half of normal infants, usually once the top and bottom two teeth have erupted. It is not clear why babies grind their teeth — it is probably because "they are there" and the infants enjoy the sound or sensation. Tooth grinding is most frequent at night, and can be very annoying or worrisome for parents. Fortunately, it is a habit that wanes with time, and it does not damage the teeth in any way. The best treatment is to ignore it.

Rhythmic movements

Some babies engage in rhythmic movements such as head banging, head rolling, or body rocking. These repetitive motions may continue for several minutes and usually occur when the child is going to sleep. Most experts believe that they are self-comforting movements. This behavior generally commences around the age of 6 months and resolves around 2 years of age. If the child is otherwise healthy and developing normally, there is no cause for concern. However, if your child has any other unusual behaviors or developmental delays, you should consult your doctor.

Exploring the genitals

Many infants discover their genitals during the second 6 months of life, usually in the bathtub or during diaper changes. They also discover that it feels good to stimulate them by touching or playing with them. You may notice that your little boy sometimes gets erections. Some little girls rub their vaginal areas against fixed objects, such as the strap of the car seat or even table legs. A form of masturbation, this self-stimulation is completely normal behavior in children of all ages. There is no reason to be concerned. When children get older, they learn that playing with their genitals should be done in a private place.

Breath-holding spells

Sometimes a child, seemingly in response to being upset or frustrated, stops breathing, turns dusky or very pale, then actually loses consciousness for a moment or two. In extreme cases, some twitching or jerking of the limbs may occur. The episodes usually last for about a minute or so. It only seems like much longer!

It's pretty scary stuff, but, in fact, breath-holding spells are both common and benign.

Did You Know?

Turning blue

Breath-holding episodes occur in about 5% of children, most often between the age of 1 and 4 years, but sometimes in infants as young as 6 months. Rarely, a painful experience or sudden startle can initiate a breath-holding spell. Breath-holding spells are not harmful unless the child injures himself while falling. Nor are they associated with neurological or psychological problems. Still, because they fear triggering a spell, parents may stop setting reasonable behavior limits for their child — which is not a good idea.

Breath-holding spells require no specific treatment, but it is wise to confirm with your doctor that any losses of consciousness in reaction to something are indeed consistent with breath-holding spells. Once you are sure that breath-holding is the cause, ignoring the behavior and not giving positive reinforcement will hasten its disappearance.

WHEN TO SEE THE DOCTOR
- If episodes are not precipitated by crying, frustration, or pain.
- If they last longer than 1 minute.
- If they occur before the age of 6 months.
- If they are severe or you aren't sure that they are breath-holding spells.

Teething time

Your child will eventually have 20 primary, or "baby," teeth — 10 on the bottom and 10 on the top. The order in which teeth erupt can vary, but the bottom central teeth, called the lower incisors, are usually the first to emerge. Often, teeth appear in pairs rather than one at a time.

First tooth

The age at which a baby's teeth first erupt is extremely variable. On average, the first tooth emerges at about 7 months, but some babies are born with a few teeth in place, while others don't get their first teeth until after their first birthday.

If a baby is born with a tooth already erupted (as is seen in one in 2,000 to 3,000 newborns), chances are that it will be poorly anchored and will need extraction to avoid the risk of choking and aspiration. If the tooth is well anchored, it can be left alone.

If no teeth have erupted, no intervention is required until at least the first birthday. Thereafter, your health-care provider may decide to check for a hormonal or vitamin deficiency.

Late eruption of teeth does not interfere with learning to chew and eat solid foods; babies can manage very well with their gums.

Teething complications

Teething has been blamed for a myriad of symptoms, including drooling, diarrhea, facial rashes, fever, congestion, sleep problems, and irritability. But teething is not necessarily the culprit behind all or any of these problems. The first teeth tend to arrive at the same time that your baby's

antibodies (which crossed over in the placenta before birth) are beginning to wane, resulting in an increase in infections, including otitis media (inflammation of the middle ear), colds, and gastroenteritis. Teething is often coincidental and not the cause of a given problem. If your infant has a fever or persistent irritability and is hard to console, for example, it would not be wise to attribute this to teething: it might be a sign of a serious infection. Likewise,

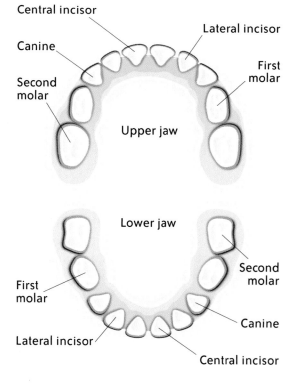

if any of the other symptoms mentioned are severe or persistent, your baby should be assessed by your health-care provider.

Treating teething symptoms

Most infants tolerate teething very well. If your baby appears to be in pain, it can be alleviated by massaging the gums with a clean finger for a few minutes. Some babies seem to get relief from chewing on a cold or hard object, such as a teething ring. Placing a clean wet washcloth or teething ring in the refrigerator can be helpful. Teething biscuits can also be effective in soothing the child, but teething gels are of questionable value — they cause numbness of the gum and may also affect the back of the mouth. Because of the risk of side effects, teething gels are not recommended by the American Academy of Pediatrics. Homeopathic teething remedies do not always clearly state what they contain and are not subject to rigorous testing. There have been reports of toxicity, including lead and mercury poisoning, so these remedies should either be avoided or used with caution. Occasionally, pain medications, such as acetaminophen or ibuprofen, are indicated.

DO'S AND DON'TS IN TREATING TEETHING

Do's
- Do massage the gum with a clean finger.
- Do let your baby bite on a cold wet washcloth or refrigerated teething ring.
- Do try teething biscuits.
- Occasionally do give a dose of acetaminophen or ibuprofen for the discomfort (but do not give on a regular basis).

Don'ts
- Don't use teething gels (there are potential side effects, and they're not very effective).
- Don't use homeopathic teething remedies (they are potentially toxic).
- Don't allow biting on cut-up vegetables, such as carrot sticks (they're a choking hazard).
- Don't feed your baby honey (there's a risk of botulism).
- Don't give your baby alcohol!
- Don't place teething rings around your baby's neck (there's a risk of strangulation).

Eruption pattern

Upper jaw

Tooth	Eruption
Central incisor	7–12 months
Lateral incisor	9–13 months
Canine	16–22 months
First molar	13–19 months
Second molar	25–33 months

Lower jaw

Tooth	Eruption
Central incisor	6–10 months
Lateral incisor	7–16 months
Canine	16–23 months
First molar	12–18 months
Second molar	20–31 months

HOW TO
Prevent cavities (dental caries)

Dental caries are not uncommon in childhood — 18% of 2- to 4-year-olds and 52% of 6- to 8-year-olds develop them. Taking good care of your baby's primary teeth is very important because they are the precursors for your child's permanent teeth. Here are some tips for preventing cavities:

- Babies and young children should not be allowed to sleep with a bottle containing milk or juice in their mouths. Even small amounts of sugar-containing fluids constantly dripping into the mouth may result in dental decay, which affects the front teeth most severely but may involve all of the infant's teeth. This is known as bottle caries. It has also been described in babies who breast-feed frequently at night, usually those who co-sleep and nurse intermittently and often.

- Fruit juices should be avoided for as long as possible because the high sugar content promotes dental decay. Give your baby fruit to eat and breast milk, formula, or water to drink.

- Teaching your baby to drink from a cup before he reaches 1 year of age helps to get him away from the constant drip of sugary material onto the teeth from the bottle.

- If your baby uses a pacifier, do not dip it in sugar or other sweet materials.

- As your child approaches his first birthday, he should have his teeth brushed twice daily.

- Your first visit to the dentist for a checkup should occur before your child's second birthday, unless other dental problems arise earlier.

Brushing your baby's teeth

Dentists recommend starting to clean the teeth as soon as they erupt. Starting early helps to ensure good dental hygiene and habits. Teeth cleaning should become part of the bedtime routine.

You can gently brush your baby's teeth with a small, soft toothbrush or wipe the teeth and gums with a clean, moist piece of gauze. Toothpaste is not necessary at this age, and if used should not contain fluoride. Another useful option is a small device that looks like a soft thimble, made of rubber with soft bristles on one side.

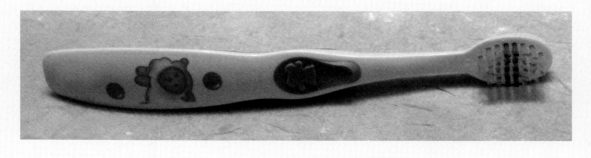

Outings

Going outside is now a true treat for parents and baby, but is still a bit complicated. A walk, run, or bicycle ride in your neighborhood should be part of your daily routine, unless, of course, the weather is extremely cold or excessively hot and humid. Always make sure to take a change of clothing for the baby and a snack and a drink for your baby and yourself.

Clothing

In general, babies over the age of 6 months do not need to be dressed much more warmly than adults and older children. Bear in mind, though, that if you are walking vigorously and your infant is sitting in a stroller, you are likely to feel warmer than he does. If it is cold outside, ensure that his head, ears, hands, and feet are covered. In wet or windy weather, transparent covers for the stroller provide good shelter from the elements. Stroller covers to protect your baby from the sun and mosquitoes are also available.

Sun protection

Sun exposure during childhood is the greatest single cause of damage to people's skin. Sunburn is associated with skin cancer and premature aging of the skin in adulthood. Cataracts in later life may also be secondary to too much sun. Most of the damage is caused by ultraviolet waves A and B (UVA and UVB). Unfortunately, sunburn is usually noticed too late, often a number of hours after exposure, when redness and pain develop. Given the risks, it makes sense to keep your baby away from excessive sunlight exposure and use sunscreen for children over the age of 6 months. Avoid prolonged sun exposure during the sunniest hours of the day: 10:00 a.m. to 2:00 p.m.

Hats with brims, long sleeves, and pants provide some sun protection. Bathing suits with long sleeves and pants, made of fabrics with higher sun protection factors than regular clothing, are very practical.

If your baby will tolerate wearing sunglasses, they will protect his eyes from the harmful rays of the sun. Make sure the label states that the sunglasses are 99% to 100% UV (ultraviolet) protective.

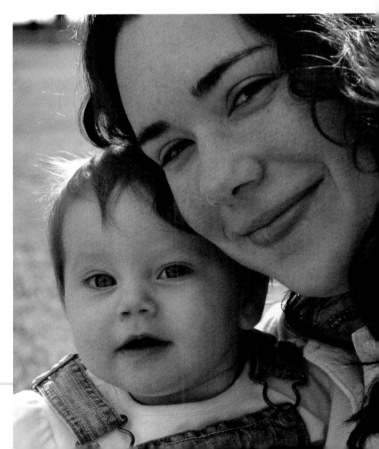

Sunscreens

Many sunscreens are available and approved for use in babies over the age of 6 months. Sunscreens have simply not been tested in younger infants, so they have not received approval for the very young. No sunscreen is 100% protective, partly because most guard against UVB rays only, but some products are more effective than others.

Some authorities recommend zinc oxide or titanium dioxide, which are inert "sunblocks," for infants in the first 6 months if sun exposure cannot be prevented.

Most dermatologists recommend sunscreens with a sun protection factor (SPF) of at least 30. The SPF indicates how long a person can be exposed to sun before the skin burns. The higher the number, the longer the effect lasts. Protection varies depending on individual skin color and age — lighter skin is more susceptible to damage, and babies are likely to burn in less than the 20 to 30 minutes it takes for older individuals.

Sunscreen should be applied liberally at least 30 minutes before you go outside and reapplied every 2 to 3 hours, especially if your baby is in the water or perspiring a lot.

Avoid products that combine sunscreen and mosquito repellent because sunscreen

Did You Know?

DEET is safe for babies

The American Academy of Pediatrics (AAP) says that DEET is safe, even in small children, *when used as directed*. According to the AAP, it can be used on babies older than 2 to 3 months in up to 30% concentration. There have, however, been occasional reports of skin and respiratory irritation and, rarely, seizures with the use of DEET.

As with sunscreen, the number on the bottle indicates the duration of effectiveness: 10% DEET provides about 2 hours of protection; 24% provides about 5 hours of protection. Use the lowest percentage that will provide protection for the time your baby may be exposed.

DEET should be applied to all exposed areas, but the eyes, mouth, and open wounds should be avoided. Don't put DEET on the hands of little children, who are likely to put their fingers into their mouths and touch their eyes. DEET can also be applied to clothing. After coming back indoors, wash the DEET off your child's skin.

Remember that DEET and other mosquito repellents are not effective against some of the other insects we frequently encounter in the summer months, including bees, wasps, hornets, and ants.

USING DEET MOSQUITO REPELLENTS
- Don't use on children under the age of 3 months.
- Read the label carefully.
- Apply sparingly.
- Do not put on the hands or face.
- Put on clothes but not under clothes.
- Wash off the skin when back indoors.

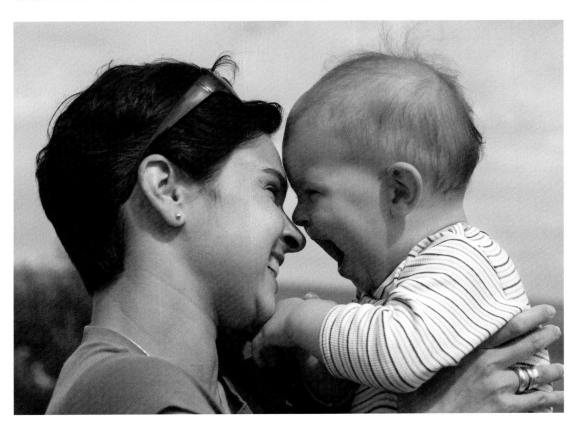

should be applied often and generously, while mosquito repellent should be used infrequently and sparingly.

Insect repellents

Mosquito bites are itchy and annoying — what's more, they occasionally become infected. Until recently, mosquito-borne diseases were extremely rare in North America; fortunately, malaria is a concern only when you're traveling in certain parts of the world. However, West Nile virus can be spread by mosquito bites between May and October, with a peak in August and September. It can occasionally cause a significant infection. Most children, if infected — which is rare — will have a mild flu-like illness, but infections of the brain have been reported to occur, so it has become increasingly important to use mosquito repellents.

The most effective way to avoid mosquito bites is to remain indoors, especially around dusk and dawn. However, when that is not a practical option, mosquito repellents and protective clothing should be worn. DEET is the most effective chemical mosquito repellent. Some natural products, such as citronella, are available, but studies have shown that these do not provide adequate protection against mosquito bites.

Remove potential breeding grounds for mosquitoes by getting rid of all standing water, for example, in outside toys, pails, and baskets.

Now the fun begins

After months of little sleep and high anxiety, you and your baby can begin to relax and truly enjoy one another's company, facing new challenges as a family and taking great pleasure in shared activities.

Reading

Reading to your baby promotes intimacy and bonding, as well as stimulating acquisition of language and intellectual skills. In the latter half of the first year, babies start to enjoy reading with their parents.

There are many ways to encourage and initiate reading with your baby. Being a good role model is the best place to start. If your baby sees you reading regularly, especially if you hold him close while you are reading, he will learn early on that reading is a positive behavior. Innumerable wonderful books are available for you and your baby to enjoy. Incorporate reading with you into your baby's daily routine, and you will set the stage for a lifelong love of reading.

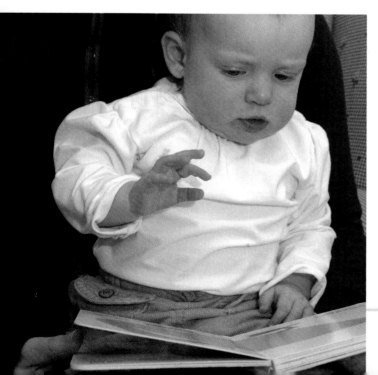

Watching television

Children in North America watch excessive amounts of television. Ultimately, this promotes a sedentary lifestyle, which contributes to obesity and its many associated health problems. We should be encouraging our children to be active "doers" rather than passive "watchers." The American Academy of Pediatrics recommends no television for children under the age of 2 years and a maximum of 2 hours a day for older children and adolescents. It's a good recommendation.

When watching television, children are repeatedly exposed to inappropriate and unrealistic depictions of violence, sexual activities, and exploitative advertising. While it is difficult to measure negative effects of television exposure in infants, some studies suggest that infants who watch television frequently are at increased risk of developing attention deficit hyperactivity disorder (ADHD).

Using the television set as a babysitter is very tempting if we tell ourselves that "TV keeps him quiet, and he only watches educational programs." Programs with names like *Baby Einstein* are enticing, conveying the impression that your baby will be developing advanced intellectual skills. But experts agree that exposure to and interaction with real people is far more beneficial, both academically and socially.

HOW TO
Read to your child

There is no "right" way to read to your baby. Reading should be an enjoyable and exciting experience for both the reader and the listener. There are, however, some practical aspects to consider when you acquire books for your little one and read from them:

- Babies' books should be sturdy and non-toxic — it is highly likely that he will chew on them, throw them, and pull them. Laminated board, vinyl, and cloth books are all good options.

- Choose books that are bright and colorful, with pictures of familiar objects.
- Babies love rhymes and songs.
- Books that stimulate their senses, such as those with peekaboo and pop-up pages and textured materials, are often great favorites.

Allow your baby to play with books on his own and to "read" to you.

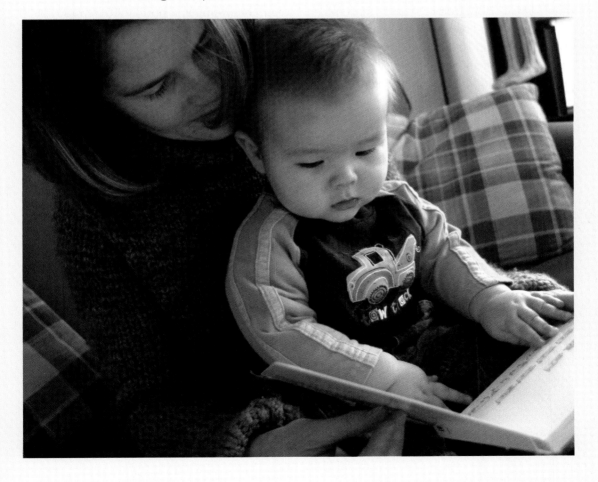

Returning to work

Parenting is work! All mothers and fathers know that taking care of an infant is pretty much a full-time job. What "returning to work" really means is going back to paid employment outside of the home — adding to your already busy schedule.

Back in the workplace, you will be frequently torn between your home and work responsibilities. Leaving your baby for several hours a day can be very difficult emotionally and, sometimes, physically. But parents who stay at home full-time sometimes feel frustrated and underappreciated.

Making a decision

Your decision to return to your previous job or start a new job rests on the specifics of your situation: your career goals, your sense of job satisfaction, financial pressures (you now have a new little person to feed, clothe, and educate), and available options for child care. Make a decision that works best for your family, and realize that there is no perfect solution.

Advance planning

To minimize stress and make the transition back to the workplace easier, advance planning is essential. Is the baby ready? Are you? Are all the supports you need in place?

Feeding

If your baby is still breast-feeding, you need to make sure he will drink expressed breast milk or formula from a bottle or cup while you are away. Many women take breast pumps to work and store expressed milk. Alternatively, slowly weaning the baby, partially or fully, from breast milk may facilitate your return to the workplace. However, abrupt weaning can be very uncomfortable, so seek advice from your health-care provider or lactation consultant.

Employer empathy

Understanding and empathetic employers and co-workers are highly desirable but not always easy to find. You may want to meet with your employer before you go back to work to discuss potential problems and solutions. For example, your work hours may now need to be more flexible because of your family obligations. You will also need to work out a contingency plan for those days when your child is ill and needs your direct care. Then there are the routine medical and dental appointments during the workday. Some people in your workplace are likely also parents and aware of the issues of working parenthood.

Family and community support

Include your partner and other supportive friends and family in the process. Paternity leave is a wonderful option for some families. Some couples can stagger their hours so that one parent is always home with the baby. Grandparents, uncles, aunts, and friends may be excited at the prospect of spending time with your beautiful baby. In our society, however, extended family members are often not available to help, so many parents have to consider other child-care options, such as in-home caregivers (nannies or babysitters) or daycare centers. There are advantages and disadvantages to both.

Child care

There are many reputable agencies to help families select and screen child-care workers. Obviously, they charge for their services. Your friends and acquaintances, especially those who have young children of their own, can be helpful resources, as can your health-care provider.

Regardless of the choice you make for child care, separation is often difficult. Innate factors, such as your baby's age and temperament, and external factors, such as familiarity with caregivers, will all affect how your child adjusts to your going back to work. In general, despite a few tears from Mom, Dad, and baby, most families settle into the new routine quite easily.

In-home caregivers

By hiring a nanny or babysitter to come to your house, you allow your child to remain in familiar surroundings and may give yourself more flexibility in your work hours. Plus, you won't always need to get the baby dressed, fed, and out the door when you are rushing to get ready for work.

However, some families feel that their personal space is invaded by having a "stranger" in their home. And an in-home babysitter is usually a more expensive option than daycare, though it becomes more cost-effective if you have more than one young child at home. Bear in mind that if your babysitter needs time off, you will have to make alternative arrangements, sometimes at very short notice. However, if your baby is sick, the babysitter will be a constant and comforting caregiver.

Be sure to hire someone reliable, who will be attentive and sensitive to your baby's needs and whose personality and approach are similar to your own. Hiring a babysitter on a trial basis is advisable to ensure that she meets your needs and expectations.

Daycare centers

In a regulated group daycare center, your baby will be cared for by trained professional child-care workers and exposed to other children, which provides opportunities for physical and social development. Daycare should provide a stimulating and enjoyable environment for children.

Most jurisdictions have stringent laws to regulate the size of daycare centers (the caregiver to child ratio), to establish safe facilities, and to ensure that staff members are adequately trained. There are also specific requirements for hygiene and sanitation. Nevertheless, the major disadvantage of daycare is the increased number of infections to which children are exposed. It is well documented that children in daycare contract more diseases than those who stay home. Most are common, minor viral illnesses, particularly gastroenteritis and colds. Daycare centers are usually very strict about excluding children who are ill with potentially

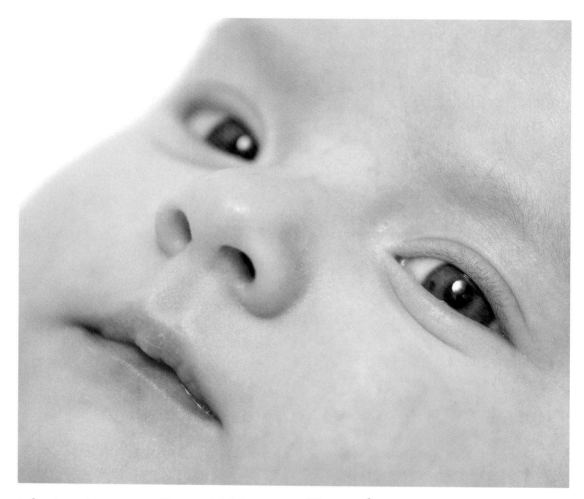

infectious diseases, so if your child does become sick, you will have to make arrangements for a parent or alternative caregiver to stay at home until he is no longer considered contagious.

When seeking out a daycare center, look for an environment in which you think your baby will thrive. Talk to parents who have children in the daycare, as well as to the caregivers who work there. Some daycare centers will allow you and your child to spend a few hours there to get a sense of whether it is a suitable place for you.

Home daycare centers

Home daycare centers are child-care programs run out of people's houses. They often have more flexible hours, and they usually take just a few children of varying ages, thus providing a smaller and more intimate environment. Because there are fewer children, the risk of infection is lower.

In many jurisdictions, home daycare centers are registered with government agencies and evaluated by the appropriate authorities on a regular basis.

Treating common conditions

Despite the many good times you will enjoy with your baby, you will still need to be vigilant in detecting, treating, and preventing some common medical conditions. For a quick reference to the symptoms and treatment of these conditions, see Part 11, "Caring for Your Sick Baby."

Food allergies

A food allergy is a reaction by the body's immune system to a specific food. To be "sensitized" to a food, a child will usually need to be exposed to the allergenic food, which, on subsequent exposures, triggers the immune system to produce a reaction that can lead to hives, wheezing, and vomiting. Serious reactions, called anaphylaxis, include throat swelling and a drop in blood pressure. These reactions can be life-threatening, and although extremely rare, can sometimes occur as the first sign of a food allergy.

Treating food allergies

Food allergies are best managed by avoiding specific foods and allergens.

To manage cow's milk allergy, for example, breast-feeding mothers are often asked to try a dairy-free diet, while formula-fed babies are usually switched to a special hypoallergenic formula.

Anaphylaxis is a medical emergency. If your baby's mouth or throat shows signs of swelling, he is having trouble breathing, and you notice a change in alertness, take him to the emergency department of your local hospital immediately.

Infants who exhibit signs of a food allergy beyond a mild skin reaction should be seen by a physician. They will be referred to a specialist, who will perform various tests, such as skin prick testing, to determine the allergen.

Did You Know?

Common food allergies

In infants, the most common food allergens are cow's milk and eggs. An allergy to the protein in cow's milk can be seen in 2% to 5% of formula-fed infants, usually starting in the first month. Symptoms may include blood in the stool, diarrhea or vomiting, irritability, and poor weight gain. Even breast-fed babies whose mothers consume dairy products can develop symptoms.

Many children, particularly those who react to milk and eggs, will "outgrow" their allergies; in the case of cow's milk, 80% to 90% of infants who are allergic to it will tolerate it by the age of 3 years.

Peanut butter, nut, and shellfish allergies generally become evident in older children as they become exposed to them. Sensitivity to nuts and shellfish tends to persist.

Depending on the circumstances, caregivers will be instructed on the use of an EpiPen (injected epinephrine to be used in case of a significant reaction). The specialist may also recommend that your child wear a MedicAlert information bracelet.

Wheezing

Wheezing is a whistling or sighing noise made by air passing through narrowed small air passages in the lungs. Usually detected by a stethoscope, wheezing may sometimes be heard by the unaided ear.

About one in 100 infants less than 1 year of age will be seen in hospital for this condition. Repeated episodes of wheezing in infancy are often a sign of asthma, which develops in about 10% of young children. Another common reason for wheezing in infants is bronchiolitis, a viral infection that causes inflammation and narrowing of the small air passages in the lungs, leading to obstruction of airflow. These extremely common viral infections occur in the winter months and usually lead to cold symptoms in adults or older children, but in young infants, who have smaller air passages, they often result in wheezing and difficulty breathing. Less common causes of wheezing include feeding difficulties and heart disease.

Treating wheezing

Any infant with signs of breathing difficulty (rapid breathing, increased effort needed to breathe) should be seen immediately by a physician. Because wheezing has a number of causes, your physician may recommend a limited number of tests. In a clinic or hospital setting, a monitor can be attached to a finger or toe to check the oxygen content of the blood. An x-ray of the chest will sometimes be warranted.

Bronchiolitis is a self-resolving condition that improves over a period of days. Infants who need more supportive care (oxygen and fluids to prevent dehydration) will require hospitalization. For infants with repeated episodes of wheezing who are suspected to have asthma, your health-care provider may prescribe medications (bronchodilators) administered through a compressor or puffer and spacer device to reverse obstruction to airflow, as well as medication to reduce inflammation of the airways (steroid medication in an inhaled or oral form).

Croup

Many parents are frightened when their infant or toddler suddenly develops a loud, barking, seal-like cough, often arriving in the middle of the night after a few days of cold

Did You Know?

Wheezing vs. congestion

The noise characteristic of wheezing should be differentiated from the noises made by congested nasal passages that occur with colds. Wheezing is typically heard when breathing out (exhaling), while nasal congestion often leads to snoring or noise while breathing in. Wheezing is often accompanied by more rapid and labored breathing than normal, which is not usually the case with nasal congestion.

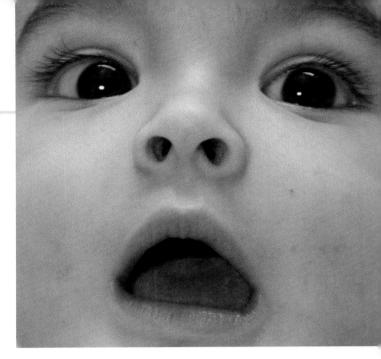

symptoms. This is croup, a common condition, usually affecting young children, caused by a viral infection that occurs most frequently in the fall months. The virus causes inflammation and swelling in the voice box and windpipe (larynx and trachea), leading to the characteristic cough and sometimes to noisy and labored breathing.

Treating croup

While croup's noisy cough can be frightening, if your child is otherwise breathing comfortably and quietly between bouts of coughing, the croup is classified as mild. Simple measures, such as bringing the child into a steamy bathroom or outside into the cool air, may be helpful.

Any child who is having difficulty breathing, however, needs to be seen immediately by a physician. Inhaled medications to reduce the swelling in the windpipe will often be used. A dose of oral steroid medication is also given to help reduce the inflammation. Most children recover quickly, but loud coughing can persist for days.

Squint (strabismus)

Squint (strabismus) is a misalignment of the eyes, caused by an eye being "turned in" (esotropia) or "turned out" (exotropia).

Misalignment of the eyes may be present continuously or apparent only when vision is focused on objects of interest. The visual system in children takes years to mature; infants in the first few months of life normally have transient misalignment of the eyes because the eyes have not yet achieved the full ability to move in concert. In addition, some children who have more prominent skin folds over the inner part of the eye may appear to have crossed eyes when the actual eye alignment is normal.

Misalignment of the eyes can be due to a variety of causes, including a disturbance in the focusing mechanisms of the eye (near- and far-sightedness), problems with the muscles and nerves that control the precise movements of the eye, cataracts, and, rarely, tumors of the eye.

Treating strabismus

Except for transient misalignment of the eyes (usually crossing), normally seen in the first few months of life, any infant with strabismus should be referred to an ophthalmologist for a detailed eye examination. Strabismus needs to be treated appropriately so that optimal visual development can occur. While adults experience double vision if the eyes are misaligned, children's brains suppress the image received from the deviating eye. This can result in the development of a "lazy eye" (amblyopia), which may become permanent if not managed appropriately before the school years.

Constipation

Concern about a baby's stools is one of the most common reasons for parents to seek advice from health-care providers. Many parents worry that their infant is constipated because the number of stools passed is less than expected. However, there is a wide range of "normal" stooling patterns during infancy. Some breast-fed infants pass multiple loose stools each day, particularly in the first weeks and months of life; others pass only one stool per week. Breast-fed babies are rarely constipated. If formula or rice cereal is introduced, stool frequency may be reduced.

The frequency of stools is not a cause for concern as long as they are soft. Constipation is characterized by the passage of hard, painful stools, often in the form of little pellets.

Rarely, constipation may be caused by an underlying medical problem. Of special concern is the newborn baby who has not passed stool. A newborn almost always passes his first stool (meconium) within 24 to 48 hours of birth. Failure to do so will prompt testing for bowel problems.

Treating constipation

Every well-meaning health-care provider and relative will have suggestions for treating constipation. Simple dietary changes, such as substituting barley for rice cereal and adding 1 to 2 ounces (30 to 60 mL) of prune juice to the diet, are sometimes sufficient. Lactulose, a non-absorbable sugar

Did You Know?

Straining

Parents often become concerned that their baby is straining and becoming red in the face while passing stools. They interpret this sometimes dramatic appearance as a sign of constipation. However, infants cannot coordinate relaxation of their pelvic muscles with pushing to evacuate their bowels. Straining results. If the passed stool is soft, you can usually be reassured that your baby is not constipated. However, if the stool is hard or a fissure develops, then the stool needs to be softened using stool softeners. Anal fissures are tears in the lining of the rectum, generally seen in the six o'clock position when looking at an infant lying on his back — at the part of the anus closest to the scrotum or labia. These are caused by the passage of hard stools.

similar to prune juice, can be prescribed as a treatment for constipation.

Mineral oil should be avoided during infancy because it can cause a serious pneumonia if aspirated into the lungs, and honey and corn syrup should not be used because of the risk of botulism. Regular stimulation of the rectum with fingers, thermometers, or suppositories is not recommended.

Otitis media (infection of the middle ear)

One of the most common infections (and reasons for antibiotic use) in young children is otitis media, an infection of the middle ear (the small space located behind the eardrum). The majority of children will have had at least one ear infection by the time they are 2 to 3 years old. Young infants, usually starting at around 6 months of age,

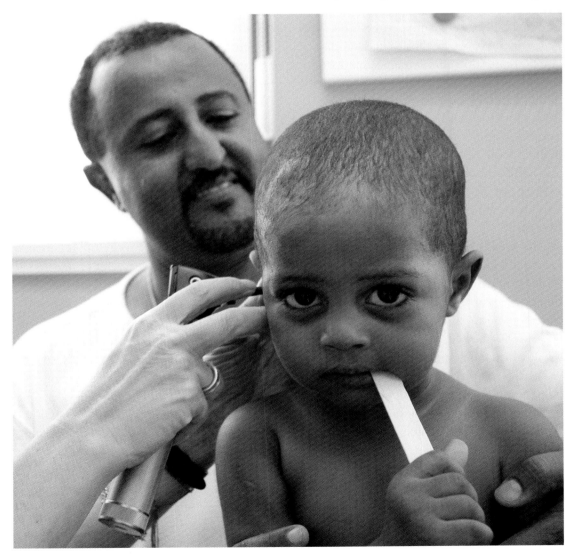

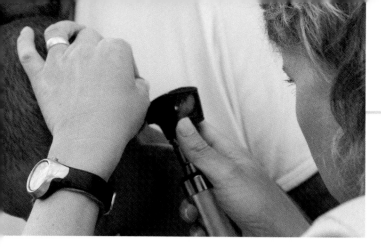

are particularly prone to these infections because they pick up a number of cold viruses, which lead to upper respiratory infections and may result in a buildup of fluid behind the eardrum that cannot drain due to a blocked eustachian tube. This fluid becomes a fertile place for bacteria and viruses to multiply and produce an infection.

Diagnosing ear infections

Most ear infections follow a common cold. Some signs that an ear infection is present include fever, fussiness, and ear rubbing or pulling. Because the pain is more prominent at night, infants with ear infections will often have difficulty sleeping and will wake from sleep.

The pressure buildup behind the eardrum sometimes causes a perforation (hole) in the drum, and fluid may be visible draining out of the ear canal. The child will often feel better as a result, because the pressure is relieved. Holes in the eardrum usually heal well on their own.

Your doctor will confirm the diagnosis of an ear infection, using an instrument called an otoscope to look for redness, swelling, or a perforation in the eardrum.

Treating ear infections

Most ear infections, especially in older children, will resolve on their own within a few days without any treatment, but an oral antibiotic is generally prescribed for children under 2 years of age. Medications for pain and fever, such as acetaminophen (Tylenol, Tempra) or ibuprofen (Advil, Motrin), might be recommended to keep your child comfortable.

Fluid in the middle ear often takes weeks to drain, but it usually does. Rarely, some children will have a persistent buildup of fluid, which can interfere with hearing. If fluid buildup is present for more than several months, your doctor might discuss putting tiny ventilating tubes in the eardrums, a simple operation performed by an ear, nose, and throat surgeon. This short procedure is usually done as day surgery. Ventilating tubes are also inserted if your child's hearing is affected or infections recur frequently.

Roseola

The most common reason for a fever in infants is a viral infection called roseola, caused by human herpes virus 6 (different from the herpes simplex virus that causes cold sores). Three-quarters of children will experience this infection by 1 year of age, most often between 6 and 9 months. The most common symptoms are high fever and fussiness. Roseola characteristically causes a blanching, flat, and slightly raised pinkish rash that typically, though not always, occurs after a few days of fever. The fever generally disappears by the time the rash is apparent, and the rash usually lasts only 1 to 2 days.

Roseola is self-limited and resolves on its own without any specific treatment, though medications, such as acetaminophen or ibuprofen, can be used for fever and discomfort.

Frequently asked questions

As family doctors and pediatricians, we answer many questions from parents. Here are some of the most frequently asked questions. Be sure to ask your health-care providers any other questions that arise. If they don't have the answers, they will refer you to a colleague who does.

Q: My 10-month-old daughter has already caught two colds since starting daycare. Is that normal?
A: For the first few months of life, babies are protected from most childhood infections by antibodies obtained from their mothers before birth. But these antibodies don't last forever. In the second 6 months of life, babies become susceptible to common childhood infections. At daycare centers, there is ample opportunity to be exposed to them. Getting colds is essentially a part of growing up. Immunity from the common childhood illnesses is acquired by infection with the viruses that cause them.

Q: Every time I leave my baby, he gets upset. How am I ever going to go back to work when my maternity leave is over?
A: It's normal for a baby to miss his mother at this age. It's also normal for mothers to be upset when this happens. After all, strong bonds have been formed between you by now. Only you know if returning to work is your best option, and, even so, it is unlikely to be a perfect one. It will be an adjustment for both of you. Take comfort knowing that, in the end, both mother and baby do adjust. The best way to handle returning to work is to ensure that your baby's surrogate caregivers are both capable and affectionate.

Q: As my baby approaches his first birthday, he looks thinner than before. Is there something wrong?
A: Probably not. Children tend to lose their baby fat at this age. They are more mobile and therefore burn more calories. Thinning out is usually a good thing — overweight children tend to become overweight adults. You should be concerned only if your baby is actually losing weight or has persisting symptoms such as prolonged cough or diarrhea.

Q: When and how do I start to bathe my baby in a regular bathtub?
A: Babies are pretty slippery when wet. While it won't harm him to slip underwater momentarily, neither of you is likely to enjoy the experience much. It's best to wait until he can sit properly on his own before switching to a full-size bathtub; otherwise, you won't have enough hands for the job. Make sure the water is the right temperature — comfortably warm to your hand but neither hot nor chilly. Bathing should be fun: a few floating bath toys will convert the bath into a delightful playground. Be prepared. Have everything you need — towels, washcloths, baby

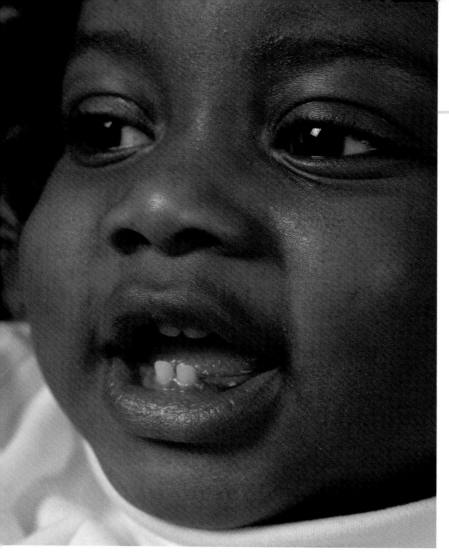

straightening them nicely. By the time they attend nursery school or preschool, children will have their full set of 20 primary teeth.

Q: What can I do for my 7-month-old, who is having a lot of symptoms caused by teething?
A: While drooling, biting, and sucking on things are certainly seen with teething, high fevers, persistent irritability, and diarrhea, despite what you may have heard, are unlikely to be related to teething and should be discussed with your health-care provider. To help with the discomfort, massage the gum with a clean finger or let your baby bite on a cold, wet washcloth or refrigerated teething ring. Teething gels are of questionable value because they don't work for long and can have side effects. The American Academy of Pediatrics does not recommend their use. Similarly, homeopathic remedies should be avoided because it is sometimes difficult to know exactly what they contain — occasionally, they can even be toxic.

shampoo — ready to go. Finally, there must always be a lifeguard on duty. Never leave a baby unattended in the bathtub, even for a moment.

Q: My baby's first tooth didn't erupt until he was 8 months old. Now his teeth seem crooked. What's wrong?
A: Nothing. Of all a baby's milestones, the eruption of the teeth often seems the most variable and least important. The lower incisors usually appear first, but, for many healthy babies, it is the uppers that start the teething experience. In the beginning, baby teeth often appear crooked after eruption. But, as the full set appears, the teeth act as splints for one another,

Q: Now that my baby can cruise the furniture, I've noticed that he appears flat-footed. How could he have developed fallen arches so soon?
A: Flat feet are normal during infancy. The muscles and ligaments that will later maintain the foot's arch are too loose and

flexible to do so at this age. They can't prevent the flattening of the foot when it is bearing weight. Over the course of several years, the joints in the foot gradually tighten, and the arch is then maintained.

Q: My daughter lost her baby hair, and it has not grown back. Should I be concerned?

Many babies lose some or all of their hair during the first few months. The hair that grows back may be quite different, both in color and texture, than the hair they were born with. Some babies remain quite bald for many months, sometimes well into the second year of life. This is most common in very fair babies.

Rest assured that your baby's hair will come in eventually, and that infantile baldness does not predict hair loss in adulthood. There are some very rare disorders that can cause baldness, which can be partial or total, so if you are concerned or the baby has other unusual features, such as very delayed or missing teeth, you should ask your doctor.

Q: I hear that obesity is a major problem in children. Should I be limiting my 1-year-old to low-fat dairy products? Is there anything else I can do to prevent him from being obese when he grows up?

A: You are correct — childhood obesity is becoming a problem; the prevalence of obesity has doubled among 6- to 11-year-olds and tripled among 12- to 17-year-olds over the last 20 years in North America. The probable cause is the underlying human tendency to store fat, which was important for the survival of early man but has now skyrocketed with too much sedentary "activity" (too much television and not enough exercise) and increased consumption of processed high-fat and high-calorie fast foods. Obese children often become obese adults, with multiple serious medical complications, so this is a serious issue.

Nevertheless, the first year of life is a time of extremely rapid growth, and your child's weight will triple over this time. For optimal growth and development, your baby's food intake should not be limited, nor should fat, an important building block, be restricted in any way.

Obesity prevention strategies are controversial. Suggestions for prospective mothers include normalizing body mass index (BMI) prior to pregnancy, not smoking during pregnancy, and maintaining moderate exercise as tolerated. If diabetes develops during the pregnancy, meticulous control of the mother's blood sugar is important. Breast-feeding is preferred for a minimum of 3 months, and solids and especially sweet liquids should not be introduced too early.

As your child gets older, do not allow him to skip meals (especially breakfast), and eat meals as a family at a fixed place and time. Do not allow television during meals! Avoid giving him soft drinks and unnecessarily sweet or fatty foods. Restrict television and video games. Keep TV out of your children's bedrooms. Be a role model by participating in regular family physical exercise, such as walking and cycling. Encourage your child's school to teach physical education.

Sam's Diary

September 8 (7 months old)

You are 7 months old tomorrow — time is going so quickly, it is hard to believe you are this "old" already. Your first couple of weeks with your new nanny, Bambi, went really well. She is really nice — she has a little girl of

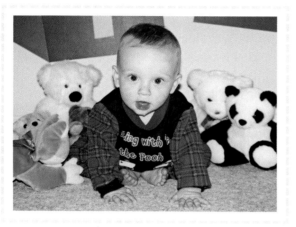

her own, and she's looked after lots of babies. You chat and laugh with her, and she's teaching you to go to sleep more easily during the day. You actually had a 2-hour nap in your crib this afternoon, which is a bit of a record. You are still waking up at irregular times during the night, and we wonder whether you are teething, but so far there's no sign of any teeth.

We've started to wean you because Mom has gone back to work, but you're still nursing at night. You're getting two bottle feeds during the day, and you take the bottle so well you've made it easy for all of us. We've also introduced you to a sippy cup with water, and holding the cup independently seems easy for you.

When Mom is at work, she misses you like crazy and thinks of you all day long; she can't wait to see you in the afternoon. You enjoy going for a run with Dad in the running stroller when he gets home from work. You are also practicing your kneeling and rocking back and forth a lot these days. You are a quick learner and love to copy your mom and dad.

September 26 (7 1/2 months old)

For the last 3 nights you have made it through the night without a feed! You have gone to sleep at 8:00 p.m. and haven't peeped until 7:00 a.m. — we are so excited and proud of you. A couple of weeks ago, Mom and Dad felt your first tooth coming through. You now have two front teeth at the bottom. The new one is quite sharp. You know something is different, as you keep rubbing your tongue over your new tooth. For quite a while now, you've been rocking backwards and forwards on all fours, and a couple of days ago you moved one arm forward — we think you're going to be crawling soon. You look so proud of yourself. You have developed the funniest expressions. Your newest one tells us when you are frustrated and upset: you put both hands on your hips, pull the funniest face, and let out a yell. You are usually fed and clean and have slept, so we guess you are just bored or annoyed. We wish you could tell us what you want!

October 7 (8 months old)

Today you started crawling really well and getting about completely on your own. You crawled to Dad, who was sitting on the couch, just to say hi, and then back to Mom when she called you. You've also learned how to sit up from lying on your stomach, which is a relief because you didn't enjoy being stuck on your tummy. We are having such fun with you! You are exploring everywhere and are attracted most by things we don't want you to touch — telephone cords and electrical sockets. It is a good thing we have childproofed the house. You are eating with your

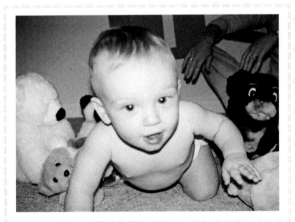

hands now, and your new favorite foods are chicken, bananas, and Bambi's chicken soup. You love trying new things. Today you had grated cheese and a baked potato for the first time. You enjoy trying to feed yourself and lurching forward for the foods you really like.

The other day, you laughed so hard that tears streamed down your face; it was delightful to watch. We were playing peekaboo with some stacking rings, and Mom put one on her head and let it drop off. Other favorite activities include lying in front of the mirror and watching your reflection, banging shapes together, being wrapped in your towel after your bath, being tickled on your tummy and under your arms, and being sung to (especially "Twinkle, Twinkle, Little Star" and "Hey, Samuel, Can You Dance with Me"). Dad and I often talk about how lucky we are to have you — we love you so very much.

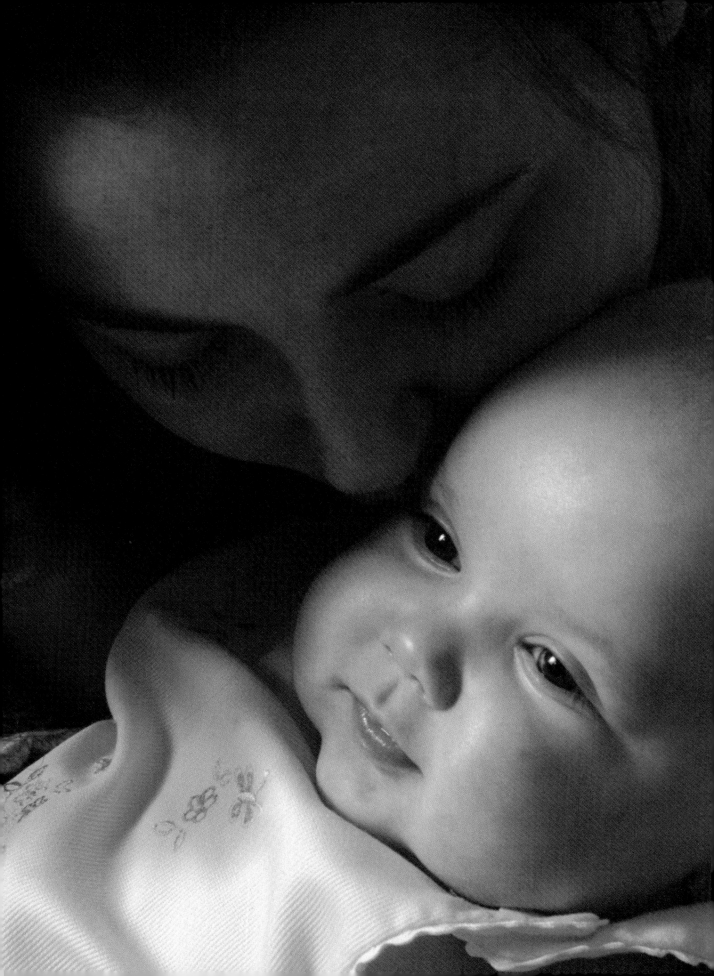

Playing with
Your Baby

The biggest toy of all

Play is the work of babies! Playing with your baby is an important part of parenting. Your baby learns to communicate and interact by playing. Play is also essential for your baby's brain development. Play is a time for you and your baby to enjoy interacting with each other, without distractions. By showing your baby that you enjoy your time with her, you create a relationship that gives her a sense of security and forms the foundation for her relationships with others.

Playtime

Despite what most baby toy companies would have you believe, the most important equipment for playing with your baby is you! Babies love to be close to their parents. Your baby will be most interested in your face and voice, especially during her early months. During this period, your baby will spend most of her playtime listening and looking. As her development progresses, she will begin to interact with her environment and become more interested in touching, feeling, and mouthing objects. And as she becomes upright and eventually mobile, her interests will evolve. Be sure to take into account your baby's stage of development and choose activities and toys appropriate for her abilities.

Where to play

Set aside a safe place, such as an activity mat, where you can spend time playing while keeping both of your hands free. Make things as easy as possible for yourself by having accessible equipment and activities close to the areas where you are likely to be playing with your baby. The early months are generally not a time to focus on keeping your home tidy. Anyone who has had children will expect to see areas with the baby's toys and activities strewn around!

Reading to your Baby

It is never too early to read to your baby. Reading on a daily basis is a great habit to get into. Reading plays an extremely important role in infant and child brain development. Even in the early stages when she doesn't understand the words, your baby will enjoy hearing your voice. Besides the tremendous stimulation it provides, reading encourages a close emotional relationship between you and your baby. Don't be perturbed if she tries to eat the books or handles them roughly — that's why you start off with durable cloth or board books. Your baby may enjoy soft cloth books in black and white or in bright colors.

Read aloud

Start reading aloud to your baby as early as possible, and certainly by the time she is 6 months old. This is a great way for Dad to get involved. In the beginning, you will likely read aloud for only a few minutes at a time, but as she starts to listen and respond, these sessions will get longer.

HOW TO
Play with your baby

Play is a little bit like exercise: you need to practice. If you really want it to work and have staying power, playing has to be enjoyable for both you and your baby. If you listen to your baby, nurture her, let her play, and let her rest, you will be giving her a stimulating start to life. Here are some "exercises" you can try:

- **Choose a time to play when your baby is awake, alert, and relaxed.** This sets the stage for fun and learning. Make sure the time is good for you, too, without the distractions of a busy agenda. You need to be relaxed to play with your baby.

- **Don't be in a hurry.** Choose one activity at a time. Be flexible.

- **Initially, keep play sessions brief — your little one has a very short attention span.** Her ability to handle new sensations is also limited, but will gradually increase as she gets older.

- **Watch for cues that your baby is interested and engaged and wants more — or has had enough and needs a break.** She will give you indications that she's had enough: she will lose attention, gazing away from you or from her activity, or she may become sleepy or cranky.

- **Don't focus on any one activity for too long.** Babies thrive on variety, just like the rest of us. Keep in mind that they don't need to be constantly entertained.

- **Don't overstimulate your baby.** In the early days, simple things such as your face, patterns of light or color, and soft noises are new and interesting. Give her time to experience and explore new things before moving on.

- **Allow your baby quiet time when she needs it.** It may be time for a nap or simply to lie awake and absorb her surroundings. Although all babies enjoy and need loving interaction, the amounts of playtime and quiet time that are right for them vary.

- **Laugh with your baby.** Laughter is a fulfilling experience that is not only fun but is also extremely healthy for both of you.

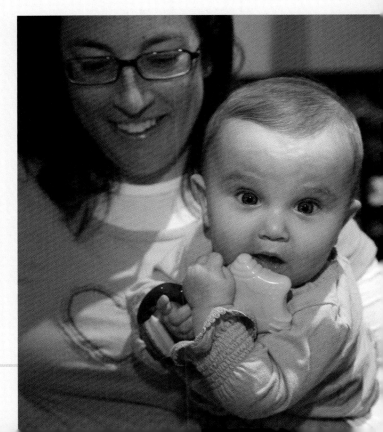

Reading together

As they get closer to 1 year of age, babies are able to hold a book and turn the pages. Start to point to things and name them. If your baby loses interest or is easily distracted, skip to a favorite page or put the book down and try again later. As she gets older, set aside a regular time each day for reading.

Visits to the public library or a local bookstore are another great habit to get into when she reaches the toddler years. You will both enjoy this outing.

Favorite stories

Most babies enjoy hearing the same story over and over again. This is normal — children learn through repetition. Books with nursery rhymes and those with familiar objects for naming are great. Songs and rhymes make words easier to remember, making the language come alive. Reading books and stories, chanting rhymes, and singing songs should become part of your baby's daily routine. This kind of play will not only help her brain develop, but will nurture a lifelong love of reading.

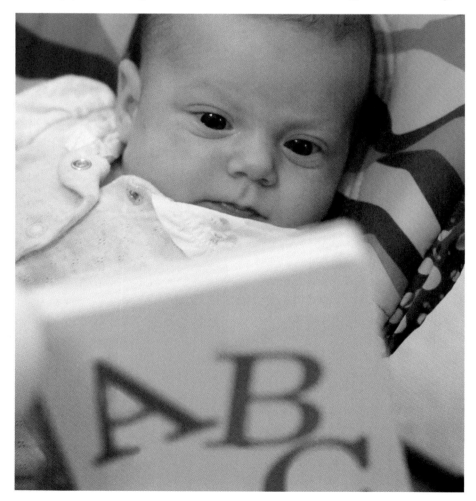

Playing during the first year

First month

During your baby's first month, most of her time and energy (and yours!) will be focused on feeding, sleeping, and growing. Even so, spending time interacting with her during awake and alert periods is important for her development and your developing relationship with her. A baby at this age might not seem to share your enthusiasm for the interaction, but she will still benefit from it.

Kinds of play

Most of your play at this stage will consist of cuddling, rocking, singing, and talking to your newborn. She may spend periods of time gazing at an object or your face. Remember that her vision is not yet fully developed. In the first month, babies find it easiest to see large objects with strong contrast, such as black and white patterns or an adult's face close to theirs. Although your baby cannot see perfectly yet, looking at faces and patterns when she is awake and alert helps her brain and vision develop.

Your baby is also learning to understand the sounds she hears. Soft cooing, talking, and singing help her with this developmental task. As she grows, you will start to see her turning toward your voice. Soon, your baby will learn to distinguish your voice from a stranger's.

Months 2 to 3

Your baby is not yet on the move and cannot talk or show you the toys she prefers. How are you supposed to play with her? In fact, there are many ways for you to interact with your baby at a level appropriate for her age and development. Your relationship with her began the moment she was born, and the way you interact with her will continue to change as she grows. Think about what stage of development your baby is at — it will guide you in your interaction and play. Follow your instincts and have fun!

Smiling

Babies usually start to smile by 6 weeks of age. Try smiling at your baby when she is alert, and look for that rewarding smile back! Teach her to interact by responding with a delighted sound or a soft touch when she smiles at you.

Did You Know?

Toys for newborns

You have probably been anticipating playing with your newborn and may have been given toys around the time she was born. However, at this age your baby is not yet developmentally ready to play with toys. Your face and voice and a mobile to look at are sufficient.

Talking

Your baby now enjoys listening to voices and is beginning to coo and make sounds. Encourage her by looking at her and slowly repeating similar sounds. Watch her watch your mouth with interest. Of course, there is no need to limit your speech to "baby talk." Talk as you would normally. Tell her what you are doing as you go about your day. Read books and sing to her. These habits will all contribute to her learning about language and about you.

Naming

Try to make a habit of referring to yourself and those around you in the third person, as Mommy and Daddy, for example. Though your baby is not yet ready to comprehend what you are saying, this will make understanding easier when the time comes.

Cuddling, rocking, and singing songs

These activities will be fun for your baby and may have having a calming or soothing effect. Choose lullabies and nursery rhymes, such as "Twinkle, Twinkle, Little Star" and "Rock-a-bye Baby."

Sitting up

As your baby's head control begins to improve, you can set her down in different positions, with assistance, providing her with a new perspective on the world. Prop her up in a sitting position or gently raise her horizontally into the air, like an airplane.

Did You Know?

Tummy time

Because "back to sleep" programs recommend that babies be put to sleep on their backs to decrease the risk of sudden infant death syndrome (SIDS), babies may spend very little time on their tummies. As a result, they may lack the opportunity to develop the corresponding muscles.

To develop these muscles, "tummy time" is an important activity for babies. While she is awake, set your baby on her tummy for a few minutes at a time, always under close supervision. Some babies will enjoy this time, while others will scream until they're picked up.

Don't force your baby into tummy time. Continue to try it regularly; eventually, your baby's head control and arm strength will allow her to feel more comfortable and happy in this position. Many parents find it helpful to put a mirror on the floor during tummy time. Lean over the mirror with your baby so that she can enjoy both of your reflections, which will gradually hold her attention for longer periods of time.

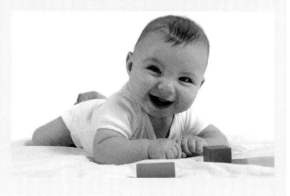

Did You Know ?

Bathing playtime
Bath time and diaper changes (which are still pretty often) are excellent opportunities to talk to, sing to, and tickle your baby. You want these activities to be fun in addition to fulfilling their function. They are also great times for other family members to get involved in playing and interacting with the baby, especially if they are unable to help with the feeding. Remember that head control is still being established, so the baby's head and neck need to be comfortably supported during any activities.

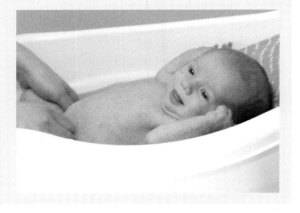

Tickling

Now that your baby is smiling more and even beginning to laugh, play tickle games by establishing an association between a rhyme and a final tickle. One easy game is to trace a circle on her tummy, saying, "Round and round the garden goes the teddy bear," then head toward her neck or underarms, "one step, two step," and add a final tickle, "tickle you under there!" With repetition, your baby will anticipate the finale and begin to laugh before she has even been tickled. "This Little Piggy" is another popular rhyme with a similar effect. She is enjoying learning about different sensations, so touch her softly, move her legs in a bicycling motion if she enjoys it, or try blowing softly on her toes. Find sensations she enjoys — you will be delighted by her response to them.

Outings

You will now be ready to get out of the house more often. Allow your baby to see what is going on in the world! Show her the grass, leaves, and flowers, and talk to her gently about what she is seeing. She will enjoy looking at patterns of light and shadows and feeling a light breeze or warm sunshine if the weather permits.

Remember to dress her appropriately for the weather and protect her from the sun, cold, and insect bites. Staying indoors can be monotonous — the fresh air and change in surroundings are good for both of you.

Safe play

At this stage, your baby's head control is still developing, so make sure you are with her during tummy time and other activities. If she falls asleep, place her on her back. Babies at this stage cannot grasp and move objects. Make sure your baby is always in a safe position, with her head and face unobstructed and away from soft blankets or toys that could interfere with her breathing. Toys should be soft, without sharp edges or small detachable parts.

Guide to

The best toys

There are many expenses involved in having children, but toys and play equipment do not need to use up your resources. A couple of bright rattles and a soft toy are nice to have, along with a mobile for your baby's crib. Otherwise, all your baby needs is a loving parent and a nurturing environment. You'll be surprised at how fascinating your fingers can be to a baby — an "open and shut" game provides endless amusement.

Given that they are rarely used for more than a few months, toys can be borrowed from friends. Garage sales are another good source of toys, particularly for older infants.

Rattles and mobiles

You will likely notice that your baby intently regards her surroundings and has begun to follow objects. Babies enjoy

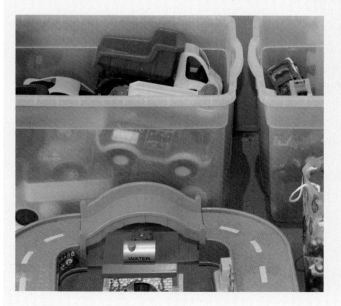

looking at bold black and white patterns, as well as bright colors. With your baby lying on her back, show her some bright toys or rattles, moving them up and down and from side to side. Move the toy slowly up away from her face, toward the ceiling. She might begin to reach for the object, though don't expect her to successfully grab it at this stage.

If you place a rattle in your baby's hand, she will learn to grasp it and eventually give it a shake. She'll be delighted with the sounds she is helping to make, and may even reward you with a smile!

Other ways to stimulate your child visually include hanging a mobile above her crib or putting black and white or brightly colored pictures on the ceiling above her change table. Just make sure that when your baby is able to sit up, around 5 to 6 months, she can't get entangled with the mobile above her crib or change table.

Activity mats and swings

Other popular items include seats that gently rock, in which the baby is harnessed securely; activity mats with toys hanging from above; and swings, which babies often find soothing. By no means are all of these big-ticket items essential. It is most practical to borrow them from friends or purchase them second-hand, as your baby may decide she is not a "swinger" or doesn't particularly like the seat. Even if she does like them, she will soon outgrow them.

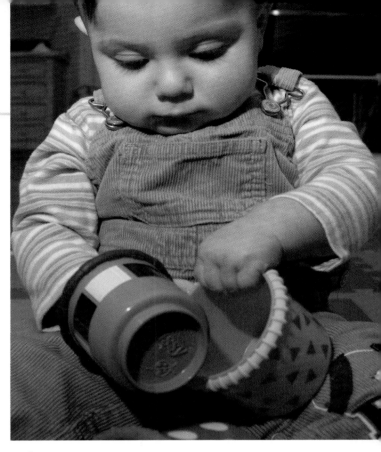

Months 4 to 6

This is a very exciting time of your baby's life. She is still an infant, and is not yet mobile, but she is becoming increasingly interactive and fun. Playing with your baby will both stimulate her development and bring you tremendous joy.

Continue to introduce your baby to the world around her during this stage. Many babies look with wide-eyed wonder at the bustle on the street or the produce in the grocery store. Talk to your baby about what she is looking at, encouraging her natural curiosity. Make a habit of describing what you are doing and seeing as you go about your daily activities.

Bear in mind your baby's developmental stage when considering appropriate toys and games to play. Her head and trunk control is increasingly strong, so she may be able to play sitting upright, with your support, as she gets closer to 6 months old. If you have a breast-feeding pillow, it can be used as a convenient support to prop her up. Otherwise, just use regular pillows.

Continue to place your baby on her tummy regularly. She'll soon be able to lift up her head and chest, which will make it a more comfortable position in which to look around and play.

Keep in mind that no equipment is essential; it is certainly not necessary to have everything. A varied and stimulating environment, provided by a loving and nurturing parent, is the only essential ingredient for happy playtime with your little one.

Object games

Try playing object games. Roll a ball on the ground and watch her as she learns to kick it with her feet or pick it up. As she learns to roll over, encourage her by showing her toys on either side; as she tries to reach out for them, she will bring her body along.

Play with your baby in a variety of positions and offer a variety of activities. This will give her the opportunity to develop different muscle groups and observe from different perspectives. She may still enjoy being under an activity arch or may prefer to be upright in a bouncy chair. Bounce her on your lap, play with her on her tummy or back, and gently fly her through the air. To encourage development of her reach and balance, hand toys to her from different angles and opposite sides of her body when she is in a sitting position.

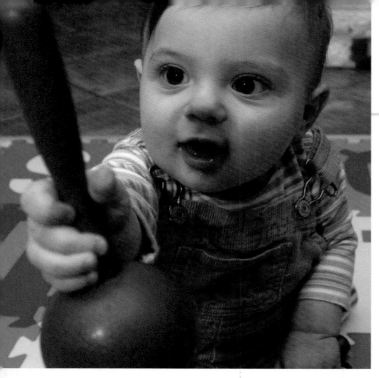

Word games

Your baby will also be vocalizing more during this stage of development. Around 4 months, you may notice that when you make a cooing sound or talk to your baby softly, she responds with a sound back. With another sound from you, she may again respond. She is learning the basics of conversation!

As she continues to develop, she will start to play with sounds. If you make a funny noise, such as blowing a raspberry, you may get a laugh from her, and she may start to try to imitate you. Through this lively interaction, you are teaching her the basics of imitating sounds — an important skill that will help her learn to talk. As she starts to babble, around 6 months of age, she will enjoy hearing you imitate her sounds. Continue to talk to her as you go about your everyday activities. The sound of your voice and the words she hears will help her continue to learn basic language skills.

Tickling games

Tickling games are even more fun now, as your little one learns to anticipate your play.

Wiggle your fingers and say, "I'm going to get you" or "Here I come," getting closer and closer until you end in a tickle and giggle! Although many babies find this fun, some find it too much or can engage in this stimulating play only very briefly. Watch for your baby's cues and choose activities she enjoys, ending when she has had enough.

Action songs

As she becomes more interested in her environment, your baby will love watching and listening to action songs. Try "Itsy Bitsy Spider" or "I'm a Little Teapot." Nursery songs, as well as children's rhymes, are often a favorite with children of this age. If you have forgotten these songs, check your library or stores that sell recordings for children. You can both listen to and learn from them.

Bathing games

Bath time can still be fun. Trickle water gently over your baby's tummy or toes and look for a delighted reaction. Try swishing the water gently and using your baby's hands or feet to gently splash the water. If your baby enjoys water play, slowly pour water from a cup and watch her look and listen to the new experience. This is a great time to start labeling body parts, telling your baby, for example, "We're washing your tummy."

Age-appropriate toys

Apart from toys to grasp, chew, and roll, very little additional equipment is needed. Provide your baby with colorful toys that she can easily grasp, pick up, and eventually transfer between her hands. Rattles,

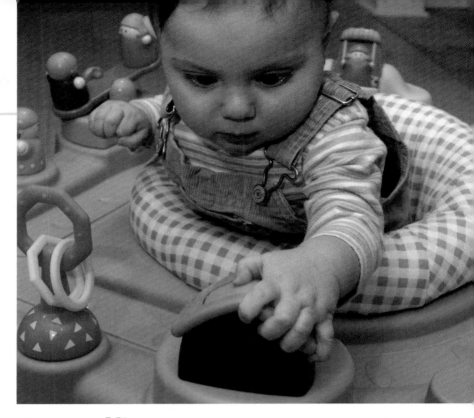

hard plastic rings that loop together, or plastic balls with holes for her to grasp are good examples of appropriate toys for this age. If your baby is teething, hard plastic teething rings can be cooled in the refrigerator and make good toys for your baby to play with and chew on. Provide a variety of textures for your little one to explore.

At this stage, your baby will start to use these toys in a more sophisticated way. Now, instead of simply gazing at and reaching out for toys, your baby can hold them. She's learning to shake a rattle, she's beginning to pick objects up, and she's likely putting everything (including her own toes) in her mouth. This is her way of exploring new things; providing that the objects are safe, this behavior should not be discouraged.

Introduce soft toys or stuffed animals, as well as objects with different gentle textures. Soft toys can get dusty and collect germs, so make sure they are washable. Try to find toys that produce gentle musical noises as opposed to loud, irritating sirens. If the noises are really obnoxious, the batteries can always be removed as a last resort! Activity centers with colorful, bright, textured toys to touch, spin, and look at are often a favorite. As you take your baby out of the home more, you may choose some toys that can be safely fastened to the stroller or car seat. Brightly colored cloth or board books with a single picture on each page are appropriate at this stage.

Mirror games

Babies generally become increasingly social during these months. They begin to recognize people, and they enjoy admiring themselves in the mirror! Many toys incorporate mirrors for babies to gaze at, but your own bathroom mirror works just as well. Hold your baby while you stand in front of a mirror, wave, and talk to her. She will likely be delighted at seeing both her reflection and yours.

Exersaucer

Your baby may be ready to play in an exersaucer during this time. An exersaucer is a stationary ring that surrounds the baby and holds stimulating toys to keep her entertained. Ensure that it is used as recommended at the appropriate height (this can usually be adjusted for your baby's growth over the coming months). Exersaucers should be used for short periods at a time — usually no more than 20 minutes. Keep it away from dangers such as hanging appliance cords or stairs.

Playpens

A playpen can provide a safe environment for an infant, but remember that it needs to meet safety standards. It should be sturdy. The slats should be close together, and mesh should have small openings. Don't put anything inside that could be used to help an older infant climb out.

Your baby needs to be out and about, exploring her environment, so use the playpen in moderation and only for short periods at a time.

Months 7 to 12

During her second 6 months of life, your baby will achieve several major milestones, which will have a tremendous impact on how she is able to play. Her newfound abilities will open up a whole new world of fun and exploration.

Major milestones

- **Sitting unsupported:** The first major gross motor milestone is the ability to sit unsupported, which is usually mastered around 7 months of age. While this opens up a bunch of new options, the next milestone is really a big one.
- **Becoming mobile:** Toward the end of the first year of life, most babies become mobile — crawling, rolling, creeping, cruising, and ultimately walking. Her mobility is going to change things dramatically for everyone concerned. If you haven't already fully childproofed your home, don't wait any longer!
- **Advanced fine motor skills:** Tremendous advances in fine motor skills also occur at this age. Your baby will progress from a coarse full-handed grasp to the much more refined pincer grasp. She will be able to pick up and manipulate small objects between her thumb and index finger. Remember that she is positioned very close to the ground, and any small objects, including choking hazards, will become potential toys to be explored and put in her mouth. So beware!

Age-appropriate activities

As a result of your baby's rapidly developing skills, appropriate toys and activities for this age group change substantially from the predominantly sensory toys recommended for younger infants. Now she will begin to enjoy activities that involve moving, banging,

---

Did You Know?

Baby walkers

Baby walkers have been banned in many countries, including Canada, because they are extremely dangerous for babies. Many children are injured every year while in a walker, usually under the close supervision of a parent. Infants in a walker can move more than 3 feet (1 m) in 1 second, and children have rolled down stairs, gotten burned, and even drowned. If you are given an old baby walker, get rid of it immediately!

pulling, squeezing, pouring, throwing, opening, closing, inserting, and removing.

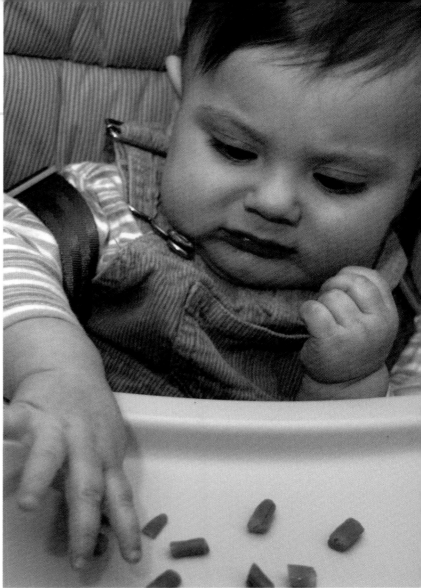

- **Interactive games:** There are many interactive games you can play with your baby. She will start to engage in activities such as peekaboo, hiding and uncovering games, imitating sounds and actions, and a great, timeless favorite — baby drops the object, adult picks it up. Most children of this age love bath time and water activities. Your encouraging words, clapping, and enthusiastic "hurrays" as you interact will encourage your baby's play and build her confidence in her growing abilities.
- **Toys:** Many age-appropriate toys are available, specifically designed by toy manufacturers for this age group. Stacking blocks, rings, or cups, objects that fit into each other, and pop-up boxes are very popular. Infants like to push and follow movable toys, such as large balls and cars. Some babies enjoy simple puzzles. Simple household items such as plastic cups, containers, and pots can provide hours of entertainment, learning opportunities, and noise!
- **Books:** Many 6- to 12-month-old children will start to develop a real interest in books. Simple, colorful illustrated books made of cloth, plastic, or cardboard are ideal, as many young children are able to manipulate the large, thick pages, and the books are relatively resistant to being torn, soaked, or chewed. Talk to your baby in simple language about the pictures in the book. Label objects and point to them. Choose books that have large pictures of other babies or familiar objects such as toys and animals, or books that illustrate familiar experiences, such as bath time or mealtime. Books with large flaps that lift up, uncovering an interesting picture underneath, are popular and encourage fine motor development.

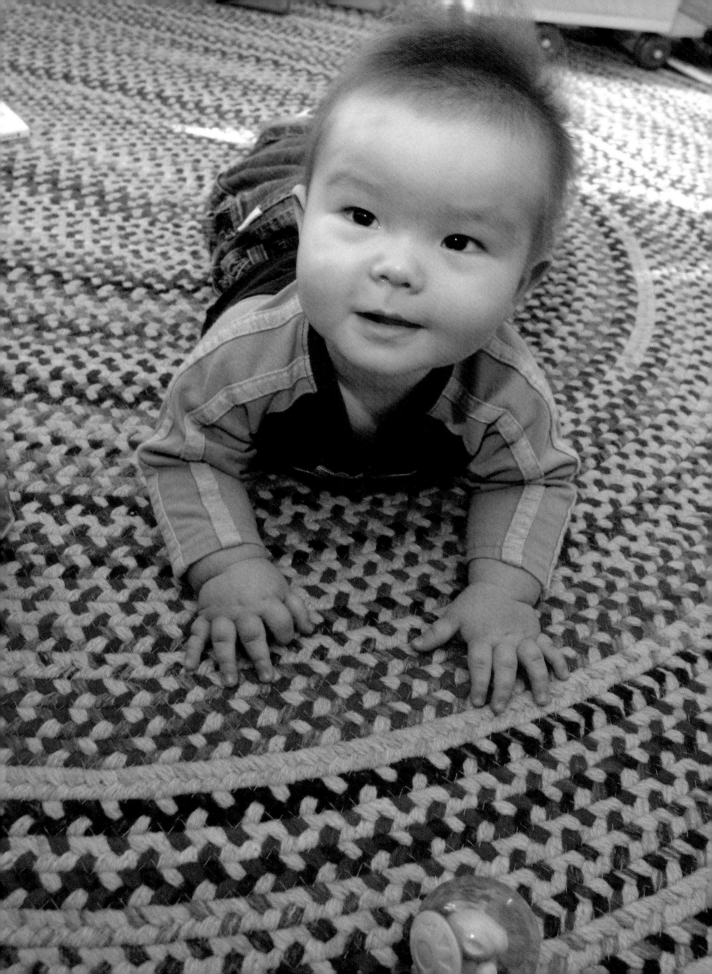

Guide to

Safe toys

Toy safety is paramount for infants, who have developed skills that allow for manipulation and motion, but have no awareness of potential harm. Toy manufacturers in North America are required to follow stringent safety laws — for example, you will notice that toys with small parts that could present choking hazards are labeled as such. Be aware that toys made in other countries may not be as strictly regulated as those made in North America.

Safety tips

Keep these safety tips in mind when you buy toys for your baby:

- **Size:** Be sure the toy is too big to fit in a baby's mouth, ears, or nose.
- **Small parts:** Avoid toys with small parts that could choke your baby. Toys intended for older children may have dangerous small pieces, so pay attention to age recommendations.
- **Solid construction:** Test toys to be sure they are well constructed and will not break easily. Eyes and noses on soft toys should be sturdily fastened. Ensure that toy boxes have a tight lid and supportive hinges.
- **Sharp edges:** Avoid toys with sharp or pointed edges.
- **Safe materials:** Make sure toys are made from a safe material intended for small babies, and avoid items decorated with paint that may chip off — it may

be toxic. Be sure any fabric used in making the toy is not flammable.

- **Hazards:** Avoid toys with strings or cords that pose a strangulation hazard. Never allow your child to play with balloons, which can cause choking and asphyxiation.
- **Walkers:** Do not use baby walkers with wheels. They can result in severe injuries.
- **Batteries:** Replace batteries in battery-operated toys frequently.
- **Cleanliness:** Be sure toys can be washed or cleaned easily.
- **Packaging:** Safely dispose of all plastic wrappings and bags.

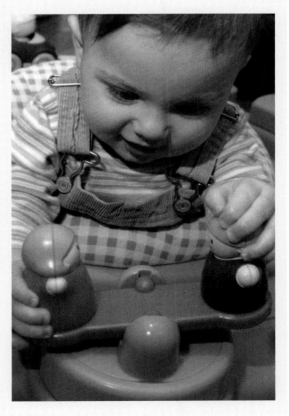

Frequently asked questions

As family doctors and pediatricians, we answer many questions from parents. Here are some of the most frequently asked questions. Be sure to ask your health-care providers any other questions that arise. If they don't have the answers, they will refer you to a colleague who does.

Q: When my sister visits, she usually brings along her own young toddler. My 11-month-old son notices her, but doesn't seem interested in playing. Is my son anti-social, or even autistic?
A: Most children don't engage in interactive play until they are beyond infancy. Most 11-month-old babies will notice and react to other children, but their play is "parallel" rather than interactive. On the other hand, it is reasonable to expect your son to notice his cousin, make eye contact, and play games such as peekaboo with adults.

Q: I understand what play is for a toddler or school-aged child, but what constitutes play for a very young infant?
A: The games that children or, for that matter, adults play clearly differ from play during infancy. But there are common themes to what is considered play that are independent of age. To play is to be pleasantly occupied; it is to be amused. Play requires involvement. That means play should be active rather than passive. And, to some degree, performance is also a key component of play.

Infants instinctively like the stimulation of their senses. Discovering sounds, be they musical or vocal, can constitute play. So can looking in a mirror. Play can also be discovery through touching objects. For an infant, the world around her is one giant playpen. If only adults could retain such joie de vivre.

Q: My 10-month-old daughter has just started to crawl. What are some appropriate games to play with her?
A: There are an infinite number of games to play with a child at this age: counting fingers and toes, playing hide and seek or peekaboo, associating words or sounds or even smells with objects, stacking two or three cubes. Of course, reading books with your child is a wonderful way to spend quieter times together. The most important thing is to make sure your child has the opportunity to explore the world around her. Finally, it's essential to appreciate that children need to be engaged, but not overstimulated.

Q: We have a 6-month-old son and would like to get a dog. Do you have any suggestions?
A: For millions of families, life is richly enhanced by the presence of a family pet. By all means, get one — just not necessarily now. Remember that puppies are babies too. Training and caring for them takes a lot of work. With a 6-month-old in the home, you are probably stretched pretty thin

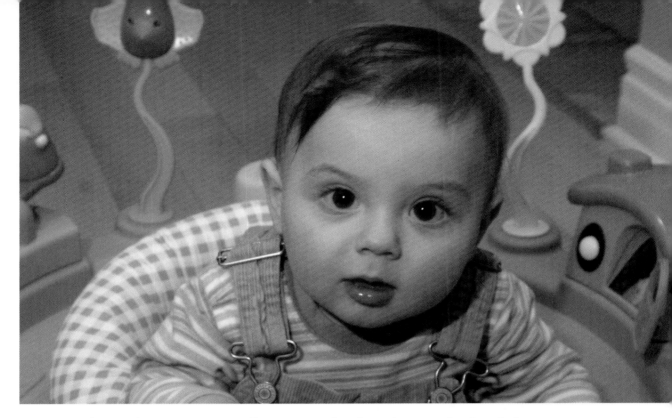

already. So first make sure you are really ready for a dog.

If, after careful reflection, you still want a dog now, here are some suggestions. Pick a breed known for its good disposition and tolerance of children. If allergies run in the family, a dog that doesn't shed is a good idea.

Try to socialize your dog with people, especially other children, and with other dogs. A well-behaved dog will be a lot easier to deal with, so enroll in a puppy obedience program.

Never leave your baby and the dog alone together. Be sure that the dog's food is out of baby's reach: turf wars can get ugly, and your baby may not appreciate the fact that tasting the dog's dinner isn't very smart. Finally, dog feces must be cleaned up immediately.

Q: Are exersaucers bad for my baby's development?
A: No. And, for busy parents, they can be very useful. Exersaucers are commonly used, safe, and practical aids to help you entertain your baby. As long as you use them in moderation and do not leave your baby in one for hours, they will not have any negative effects on your baby.

Q: I speak English and my husband speaks French. Is it a good idea to expose our baby to both languages from the beginning? I've heard different opinions.
A: You've heard different opinions because it is a matter of personal choice. Babies and young children are very quick to pick up languages, and even though they may mix them up a little initially, they will ultimately master both of them. A second language is often part of a family's history and culture, and this will be an important part of your baby's life in the future. Whether you start from birth or wait until your child is a few years old, use the second language as you do the first — interspersed in the regular activities of day-to-day life, including play and reading.

Sam's Diary

November 4 (9 months old)

You are so proud of yourself — you now know how to clap. You clap when you hear the song "When You're Happy and You Know It." The other night, you surprised us by clapping with the audience when a contestant got the correct answer while you were watching *Jeopardy* with Dad! You can wave hello and goodbye, and you enjoy knocking on the front door with the knocker. Your fourth tooth has just come through, and you are a bit sick with a cold. You don't like having your nose cleaned, but you

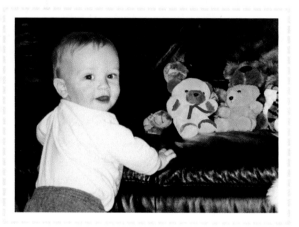

breathe better when it isn't all blocked up. You are also not keen on having your diaper changed or getting dressed. You are a strong little man and put up a good fight.

December 9 (10 months old)

We are on vacation, having a wonderful time visiting with both sets of grandparents and your 103-year-old great-granny, Tilly. You've spent hours "talking" to her, and we are capturing it on video so you will remember her when you are older. We think you like her smiley, wrinkly face, and she is crazy about you. You are also having fun with all of the aunts and uncles you are meeting for the first time. You are thriving with all the attention and delighting people wherever you go. You particularly like to sit with your grandpa watching the cars, and you enjoy letting your granny bathe you and sing to you. You loved the tape recorder we bought for you and listened to all your favorite songs on the airplane. You were too big for the SkyCot, so you slept on Mom and Dad and played beautifully when you were awake. Quite a few of the passengers commented on how good you were, considering you were on the plane for 14 hours.

You are now pulling up to stand and have started to walk while holding on to furniture. You also understand so many things — you look for and fetch your ball when we ask, and you hand us things when we say "Ta." You had your first visit to a real beach and loved the soft white sand and the sea. Unfortunately, you're not that crazy about wearing your sun hat and managed to get out of wearing it for a while by dropping it in the sea.

January 9 (11 months old)

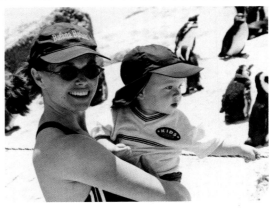

Last week you climbed up the stairs on all fours, with Mom behind you, and you were very impressed with yourself when you got to the top. You have also started to stand all alone for a few seconds before sitting down. You are happy to walk behind your toy car or push a chair, and yesterday you walked with Dad, holding on with just one hand. When you read this, I'm sure it will be strange to think that you haven't always walked. Each new milestone is exciting, and more so because you are so

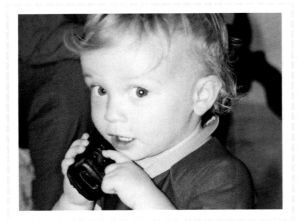

pleased with yourself. You still love reading and will often pick up a book, then motion that you want to climb onto our laps. Reading is a special time — you turn the pages beautifully and will often "read" aloud yourself. Yesterday we all went to the library. After spending some time reading and watching the other kids, we took out a bunch of new books to read at home.

You love to talk on the telephone. When you hear it ring, you put anything to your ear and start talking away. You are going through a really affectionate stage and will often come for a tight squeeze with your little hands around our neck and your head on our shoulders.

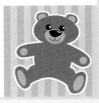

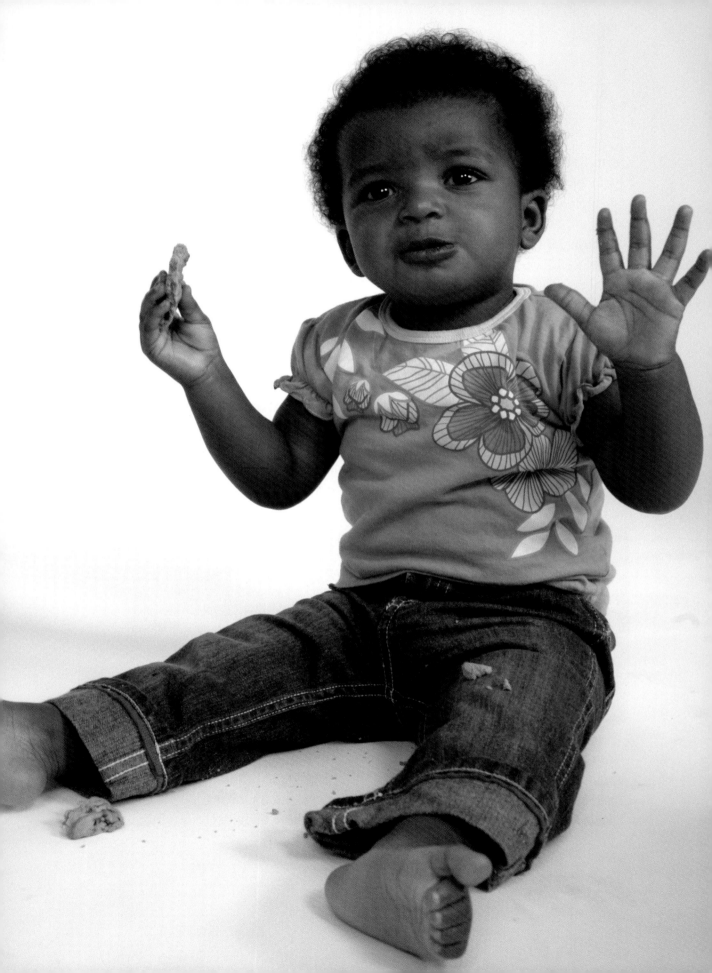

PART 10

Protecting
Your Baby

Prevention is always better than cure

One of a parent's worst nightmares is that their infant will injure himself, and for good reason: injuries are the greatest cause of death and disability for children in North America. The numbers are staggering — in Canada alone, 900 children die every year from their injuries and over 40,000 are hospitalized. In the United States, approximately 5,000 children die each year from accidental injuries — 40% occur at home. Thousands more infants and young children require visits to the emergency room or a physician's office because of various accidents.

It doesn't have to be that way. Common sense, in the form of appropriate supervision, advance planning, and "childproofing" your home, will prevent most accidents. When accidents do occur, you can prepare yourself and even save your child by learning first aid.

New motor skills

Infants achieve two significant developmental milestones during the second 6 months of life: first, increased mobility in the form of rolling, creeping, crawling, or walking; and second, finger dexterity — the pincer grasp — which enables them to pick up small objects. While these milestones are wonderful achievements, allowing your child to explore his exciting new world, they also present opportunities for accidents and injury. Children generally acquire motor skills long before they have the intellectual ability to recognize danger. For this reason, it is very important to make sure that your child's environment is rendered as safe as possible.

A growing number of businesses specialize in providing child safety advice and devices. If it's practical, visit one of these stores before your baby's arrival or before his graduation from babe-in-arms to inquisitive, mobile little person. You might not prevent all of the bumps and bruises of infancy, but you can try to reduce the likelihood of serious injury.

Did You Know?

Common accidents

Suffocation and choking are the injuries that most often result in death in the first year of life. Falling is the one that most frequently results in hospitalization. Other common accidents include burns, drowning, and poisoning.

Many of these injuries occur in the home.

Childproofing basics

Even the most obsessive parent will not be able to supervise every second of a baby's first year. Bearing this in mind, the three most important factors influencing accidents are your baby's age, temperament, and environment. Because you have little control over the first two factors, most of your efforts should be geared toward removing hazards from your baby's surroundings.

See like a child

To minimize the risk of accidents, try to see the world through the eyes of an inquisitive infant. Get down on all fours and see what you could potentially pull down or grasp. You also need to anticipate the dangers that might accompany each new developmental milestone. For example, you won't want to remember that the first time your baby rolled over was when he fell from the changing table!

Look for hazards

Pay attention to hazards that can injure your baby, such as sharp corners, cords for blinds or curtains, and electrical outlets and wires. Staircases can be extremely dangerous. Small objects, including toys with small pieces, small batteries, jewelry, and stones, are potential choking hazards; make sure they are inaccessible.

Remove temptations

When your baby starts to move around in the second 6 months, be aware that he is not developmentally capable of remembering that you told him not to play with the electrical cord, even if you have told him 20 times. He is not being "naughty"; he is merely behaving like any other inquisitive 9-month-old. It is your job to remove any dangers and temptations.

Beware of imitation

As much pleasure as you will get when he copies your "pat-a-cake," he is equally likely to copy other activities that could be dangerous. For example, he may attempt to swallow tablets or use a razor to shave his legs.

Don't be distracted

Studies suggest that babies are most at risk when you are distracted, they have acquired a new skill, they are tired and hungry, or they are out of their regular environment.

Supervise

Certainly childproof your baby's environment as meticulously as possible, but there is no substitute for vigilance and supervision. Unless they are asleep in their cribs, infants should not be left alone. Parents should never leave their baby alone in the bathtub or near water. Children can drown in only a few inches or centimeters of water. Nor should babies be left unsupervised with young children, who are notorious for poking and prodding or trying to feed the baby inappropriate food as soon as the adult leaves the room.

No hot drinks

Never drink or hold hot liquid when holding your child — a spill could scald your baby. Using a cup with a lid can be helpful. And never leave glasses or cups of alcohol lying around the house.

Making your home safe for your baby

Childproofing your home will not only protect your child from injury, but will also increase the pleasure you derive from your baby's increasing mobility and independence because you won't have to worry about his safety. Here are some guidelines for making your home safe for your baby, room by room.

Bedroom

Although the bedroom is a place of comfort, it can also be a dangerous place if cribs, change tables, and other furniture are not safe. Follow these guidelines for furnishing your child's bedroom safely.

Safe cribs and bedding

SAFETY STANDARDS
When buying a crib, whether new or used, make sure it meets current safety standards. Cribs made before 1986 are generally not considered safe.

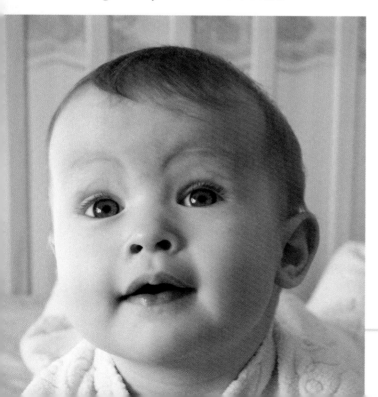

MATTRESSES
A mattress should be firm and should fit snugly into the crib, with no room for tiny limbs to get stuck. Set the mattress lower when your baby starts to sit and at its lowest position when he can stand. Never leave the side of the crib down — he should never be allowed to roll out or be tempted to climb out.

BEDDING
When you put your baby down to sleep, he will need a sheet, but no pillows, bumper pads, comforters, stuffed toys, or soft objects, all of which have been shown to increase the risk of sudden infant death syndrome (SIDS).

LOCATION OF CRIBS
Cribs should be placed away from the window, clear of blind or curtain cords, which can strangle an older baby.

MOBILES AND GYMS
If you use a crib mobile, ensure that your baby cannot reach it. Crib "gyms" should be removed when he can get up on all fours.

Did You Know?

SIDS prevention

Most parents want to decorate the crib with baby gifts, but when it is time for sleep, take all the pretty things out. To minimize the risk of sudden infant death syndrome (SIDS), put your baby to sleep on his back, lightly clothed, with only a sheet for bedding. Do not overheat him. Avoid bedding that could interfere with the air circulation around your baby's head.

The risks increase if you bed-share with your baby, especially if you or your partner smokes, is significantly overweight, or has consumed alcohol, drugs, or any medications that would make you drowsy.

Diaper changing tables

Never leave your baby unattended on a changing table or bed — you never know when he will decide to roll for the first time. Keep diapers and a fresh set of clothing within easy reach, and always keep one hand on the baby. Don't let your baby play with the baby powder container — particles can be inhaled if he opens it. Keep his hands off disposable diapers; a baby can choke on pieces of the plastic lining.

Window blinds

When your infant starts to move around, make sure all window blind and curtain cords are clamped far out of reach.

Wastebaskets

Wastebaskets should either be covered or out of reach of prying little hands.

Toy boxes

Toy boxes can be dangerous. Injuries are occasionally caused when the lid falls on the child's head or body, and children can get stuck inside. The safest ones have no lid. Better yet, store your child's toys in open and easily accessible places.

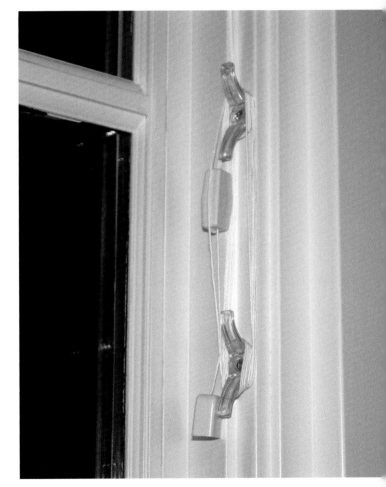

■ All curtain and blind cords should be clamped to the window frame, far out of your child's reach.

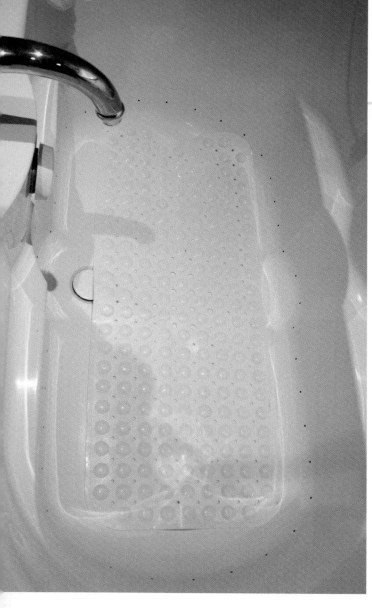

■ Non-slip mats make bathing safer.

Bathroom

Most important of all — never, ever leave your infant or toddler unsupervised in the bath. Children can drown in as little as 1.5 inches (4 cm) of water. If you have to answer the telephone or doorbell, wrap your child in a towel and take him with you.

Non-slip mats and tap covers

Use a non-slip mat on the bottom of the bathtub. Protective covers for the spout of the tap are also available.

Bath seats and rings

Although infant bath seats and rings may be helpful, be very careful when using one. Many infants have drowned while placed in their bath seat. They are not recommended. In any event, always watch your baby very closely in the bath.

Locks

A lock on the outside of the bathroom door to keep out little people who don't need to be in there can be helpful. Do not use a locking mechanism that allows children to lock themselves inside the bathroom.

Did You Know?

Water temperature

Water heaters in North American homes are often set to 140°F (60°C). At this temperature, severe burns can occur within 1 to 5 seconds of contact with water! To prevent scalding burns, set your home water heater to no more than 120°F (50°C). At temperatures below 120°F (50°C), water will take 2 to 10 minutes to cause a severe burn, which gives you much more time to prevent scalding by getting your baby out of the water.

A single tap for both hot and cold is best, but if they are separate, get into the habit of switching the cold tap on first.

Toilet lids

Infants and young toddlers are fascinated by the toilet — that is, until you want them to use it during toilet training! To prevent your child from playing in the toilet or even falling in, purchase a latching mechanism to keep the lid closed.

Medicine cabinet

Make sure your medicine cabinet is out of reach and has a child-resistant lock to keep inquisitive fingers out. Even though all medications should have a safety cap, they still need to be locked away. Do not leave any type of medication, even vitamins, outside of the locked cabinet, and especially not in purses or bags. Don't refer to your child's medication as candy — they may seek it out. Soaps, shampoos, perfumes, and deodorants should also be kept out of reach.

Kitchen

The kitchen is another potentially dangerous room for your baby, not only because of cooking appliances, but also because you are often preoccupied with cooking when you're in there. That's when accidents can happen.

Stoves and ovens

Pots on the stove should be on the rear plates, with the handles pointing inward — pulling up on the handle of a pot or pan can result in a tragic scald burn. The oven door should be well insulated (the same is true for the glass fronts of fireplaces) and should never be left open.

Cupboard locks

All dangerous objects, including kitchen cleaners and sharp utensils, should be kept in a cabinet out of reach and protected with a child-resistant lock; in fact, it's a good idea to put child-resistant locks on all of your kitchen cabinets. Place dangerous items in the upper cabinets and safer items in the lower, more reachable cabinets.

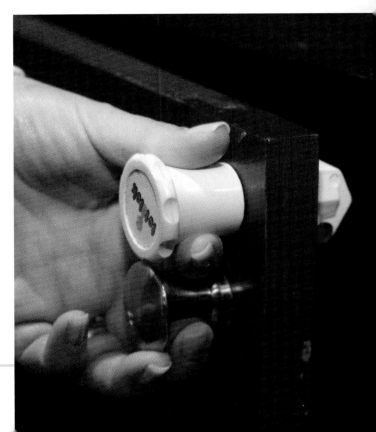

Toys

Keep a large container of toys in the kitchen to distract your baby while you're cooking, and create a "safe" zone — for example, a playpen, high chair, or exersaucer. Small refrigerator magnet toys are a potential choking hazard, so avoid them.

Table mats

Use table mats or placemats instead of tablecloths, which can be pulled down, with all of their contents landing on top of your child.

Laundry room

The laundry room should be off limits; nevertheless, ensure that the washer and dryer doors are always closed and that all detergents and bleach are kept in secured cupboards, well out of reach. Switch off and put away the iron when you are done with it.

Further precautions

With some advance planning, there are many other steps you can take to make your home as safe as possible for your child.

Electrical sockets

Plastic covers inserted in all unused electrical sockets will prevent your baby from sticking his fingers or other objects into them. Appliances not in use should be unplugged, and any electrical cords kept far out of reach.

Heat sources

Avoid using space heaters if possible and keep all heaters out of reach of children. All heat sources, including hot water or

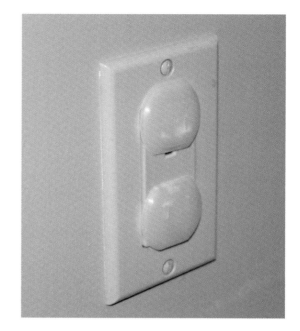

steam radiators, baseboard heaters, and air vents from furnaces should be checked to see how hot they can become; if necessary, they should be screened off. Matches and lighters should be locked away. Installing a fire extinguisher in the home is highly recommended.

Smoke and carbon monoxide detectors

Smoke and carbon monoxide detectors should be installed on every level of the home, at a minimum. They need to be carefully maintained and regularly checked. Many people remember to change the batteries at least twice a year by doing so when they are putting their clocks forward or back in the spring and fall.

Furniture

Sharp edges on furniture are particularly dangerous when your baby starts to crawl

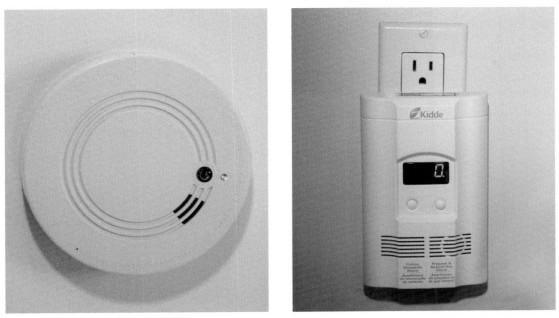

■ Smoke alarms and carbon monoxide detectors are essential safety devices on every level of the home.

and cruise around. Coffee tables are notorious for this problem. Edges can be covered with protectors (or remove the offending furniture altogether!)

Carpets

When your baby starts to stand up and cruise, place a non-slip lining underneath your mats and carpets.

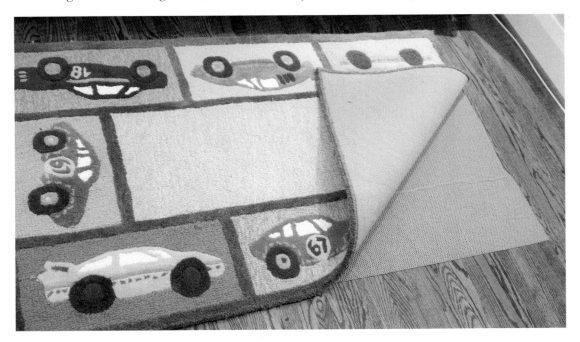

Did You Know?

Stairs

Stairs are particularly hazardous for babies at this age. Gates need to be placed both at the top and the bottom before your baby starts crawling. Make sure your gates meet current safety standards and are properly secured. Note that the older accordion type of gate is not safe — a child can get his head stuck trying to get through it. The gate at the top of the stairs needs to be secured to the wall so that it will not give way if pushed.

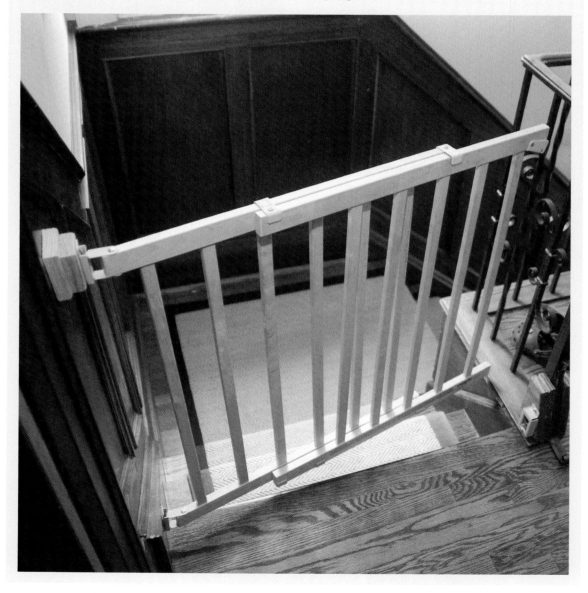

Guide to

Poisonous plants

Here is a short list of common poisonous houseplants. Check with a poison control center for more information and follow their first aid advice if your child does taste one of these plants. The best policy is to remove these plants from your house:

- aloe vera
- azalea
- chrysanthemum
- croton
- cyclamen
- English ivy
- hydrangea
- philodendron

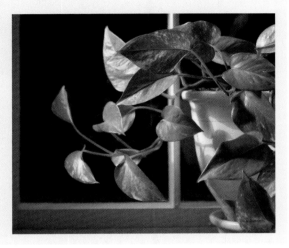

Appliances and bookcases

Heavy appliances such as televisions should be carefully secured and preferably placed out of reach. Special guards are available to place in the VCR and DVD player to keep little fingers out. Bookcases and dressers can be screwed in to the wall so they don't topple over onto the child.

Window hardware

Windows should have safety catches and screens attached. All blind and curtain cords should be carefully wrapped or clipped out of reach to prevent strangulation.

Doors and screens

Be sure to keep all doors and screens secured with child-resistant locks. Glass doors should be marked with decals to prevent your child from walking into them.

Trash cans and plastic bags

Trash containers need childproof lids. Never leave plastic bags lying around: your child might place one over his head, causing suffocation.

Weapons

Do not keep weapons in the home. If you must, ensure that firearms are not loaded and are carefully locked up.

Better safe than sorry

If it seems as if all these precautions are more likely to make you neurotic than protect your baby, be assured that's not the case. Once protective devices are in place and the recommended safety practices become routine, it becomes much easier — and less stressful — to care for your curious baby.

Parents will always need to be attentive, but they can take comfort in the knowledge that they have provided a safe environment for their child to explore the exciting world around him.

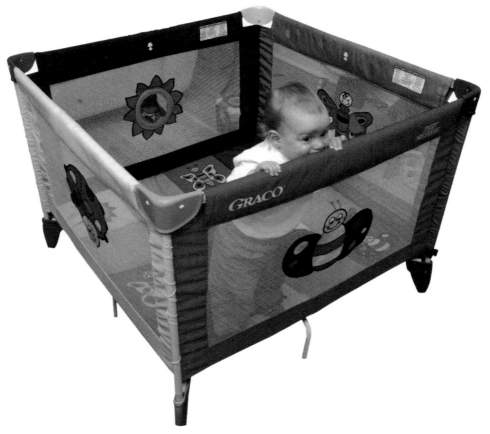

Baby "equipment"

Precautions also apply to baby equipment — walkers, swings, pacifiers, and toys.

Baby walkers

Do not use baby walkers. As a result of many injuries and some deaths from falls down stairs, they have been banned in many jurisdictions.

Playpens

Playpens should always be opened completely so they don't collapse later with the baby inside. The mattress should fit the base snugly. The openings in the mesh sides should be too small for your baby to get anything caught in them. When your baby is able to sit up, remove any toys that are strung across the playpen so he cannot strangle himself on them. Make sure your baby cannot climb out of the playpen.

Jumpers and exersaucers

Jumpers and exersaucers entertain your baby and provide a bit of a break for you. Be careful to fasten jumpers securely in such a way that your baby cannot bump up against anything. Exersaucers should be placed far away from any dangers, such as window cords and stairs.

Toys

Toys need to be age-appropriate — check for this on the packaging. No toy small enough to fit in your baby's mouth is safe! Make sure your young baby's rattle has no detachable parts. Check from time to time to make sure the eyes and nose on his soft toys are still firmly attached. Latex balloons are dangerous — if one pops, the plastic can be inhaled, suffocating the child.

Tiny objects seem to act as magnets for little hands and can cause your baby to choke if he swallows one. This is a particular danger in homes with older children, where small toys tend to be littered everywhere. Teach older siblings to pick up all the pieces of their toys. If they can't clean up all by themselves, make sure to help them. When a toy involves small pieces, it's better if your older child plays with it on the kitchen table or anywhere above your baby's reach.

Pets

Children are more commonly bitten by pets than adults are. The arrival of a new baby on the scene is a time for extreme caution, even with a trusted gentle canine or feline member of the family. Do not leave your child alone with your pet until much later. Bites can occur during play. When your baby becomes mobile, keep him away from the cat's litter box because the litter is a possible source of infection (for example, toxoplasmosis) and is a potential choking hazard

Learning first aid

Despite your most conscientious efforts to childproof your home and supervise your baby, injuries can occur at any time and at any age. Having a prepared plan of what to do in an emergency will certainly beat making decisions when you're upset and panicky. It's wise to have a list of emergency telephone numbers, including your local poison control center and family physician's office, clearly posted in a couple of places.

Basic life support

We strongly advise new parents to learn basic lifesaving techniques by taking a basic life support (BLS) course that deals with infants (less than 1 year) and young children (1 to 8 years of age). Try to take this course before your baby arrives, because it will be tough to find the time afterwards. Reading about it is not a good substitute. You need to practice on mannequins until you feel confident that you can perform the necessary techniques.

Knowing how to respond to an emergency can save a life. The techniques you are taught will allow you to remain calm and provide appropriate first aid to your child while help is on its way.

Choking

Unfortunately, choking is still the most common accidental cause of death in infancy. It is not unusual for babies to choke. In fact, more than 90% of deaths from foreign body aspiration occur in children under 5 years of age, and 65% of the victims are infants. Parents need to be prepared to help children who are choking.

Solid objects, such as toys or coins, are not the only cause of choking. If milk or food goes down "the wrong way" into the windpipe and lungs rather than into the esophagus and stomach, it can lead to choking. Usually, this will be followed by a coughing spell with some gagging until the windpipe has been cleared.

Symptoms of serious choking

The characteristics that distinguish choking from other coughing and gagging episodes, such as croup, are the sudden onset and the absence of the typical cold symptoms and other signs of being unwell that often precede a respiratory tract infection.

While babies will be able to clear the obstruction most of the time by coughing and gagging, occasionally they will not be able to. Then the coughing will become weaker, breathing will become extremely difficult, and the face may turn a bright red to blue color. The baby may be gasping for air. This is a medical emergency, requiring immediate first aid treatment (see pages 378–79) and possible emergency department care.

Did You Know?

Cardiopulmonary resuscitation (CPR)

In a basic life support (BLS) course, you will learn how to administer first aid in several emergency situations, including burns and cuts, and how to perform basic cardiopulmonary resuscitation (CPR). In adults, CPR is usually instituted because the heart stops pumping and no pulse can be felt — in other words, because of cardiac arrest. Infants and children differ in that they are far more likely to stop breathing before the heart stops beating. There are many reasons why a baby might stop breathing, such as choking, drowning, suffocation, and poisoning. If CPR is quickly begun, it is quite possible that a child will start breathing again before he goes into cardiac arrest.

Burns

There are many ways in which a baby can accidentally get burned: pulling a pan of hot liquid down on top of himself, touching a glass fireplace protector, a heater, or an oven door, or getting caught in a house fire. Once again, these serious injuries can be prevented with some straightforward childproofing techniques.

Burns are classified according to severity and depth. First-degree (superficial) burns cause redness and mild swelling. They can be very painful, as in the case of a mild sunburn. Second-degree (partial thickness) burns usually cause blistering, swelling, peeling, and severe pain. Third-degree (full thickness) burns are the worst, affecting the deeper layers, giving them a white or charred look. If the nerve endings are damaged, they may be painless.

How to treat burns

- If it is anything more serious than a mild first-degree burn, call your family physician and, depending on the severity, have your baby seen in the emergency department or doctor's office.
- Cool the area as soon as possible, because the burn will continue until the skin is cooled down. Cold water (but not ice water) is easiest to use — either dip an extremity into a bowl of cold water (for at least 10 to 20 minutes) or wet a sheet and wrap it around the burnt area. *Note:* Do not use ice — it can cause further damage to the tissues.
- Remove any constricting clothing before the swelling starts, but if clothing is stuck to the burnt area, do not pull it off.
- Don't apply butter, creams, grease, or powder — these can make the burn worse, despite what our grandmothers told us.
- Cover the burn with sterile gauze (if you have it in your first aid kit) or a clean sheet or towel.
- Give the child acetaminophen or ibuprofen for pain relief.

HOW TO
Prevent and treat choking

Minimize risk

As always, prevention is the best treatment. To minimize the risk of a serious choking episode, follow these steps:

- Grate, blend, mash or chop your child's food into very small pieces (less than ½ inch/1 cm).
- Slice round, firm foods, such as hot dogs or grapes, down the middle or into very small pieces.
- Remove small objects and pieces of toys from the baby's surroundings. Pieces of broken balloon, button-type batteries, small coins, and pop-tops are likely to cause major problems.
- Remove toys marked "Not for children under 3 years" — they are usually a choking hazard.

First aid for choking

Despite your efforts to minimize the risk of choking, it can occur. Here are the first aid steps to follow:

Step 1

If a baby is choking but remains conscious, first decide whether he needs help. If he is coughing and still breathing adequately, it is best to see if he can cough up the object he has choked on.

Note: If you start to perform CPR on a baby who is breathing and coughing effectively, you could do more harm than good.

If you see that the baby cannot breathe or cough or is gasping for air, or you hear a faint whistling sound and his face is turning bright red to blue, proceed to Step 2.

Step 2

If anyone else is around, tell them to call 911 and ask for immediate help. If you are

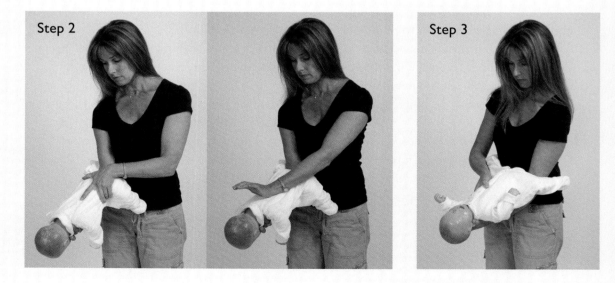

alone, carry the baby to the phone and call 911 while you proceed with first aid.

Straddle the baby over your forearm, face down, using your hand to stabilize his head and neck. The head should be lower than the body. If the baby is close to 1 year old, it may be easier to lay him over your lap, once again supporting his head and neck, with his head lower than his body.

With the heel of your other hand, give five firm blows between the baby's shoulder blades to try and push the obstruction out of the airway.

If this is unsuccessful, proceed to Step 3.

Step 3

Roll the baby over onto his back on your other forearm or on any firm surface. Using two fingers positioned over the middle of the breastbone, about one finger's width below the baby's nipples, rapidly push straight down five times. The breastbone should move about ¾ inch (1.5 to 2 cm) down with each thrust.

If he is still not breathing, proceed to the Step 4.

Note: Abdominal thrusts are not recommended for infants because they may damage the relatively large and unprotected liver.

Step 4

Open the baby's airway by pushing the chin up gently, supporting the bones at the back of the jaw with one hand. With the other hand, push down gently on the forehead.

If you can clearly see the object blocking the airway, try to remove it with your finger. If you cannot see any object at the back of the throat and the baby is not breathing, proceed to Step 5.

Step 5

Take a breath, put your mouth tightly over the baby's nose and mouth, and give two breaths. You should breathe with enough force to see some movement of his chest.

If there is no movement of the chest, try to open the airway again by pushing upward on the chin and slightly downward on the forehead as described in Step 4.

If your baby has not resumed breathing, start again at Step 2 and continue to Step 5 until help arrives.

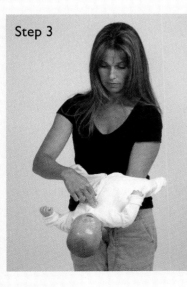

Step 3

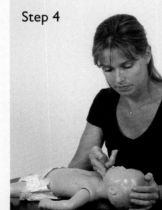

Step 4

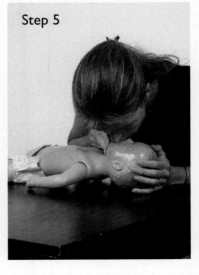

Step 5

HOW TO
Administer CPR to your baby

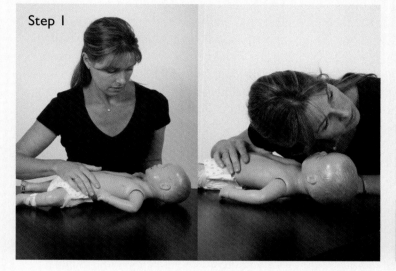

Step 1

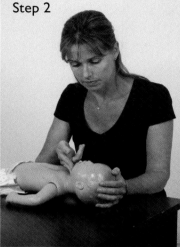

Step 2

Step 1
To establish whether the baby is breathing, open up his clothes to see whether his chest is moving up and down. You can also listen and feel over his mouth.

If you cannot see or hear any sign of breathing within 10 seconds, ask someone to call 911, or place the call yourself.

Place the baby on a firm, flat surface such as a table or the floor.

Step 2
Begin with A = airway. Open your baby's airway by pushing his chin forward slightly with some gentle pressure behind the jaw bone. With your other hand, push his forehead down very gently. This should clear the tongue from the back of the throat, and he may resume breathing.

Check to see if he has choked on something; if something is clearly visible, remove it with your fingers.

The ABCs of CPR

If your baby has stopped breathing as a result of drowning, suffocation, or poisoning, follow these steps based on the ABCs of CPR, where A = airway, B = breathing, and C = circulation. (If you know that he choked on something, follow the protocol for choking.)

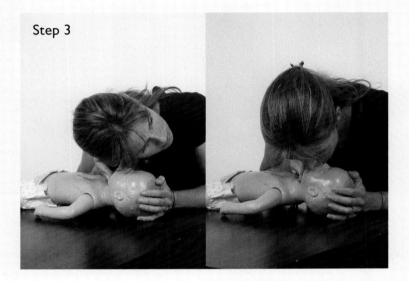

Step 3

Step 3

While maintaining the open airway, take no more than 10 seconds to check whether the baby is breathing. Look for chest and stomach movement, listen at the nose and mouth for exhaled breath sounds, and feel for exhaled air on your cheek.

If he is still not breathing, move quickly to B = breathing. Take a big breath and place your mouth tightly over his nose and mouth. Give two slow breaths (1 to 1.5 seconds per breath), which should be strong enough to move his chest.

If you see his chest rise, give him about 20 breaths per minute, or one breath every 3 seconds, until he begins to breathe by himself.

If his chest doesn't move, go back to Step 2 and make sure his airway is open. You may be pushing too much on his forehead, which could result in his neck extending too much, causing an obstruction to the airway.

If an obstructed airway is not a problem, go on to Step 4.

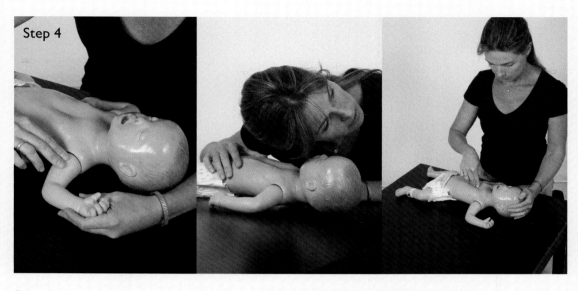

Step 4

Step 4

Proceed to C = circulation by feeling for the brachial pulse. To locate it, place your thumb on the outside of your infant's bare arm, just above the elbow. Press gently with your middle finger and index finger on the inside of the arm between the elbow and the shoulder, feeling for a pulse.

Many people (including health-care professionals) find this difficult to do reliably. If you are not comfortable with it, spend less than 10 seconds on it or go straight to looking, listening, and feeling for signs of breathing or movement.

If you cannot feel a pulse and he is not breathing or moving, you will need to restore circulation by means of chest compressions. Place two fingers over the center of the breastbone, about one finger width below the nipples, and push down about 100 times per minute. Your fingers should compress the breastbone by about one-third of his chest depth with each compression. For good compressions, push hard and fast, release completely between compressions to allow the chest to relax fully, and minimize interruptions between compressions.

After every 30 compressions, open his airway, place your mouth tightly over his nose and mouth, and give two breaths, with as short a pause in chest compressions as possible.

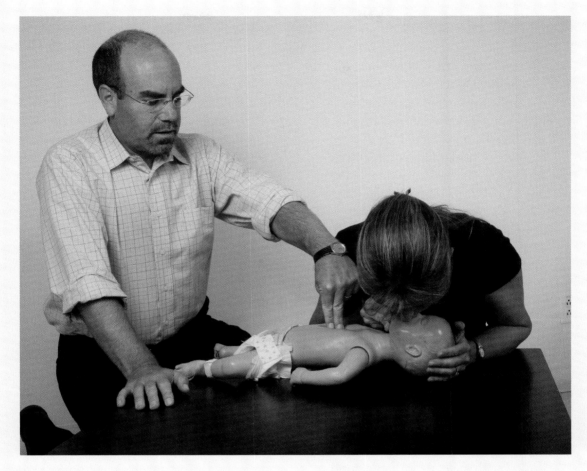

If two people are available who are trained in CPR for babies, then one should perform chest compressions while the other maintains the airway and performs ventilations by giving two breaths for every 15 chest compressions.

If you are by yourself, continue CPR with as few interruptions of chest compressions as possible until help arrives.

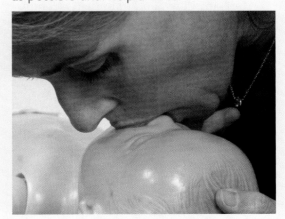

Cuts and bleeding

Bleeding from cuts and other injuries is uncommon in the first year but becomes more common as your baby becomes more mobile and adventurous. Cuts on the forehead and chin are not uncommon and can bleed quite a bit!

To prevent cuts and bleeding, follow the advice for childproofing your home, including covering the sharp edges of furniture (particularly coffee tables), securing heavy objects, such as bookcases and television sets, and locking all sharp instruments in a cupboard equipped with a child-resistant lock, preferably out of reach.

How to treat cuts and bleeding

- Cover the wound with a clean cloth and apply pressure for a few minutes to stop any active bleeding.
- Rinse the wound with water, washing out any gravel or dirt.
- If bleeding is ongoing, cover the wound with a clean cloth and apply firm pressure while elevating the area above the level of the heart. If the wound is on an extremity, lay the baby down and hold the extremity up. If it is on the head or face, sit the baby upright. If the area of the wound cannot be raised above the level of the heart, simply continue to apply pressure.
- If the wound is very dirty, with foreign material embedded, it may need to be carefully cleaned. If the wound is gaping, or bleeding continues, stitches may be required. Seek medical attention immediately.

- All wounds caused by a bite (animal or human) that breaks the skin should be seen by a doctor.

Poisoning

Over a million children under the age of 6 are exposed to poisons every year. Many poisonous substances can be found in kitchens, bathrooms, and laundry rooms — and even in household plants. Poisons can be swallowed, breathed in, or absorbed through the skin. Keep the telephone number of your local poison control center readily available in case you suspect that your baby has been exposed to something poisonous.

Keep all medicines and other potential poisons in their original containers. Take your medicine out of sight of your infant, and discard any leftover prescription medications down the drain (not in the wastebasket). Never put poisonous products in containers used for food or drink, such as empty drink bottles. Be particularly vigilant when away from home, at the grandparents' house, for example.

Poisoning symptoms

The symptoms of poisoning exhibited by the child will vary depending on the substance he is exposed to, but may include

- stomach upset with pain, vomiting, and diarrhea
- drowsiness
- convulsions and loss of consciousness
- drooling
- difficulty breathing
- redness or burns in or around the baby's mouth

HOW TO
Treat poisoning

- If your child can't be roused and isn't breathing, begin CPR and call 911 immediately.

- Look for a source of poison in the near vicinity (for example, a medication container or a chewed houseplant), then call the poison control center and provide them with the names of any substances you think may have been ingested or inhaled.

- If anything is still in your baby's mouth, remove it immediately, but don't throw it away — it may help identify the type of poison.

- If you suspect that your baby has swallowed a chemical poison, wash his lips with water. Do not give him more than a few sips of water before getting advice from the poison control center or your health-care provider.

- If you think your baby has spilled a chemical on his skin, remove his clothes and rinse the skin with lukewarm water for at least 10 minutes.

- If you think he may have inhaled poisonous fumes, move him out into the fresh air.

- If a poisonous substance has splashed in his eye, rinse the inner corner of the eye with lukewarm water for as long as you can (up to 15 minutes).

- If your child vomits, try to keep a sample to take with you to the hospital. Do not give your child anything to make him vomit. If he has ingested a caustic substance (contained in many detergents and kitchen cleaners), inducing vomiting may cause more damage. (Note: Syrup of ipecac is no longer recommended under any circumstances — if you have any at home, get rid of it.)

- If your child cannot be roused but is breathing normally, place him on his side to ensure that he doesn't choke if he vomits.

Household poison hazards

Keep these products locked in a high cupboard, out of sight and out of reach:

- All medicines, especially iron supplements, vitamins, aspirin, and acetaminophen

- Cleaning products, including drain cleaner, furniture polish, dishwashing soap, and bleach

- Pesticides and herbicides, such as weed killer, ant traps, and mouse and rat poison

- Motor vehicle products, such as gasoline, antifreeze, and windshield wiper fluid

- Paint, paint thinners, glue, kerosene, and other solvents and fuels

- Mothballs

Frequently asked questions

As family doctors and pediatricians, we answer many questions from parents. Here are some of the most frequently asked questions. Be sure to ask your health-care providers any other questions that arise. If they don't have the answers, they will refer you to a colleague who does.

Q: My parents have a condo with a swimming pool. What precautions should we take when our 8-month-old boy is around the pool?

A: When it comes to water safety, you can never be too careful. Drownings do occur in the first year of life, and not just because of boating accidents; a swimming pool can also be the scene of tragedy. For an infant, even a bathtub can be dangerous. Kids have also accidentally drowned in ponds and buckets.

The moral of all this is obvious: infants need to be watched constantly when they are near water. It takes only a few seconds for a curious crawler to enter a pool and stay submerged beneath the surface without even struggling. A momentary diversion can lead to disaster. Caregivers, be they professional lifeguards or grandparents, must know this and behave accordingly.

Q: Are infant bath seats and rings safe?

A: In the United States, there have been more than 100 deaths and many more reported near-miss drownings during the last 20 years related to the use of infant bath seats or rings. Accidents typically occur when the seat becomes unstable and tips over or the baby slips through or climbs out while the caregiver has briefly left him unattended or in the care of a sibling. For this reason, many authorities discourage their use. If you use one, it is essential that you maintain close, constant supervision for the entire time your baby remains in the bath.

Q: Where is the safest place to seat my infant on an airplane?

A: Not on the aisle. Scalding liquids spilled by passers-by create a real risk for serious burns. Those aisles are quite narrow, and an outstretched arm can easily be trapped and injured by a passing service cart or an unsteady passenger. Your baby is better off in a window seat, or even the middle seat.

The American Academy of Pediatrics recommends that infants who fly do so in a ticketed seat, placed in a car seat for restraint. Air travel with a young family may seem cumbersome and labor-intensive if you're used to traveling solo with a small carry-on. But that car seat may well prove helpful during a turbulent flight.

Q: At what age is ear piercing safe?

A: The risks involved with ear piercing are minimal, even when it's done during infancy. However, infection sometimes does occur at the site of the piercing, particularly if it is done by unskilled personnel. Furthermore, the procedure is painful, at least momentarily. But there is a greater issue that thoughtful parents need to consider: ear piercing has no medical value; it is strictly a cosmetic procedure. Consider waiting until your daughter can understand the advantages and risks of ear piercing, and then let her decide for herself what she would like to do.

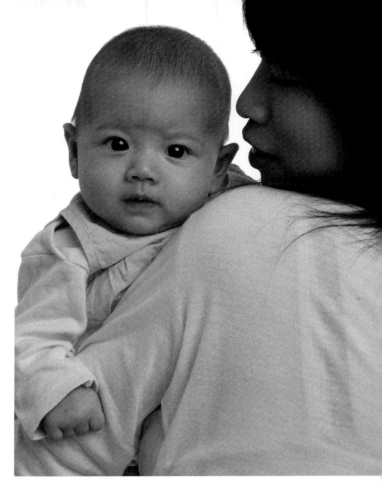

Q: My 10-month-old daughter was crawling on our deck and got a large sliver in her hand. What is the best way to remove it?

A: First, get ready all the things you are likely to need: gauze pads (or cotton balls), a sewing needle, tweezers that still pinch tightly, antibiotic ointment, and a Band-Aid. Because babies don't appreciate the advantages of sliver removal, an assistant, if available, will be a good idea.

Cleanse the area with soap and water. Using the needle, further expose the protruding end of the sliver as best as you can. Grab that end with the tweezers and pull out the sliver. Afterwards, liberally apply antibiotic ointment and cover the sore with a Band-Aid.

Sometimes, a sliver will be quite superficial and lie parallel to the skin's surface. In that case, you can easily expose the splinter by using the needle to stroke the skin directly above the sliver. Then, remove it with the tweezers.

If the sliver appears to have lodged very deep and is unlikely to be easily removed, consult a health-care provider.

If your baby has multiple tiny (1 to 2 mm) slivers that are very superficial, it might be best to leave them alone, although you should still apply antibiotic ointment. The potential tissue damage caused by the attempt to remove the slivers may cause your baby greater distress than the slivers themselves. They will grow out in time.

Q: Upon entering the kitchen, you find your 1-month-old son wheezing and choking on a grape he found on the floor. What should you do?

A: The techniques for helping a choking infant were discussed in some detail earlier in this section. You probably read them. And, we'll bet, you also understood them. But … when faced with your own precious baby choking, would you actually possess the skills to save him? Likely, not. Resuscitation techniques cannot merely be read once. They must be carefully studied, memorized and practiced over and over. Take a certified CPR course and, a year later, take it again. You will never regret your decision.

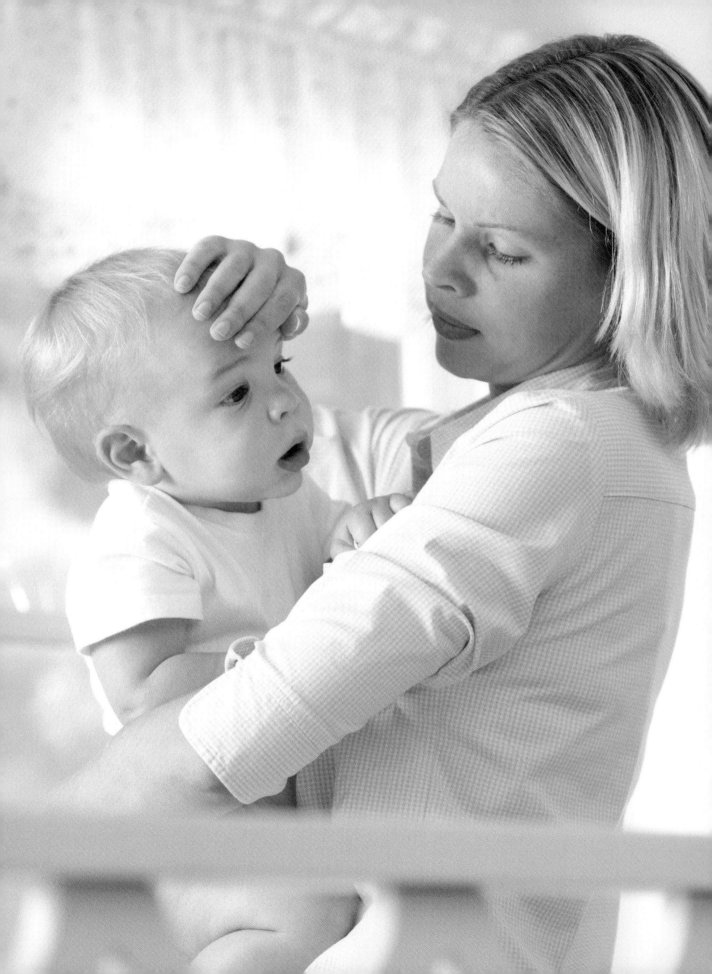

Caring for
Your Sick Baby

390 Caring for Your Sick Baby

Recognizing signs and symptoms of illness

Despite your best efforts to protect your baby from injury, feed her appropriately, and attend to all her needs, she may become ill. Caring for a sick child is, without a doubt, the most distressing part of being a parent.

Recognizing the signs and symptoms of common illnesses can help reduce this stress and, more importantly, help you care for your sick baby. Fever, vomiting, rashes, persistent coughs, and failure to thrive are common symptoms that are usually self-limited, with only minor consequences. However, because they may sometimes indicate an underlying, possibly serious illness, they are given special attention here. While you can treat some illnesses at home, others need to be addressed by health-care providers in their medical offices and clinics. Emergency situations, of course, require immediate care in a hospital; be especially alert for "red flag" signs and symptoms.

General signs and symptoms of illness

There are several behavioral symptoms and medical signs that may indicate that your baby is not feeling well:

- Your baby is not acting "like herself."
- Your baby is feeding poorly.
- Your baby is lethargic, less interactive, or less playful than usual.
- Your baby is irritable, whiney, clingy, or crying more than usual.
- Your baby is more sleepy than usual.
- Your baby is running a fever greater than 99°F (37.2°C) axillary (under the arm) or 100.4°F (38°C) rectal.

Urgent attention required

If your baby shows these red flag signs and symptoms, seek immediate medical attention from a health-care provider:

- Fever in the first 3 months of life
- Refusal to feed and/or vomiting with decreased urination (wet diapers) and dry eyes, dry tongue, and lack of tears (suggestive of dehydration)
- Lethargy, with decreased consciousness
- Irritability or crying that is out of character and cannot be consoled
- Very rapid breathing or increased effort to breathe, suggested by flaring of the nostrils or "in-drawing" of the skin between the ribs or below the ribcage with each breath
- Abnormal jerking movements of the limbs, especially if they cannot be stopped by holding the limb (suggestive of a convulsion or seizure)
- Flat reddish purple spots or rash on the skin that doesn't lose color when you press down on the skin with your finger

Taking care of a fever

At some time, every child will experience fever. Fever is the most common reason for a child to be brought for emergency care. While most fevers are the result of a self-limited and benign illness, almost all parents will at some point worry that a more serious disease is causing their baby's fever. Your anxiety will be reduced if you understand how fevers develop and know how to take your child's temperature.

Fever facts

Although the experience of fever is universal, there are many misconceptions about its implications and management. Even the seemingly simple question of what constitutes a fever can be less straightforward than it first appears.

Most fevers are caused by self-limited viral infections. Fevers are normal — indeed, they are an important part of the body's natural immune response to infection.

"Normal" temperature

Technically defined, a fever is an elevation in body temperature; however, "normal" body temperature varies according to where it is measured and when it is measured, as well as by the surrounding environment and your child's clothing. Fevers are diagnosed by taking a child's rectal, axillary (underarm), oral, or tympanic (ear) temperature and determining if it is above "normal."

Convulsions

While many parents are concerned about the potentially harmful effects of an elevated body temperature, they are especially frightened by fever-induced convulsions. Called febrile seizures, these convulsions are relatively common — about one in 30 children between 6 months and 5 years of age will have a febrile convulsion. These events, while scary, almost always have minimal consequences for the child.

Complications

Fever caused by uncomplicated infections does not cause brain damage, hearing loss,

Measuring your child's temperature

Route measured	What is a fever?
Rectal	> 100.4°F (38.0°C)
Axillary (under arm)	> 99°F (37.2°C)
Oral (under tongue)	> 99.5°F (37.5°C)
Tympanic (ear)	> 99.5°F (37.5°C)

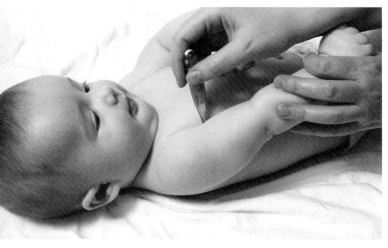

or blindness, as some people believe. Nor does the height of a fever indicate the severity of illness. In fact, some serious infections may be accompanied by a minimally elevated or even lower-than-normal body temperature.

More important than the height of the fever is your baby's behavior. While most feverish babies are cranky and clingy, with decreased appetite, be especially concerned if your baby does not show interest in or awareness of her surroundings, does not make appropriate eye contact, or is inconsolable. Contact a health-care provider immediately if these behaviors accompany a fever.

Fever in young infants

Fever in young infants, particularly those under 3 months of age, is cause for concern, in part because the child's immune system is immature and in part because the child has few ways to exhibit signs of serious illness. While more than 90% of feverish infants under 3 months of age have a self-resolving, uncomplicated viral infection, health-care providers will frequently perform a number of tests to look for potentially serious infections, such as meningitis, bacteremias (bloodstream infections), and urinary tract infections.

Reducing risk

Your baby is at a slightly increased risk of infection in the first 2 to 3 months of life because her immune system is still developing. Nonetheless, she has the benefit of much of your immunity because your antibodies crossed through the placenta into her bloodstream during fetal development. By giving her the recommended immunizations at the recommended times, you will help her to develop her own immunity to some rare but potentially devastating diseases.

Fever red flags

See a health-care provider immediately if your baby has these signs and symptoms in addition to a fever:

- She is less than 3 months of age.
- She does not interact appropriately.
- She is difficult to rouse, poorly responsive, or limp.
- She is inconsolable or appears to be in pain.
- She refuses to eat and drink.
- She is behaving as if her neck is stiff.
- She is having difficulty breathing.
- She has developed purple "spots" or bruises on her skin.

Also seek help if the fever has persisted for 2 to 3 days and your instincts tell you that your baby is "not herself."

Guide to

Taking your baby's temperature

The type of thermometer and the route you should use to measure a child's temperature depend on her age, the circumstances, and the equipment available:

TYPE OF THERMOMETER

- **Mercury:** Mercury thermometers are not recommended because of the potential for mercury exposure if the thermometer breaks. In addition, they have to remain in place longer before they record the correct temperature.
- **Digital:** Digital thermometers are safe, easy to use, and inexpensive. They are ready to read in less than a minute, which is helpful with a squirmy baby.
- **Tympanic (ear):** Tympanic thermometers are convenient, but are less reliable in children under 2 years of age. They give a reading in a few seconds, but are much more expensive than simple plastic digital thermometers.

ROUTE

- **Rectal:** Rectal temperature measurement is the most accurate method for young infants and is therefore the preferred route in the first 3 months.
- **Axillary (under arm):** Axillary temperature measurement is convenient but is also the most unreliable. To take your child's temperature this way, place the tip of a digital oral or rectal thermometer in the armpit, and tuck the child's arm snugly against her chest.
- **Oral (under tongue):** By 4 to 5 years of age, children will usually cooperate with oral temperature measurement, which requires keeping the thermometer under the tongue.
- **Tympanic (ear):** Tympanic thermometers must fit easily inside the child's ear canal.

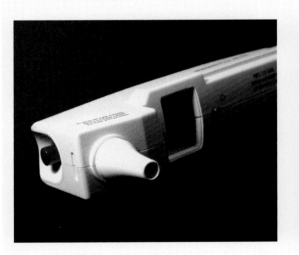

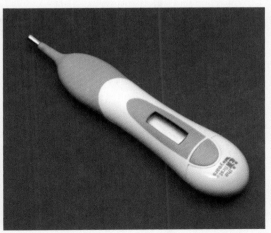

HOW TO
Manage a fever

Remember that most fevers in infants are caused by benign, self-limited viral infections that your baby can and will fight off by herself. Most fevers due to viral infections can be managed at home.

1. Determine if a fever is, in fact, present by taking your baby's temperature.

- **Axillary method:** Most parents use a digital thermometer with the bulb placed under the undressed baby's armpit. Hold the thermometer in place until it beeps, which is usually less than 1 minute. This method is convenient but somewhat unreliable; therefore, in the first 3 months of life, when the presence of fever may cause your physician to consider performing a number of different tests, it is often recommended that you take a rectal temperature, which is far more accurate.
- **Rectal method:** Place the baby on her back and lubricate the bulb of the thermometer with petroleum jelly (Vaseline). Lifting her legs up against her tummy, pinch the thermometer $\frac{1}{2}$ to $\frac{3}{4}$ inch (1 to 2 cm) from the tip of the bulb and gently insert it into the anus up to your pinched fingers. Parents are often nervous about this technique, but it is really very safe for young babies.

2. Seek urgent medical care from a health-care provider if your baby has a fever in the first 3 months of life or if a fever persists for more than 2 to 3 days.

3. Consider the following factors if your baby has a fever but is more than 3 months of age and seems relatively well, showing a willingness to feed and interact with you:

- **Infections:** Has anyone in close contact with your baby been sick with a fever, cold symptoms, or some other type of infection? If so, your baby may have developed a similar illness from contact or airborne droplet spread.
- **Common cold:** Does your baby have a runny nose, nasal congestion, or cough? These symptoms are suggestive of a common cold or an upper respiratory tract infection. For cold treatments, see page 274 and the "Quick guide to common health conditions," page 417.
- **Bronchiolitis:** Is your baby wheezing (a high-pitched musical noise heard when breathing) or showing any signs of difficulty breathing? These signs could include rapid breathing or increased effort with each breath, manifested by flaring of the nostrils and "in-drawing" of the skin between and below the ribs with each breath. Difficulty breathing is suggestive of bronchiolitis, which may start out with cold symptoms. It is very common in babies in the winter. For bronchiolitis treatments, see page 332 and the "Quick guide to common health conditions," page 415.
- **Croup:** Does your baby have a barking, seal-like cough that occurs after a few days of cold symptoms and is worse in

the middle of the night? This is likely to be croup, which occurs most often in the fall and spring. For croup treatments, see page 333 and the "Quick guide to common health conditions," page 418.

- **Gastroenteritis:** Is your baby vomiting or feeding poorly, or does she have diarrhea (frequent loose stools)? These symptoms are suggestive of gastroenteritis. The most common cause is a virus called rotavirus, which occurs in the winter, although other viruses can cause gastroenteritis in the summer. It is particularly important to look for signs of dehydration. For gastroenteritis treatments, see page 275 and the "Quick guide to common health conditions," page 419, under Diarrhea and vomiting.

- **Otitis media (middle ear infection):** Is your child waking in the night crying with what seems like pain, or is she rubbing or pulling on her ear? Otitis media starts to become common after the age of 6 months, although it can occur in younger babies. It is usually seen in a baby who has had a cold. Your health-care provider can diagnose this condition by examining the eardrum. For otitis media treatments, see page 336 and the "Quick guide to common health conditions," page 426.

- **Roseola:** Does your baby have a high fever and fussiness without any other symptoms? This could be roseola, but you won't know until the fever breaks after a few days and a pinkish rash, which blanches, appears just as she is getting better. Roseola is most commonly seen in babies between 6 and 9 months of age, although it doesn't always present with a fever. Three-quarters of all babies will have had it by the age of 1 year. For roseola treatments, see page 336 and the "Quick guide to common health conditions," page 428.

4. Comfort and cool your baby. Dress her lightly in a diaper and vest to allow body heat to escape.

5. Do not give your baby a cold water bath or sponge her with alcohol. The cold water is likely to be uncomfortable and can make her shiver; the alcohol can be absorbed into the body through the skin.

6. Offer your baby frequent feedings because fever causes increased loss of water.

7. Administer over-the-counter medications. The primary function of medication is to provide comfort for the child, not to eliminate the elevated body temperature. Acetaminophen (Tylenol, Tempra) and ibuprofen (Advil, Motrin) are safe and effective treatments for fever. There isn't much difference among these medications, which come in drops, syrups, suppositories, and chewable tablets for older children.

Dosage: The dosage varies depending on your baby's weight. Don't wait until 3:00 a.m. to work out what the appropriate dose is — check it out ahead of time!

Caution: Aspirin (ASA) should not be given to children because of the risk of Reye's syndrome, a serious condition that can cause liver and brain injury.

Understanding vomiting

Almost every infant vomits at some point. Vomiting should be distinguished from spitting up, or reflux, a normal, effortless regurgitation of stomach contents that occurs most often during and after feeding. Vomiting is a forceful expulsion of stomach contents. Babies may vomit through the nose as well as the mouth. While it certainly isn't pretty, vomiting through the nose does not mean the condition is more severe. Be aware that vomiting may lead to dehydration.

Causes of vomiting

Infants, and children in general, are more prone to vomiting than adults, and they can vomit for a wide variety of reasons. For example, babies tend to vomit if they have a forceful cough. The most common cause of vomiting is an acute infection, such as a viral intestinal infection or a urinary tract infection. Other causes of vomiting include allergies to milk and obstructions to the stomach and intestinal tract.

Dehydration

Whatever the cause, if your child is vomiting persistently, she may become dehydrated due to the loss of fluids from the stomach. The younger she is, the more quickly she will become dehydrated if she cannot keep her fluids down. If you notice a decrease in the amount of urine in her diapers, and she is becoming listless and has a dry tongue, sunken eyes, and decreased tears, seek medical attention immediately. If she is breast-feeding, continue feeding her normally. If she is formula-fed or on solids, consider supplementing with an oral rehydration solution (Pedialyte, Gastrolyte, Oralyte, or Rehydralyte), available at most drugstores. Small amounts (½ to 1 oz/15 to 30 mL) given every 10 to 15 minutes seem to work best. The solution can be given by syringe, spoon, bottle, or cup, depending on what your baby is willing to take. Introduce her regular diet once she appears to be adequately rehydrated.

Vomiting red flags

- The vomit contains blood. If you see lots of fresh blood (this is very unusual), seek immediate medical attention. If you see tiny bits of blood or pieces of digested blood that resemble coffee grounds, mention it to your health-care provider right away.
- The vomit contains bile. Bile is dark green (not yellow) and could indicate an intestinal obstruction.
- The vomit (particularly in the first 2 months of life) is projectile, traveling up to 3 feet (1 m). This suggests an obstruction at the outlet of the stomach, called pyloric stenosis.
- Your baby has a dry mouth or is not wetting her diapers. These signs could indicate dehydration.
- Your baby is listless and is not interested in feeding or her environment. This indicates dehydration or an infection.
- Vomiting is persistent and your baby is unable to keep anything down.

HOW TO
Manage vomiting

If your child has vomited just once and looks fine afterwards, continue with normal care. Vomiting that doesn't recur is unlikely to be a cause for concern.

If the vomiting recurs, you'll need to determine the cause and follow the treatment procedures for the condition causing the vomiting. Be alert for red flag signs and symptoms that require urgent medical attention.

Gastroesophageal reflux

Many young babies spit up on a fairly regular basis due to gastroesophageal reflux (GER). Some babies even vomit forcefully an hour or two after finishing their feed. If this has been happening for weeks or months, but your baby seems contented and has continued to gain weight and develop appropriately, intervention is not likely to be necessary; nevertheless, you should mention the persistent vomiting to your health-care provider. If your baby is not gaining weight or seems uncomfortable when feeding (as though she is experiencing heartburn), discuss her persistent vomiting with your health-care provider without delay. There are a number of interventions that will improve gastroesophageal reflux. This recurrent condition tends to get better as your child gets older. For gastroesophageal reflux treatments, see page 217 and the "Quick guide to common health conditions," page 429, under Spitting up.

Gastroenteritis

Is there an associated change in your baby's stools? The second most common cause of vomiting in infancy is viral gastroenteritis. The typical course begins with 1 to 2 days of vomiting, when it seems as if everything that goes into the stomach comes right back out again. The vomit usually resembles whatever has been ingested, and may become yellow when the stomach is empty. It may be accompanied by a low-grade fever, as well as signs that your baby is not her normal happy and energetic self. As the vomiting starts to settle, diarrhea will likely begin, with an increased number of smelly and very watery stools. Often, someone in close contact with your baby will have had an upset tummy in the last few days. For gastroenteritis treatments, see page 275 and the "Quick guide to common health conditions," page 419, under Diarrhea and vomiting.

Gastroenteritis is generally self-limited, meaning that your child will get over it by herself, without medication. In fact, medications to treat vomiting and diarrhea, although often used in older children and adults, are generally contraindicated in infants. Acetaminophen (Tylenol, Tempra) can be used if she appears to have tummy cramps or the fever seems to be bothering her. You may have to consider giving it as a suppository if she isn't keeping anything down.

Infection

Is the vomiting accompanied by other signs of an infection? For example, is your baby lethargic or crying when passing urine? A change in the smell or color of the urine may suggest a urinary tract infection, although dehydration can also make the urine darker and smell a bit "stronger."

For urinary tract infection treatments, see page 223 and the "Quick guide to common health conditions," page 431.

Urgent care: A baby who has a fever, is inconsolable, or is very listless and "not herself" may have a serious infection, such as meningitis. If she is coughing and having trouble breathing, the vomiting may be a result of pneumonia or bronchiolitis. (It is not unusual for a baby to empty her stomach as part of a forceful cough.) In either case, see your health-care provider immediately.

Intestinal obstruction

If the vomit is dark green (bile-stained), rather than bright yellow, see your health-care provider immediately. Your baby's bowel may be blocked below the point where the gallbladder empties bile into it. Although it's very unusual, intestinal obstruction can occur in healthy infants when a loop of bowel becomes twisted (volvulus) or telescopes into the segment in front of it (intussusception). Intussusception may be associated with blood in the stools, which can look like red currant jelly. The baby may become pale and limp, and may have recurrent bouts of severe abdominal spasms, during which she draws up her legs. Intestinal obstructions are more common in children who have a history of bowel problems, particularly if they have had abdominal surgery, which can result in scar tissue.

Pyloric stenosis

If the vomiting is projectile, traveling up to 3 feet (1 m), your baby may have an obstruction at the end of the stomach, a condition called pyloric stenosis. It is usually seen in the first 2 months of life, particularly in boys and in babies with a family history of this condition. The vomiting tends to get worse over the course of days, to the point where nothing stays down. Because the obstruction occurs before the gallbladder empties into the intestine, the vomit does not contain bile. For pyloric stenosis treatments, see page 218 and the "Quick guide to common health conditions," page 428.

Gastritis

Is there any blood in the vomit? Blood can look bright red, or darkish purple if clotted. Once it has been in the stomach for a while and is a bit digested, it resembles coffee grounds. There are several ways that blood might get into the stomach: it is not unusual for the stomach lining to ooze blood when inflamed or irritated (gastritis); the lining of the esophagus (gullet) may become inflamed in babies with GER and can be torn slightly by forceful vomiting; and breast-fed babies can swallow blood while feeding if the mother's nipples are cracked or raw. There is no need to panic if you see small quantities of blood or "coffee grounds," though you should report it to your health-care provider as soon as possible.

Urgent care: If you see lots of fresh blood, seek immediate medical attention.

Food allergies

Allergies to specific foods are quite common in infants. Perhaps the most common is an allergy to cow's milk protein, which can be seen not only in formula-fed babies, but also in breast-fed infants (a mother who is ingesting dairy products passes the protein on to her baby in her breast milk). Although diarrhea is the most common symptom, vomiting may also result. In addition, you may see blood in the stool, irritability, and poor weight gain. Discuss these symptoms with your health-care provider.

Dealing with rashes

Skin rashes in infants come in all forms, from raised bumps to flat blotches. Most are transient and harmless. Occasionally, a rash can be a sign of a serious condition (for example, an infection) that needs immediate attention.

Causes of rashes

Rashes can result from a multitude of causes:

- Transient skin conditions common in early infancy, such as erythema toxicum, baby acne, and heat rash
- Irritants to the skin (diaper rash is an example of a rash caused by an irritant)
- Chronic skin conditions, such as eczema and seborrheic dermatitis
- Allergies
- Infections

Rash red flags

See your health-care provider if your baby's rash has the following characteristics and your baby appears generally unwell:

- The rash is non-blanching (when you press on the skin with your thumb, the rash does not fade, or "blanch"), particularly when accompanied by fever. This type of rash (petechiae or purpura) is caused by bleeding into the tissues below the skin and can appear as flat reddish pinpoints or larger purplish bumps. It can be a sign of a serious infection, such as meningococcemia.
- The rash looks infected (it is red, hot, swollen, and painful).
- Widespread hives are present. Hives can be a sign of an allergy to foods, medications, inhaled allergens (such as animal dander), or something in contact with the skin. Hives appear as raised pink-red welts. They usually disappear within hours, so circling some of the marks with a pen and observing them to see whether they disappear can be helpful in diagnosis.

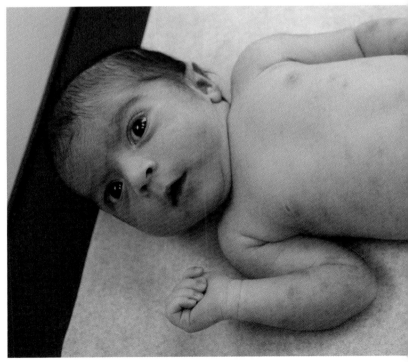

■ Erythema toxicum: A normal newborn rash.

HOW TO
Manage rashes

Transient skin conditions

Many rashes commonly seen in newborn children require no intervention. Your health-care provider can help you recognize these rashes:

- **Erythema toxicum:** These yellowish white pimples on a red background appear all over the body. They usually occur in the first week and tend to come and go in groups over a matter of hours. No treatment is required.

- **Infantile acne:** Very similar in appearance to the acne seen in teenagers, infantile acne tends to disappear after the first few months of life (and causes much less angst!). No treatment is required.

- **Milia:** This rash manifests as tiny white bumps over the bridge of the nose and cheeks, and disappears within a few weeks. No treatment is required.

- **Heat rash, or prickly heat:** These reddish bumps and blotches usually appear on areas that tend to be covered and therefore get sweaty, such as the upper back, chest, and neck. To prevent heat rash, avoid overbundling your baby or exposing her to excessive heat and humidity. Cotton clothing allows heat and moisture to escape more easily.

- **Mongolian spots (birthmarks):** A type of skin pigmentation usually found across the buttocks and lower spine, especially in dark-skinned babies, these spots are flat, bluish gray in color, and resemble a bruise, except that the color does not change. They tend to disappear after a few years of life. No treatment is required.

Diaper dermatitis

The two most likely causes of a rash in the diaper area are fungal (yeast) infection and irritation from contact with urine or stool. These rashes can look quite similar and are often found together. A fungal infection is more likely if the skin between the groin folds is affected, as yeasts thrive in dark, moist, enclosed spaces and this skin does not come into contact with urine or stool. A baby with fungal diaper dermatitis will sometimes have white patches in her mouth (thrush) and small red patches of rash just outside of the diaper area (satellite lesions).

Treatment involves leaving the area open to the air and frequent diaper changes to minimize contact with irritating substances. If the rash isn't improving, your health-care provider can prescribe a topical cream, either a mild anti-inflammatory steroid (for example, 1% hydrocortisone) for irritant diaper dermatitis or an antifungal cream (for example, nystatin) for yeast infections — or a combination of both — to be applied to the rash two to three times daily for 5 to 7 days.

Eczema and seborrheic dermatitis

These two common rashes tend to wax and wane throughout the first year of life. In the case of eczema (atopic dermatitis), infants are usually affected on the face, especially the cheeks, although the outside of the knees and elbows can also be involved. The skin tends to be very dry and is often red, scaly, and itchy.

Eczema is particularly common in families with a history of allergies. Eczema resolves spontaneously in up to 50% of children by school age, but there is no cure. To prevent flare-ups, avoid irritants (for example, perfumed soaps, fabric softener, woolen garments) and use hypoallergenic soaps and moisturizers to trap moisture in the skin. During flare-ups, a mild corticosteroid cream is often required for the inflamed areas.

Seborrheic dermatitis is often seen in the first few months of life, usually on the scalp (cradle cap), although it can also affect the skin over the eyebrows, behind the ears, on the neck, and in the diaper region. The rash tends to look greasy, with yellowish scales over reddened skin. It is not usually itchy, and infants generally outgrow it. If it is mild, it will resolve spontaneously, without treatment. In more severe cases, a special shampoo or a corticosteroid lotion can be used.

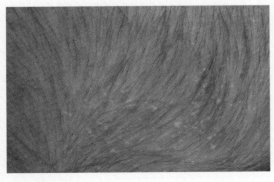

■ Cradle cap

Allergic reactions

Less commonly, allergic reactions can cause a rash in infants. Hives can be a sign of an allergic reaction to foods, medications, inhaled allergens (animal dander), or something in contact with the skin. Hives appear as raised pink-red welts; they usually appear and disappear within hours and are generally itchy. If the cause of the reaction is clear, remove the allergen.

It is very common for a rash to appear while a baby is taking antibiotics (although it does not usually take the form of hives). This does not necessarily mean that your baby is allergic to that antibiotic. When a viral illness is mistakenly treated with an antibiotic, the appearance of a rash is often related to the natural progression of the viral illness; the antibiotic is just an innocent bystander. Ask your doctor whether your baby is still able to take that antibiotic.

Viral infections

If, in addition to a rash, your baby has a fever or cold symptoms, is feeding poorly, or is irritable, the rash is likely related to a viral infection, especially if it is a non-specific, pinkish, generally flat rash that blanches when pressure is applied. This type of rash can occur anywhere on the body.

How quickly you seek medical attention depends on how unwell your baby looks. Deciding whether she is contagious is not always easy. If she has a fever, cough and cold symptoms, or diarrhea and vomiting, chances are she is still contagious, but babies are often most contagious before the rash appears.

Handling coughs

The lungs are made up of many tiny branching airways, and a cough is usually an airway's reflex response to irritation. Most coughs are caused by fairly harmless and self-limited viral illnesses, but some can be a sign of a more serious condition that may need specific therapy and urgent attention.

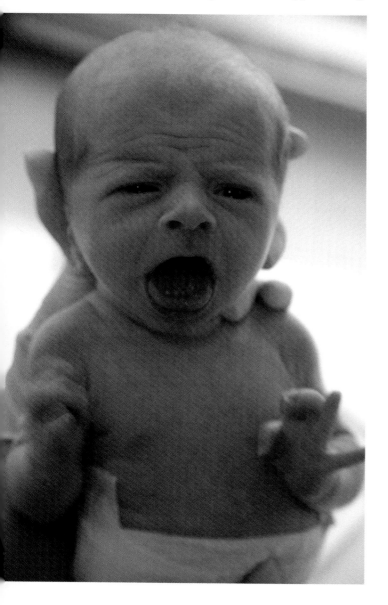

Coughing red flags

- Your baby is having trouble breathing even when not coughing. Breathing difficulties may include rapid breathing or breathing that requires extra effort (sucking in of the skin between the ribs or flaring of the nostrils with each breath). Trouble breathing could indicate bronchiolitis, pneumonia, or asthma.
- The cough is associated with wheezing (a high-pitched musical sound on breathing out). This could suggest bronchiolitis or asthma.
- The cough is associated with a "whoop," or your baby's lips turn blue during a coughing spell ("blue spell"). These signs could indicate whooping cough (pertussis).
- The cough occurs after a choking episode and doesn't settle down quickly. This suggests that your baby has aspirated a foreign material (food or toy) into her lungs.
- The cough is associated with fever, vomiting, or listlessness, and your baby is not her normal self. These symptoms suggest bacterial pneumonia.
- The cough is not getting better after a week, or is worrying you for any reason.

HOW TO
Manage a cough

Common cold

Most coughs in infants are part of a common cold or upper respiratory tract infection. Children may get up to 8 to 10 colds every year in the first few years of life. In addition to the cough, they may have nasal congestion and discharge. Young infants may have noisy breathing and even difficulty feeding because of a blocked nose. Most symptoms will resolve within about a week.

Over-the-counter cough syrups and decongestants are not generally recommended for infants — they do not seem to work well, and they may have side effects. A bulb nasal suction with saline nose drops may help to relieve some of the nasal obstruction in very young infants, especially if the blocked nose is resulting in difficulty sleeping or feeding. If the cold is running its course and gradually improving as expected, an infant will not need to see her health-care provider. For cold treatments, see page 274 and the "Quick guide to common health conditions," page 417.

Bronchiolitis, asthma, and wheezing

If your baby is wheezing (making a whistling noise when she breathes out), she may have bronchiolitis, a viral infection that gets into the chest, or she may be experiencing bronchospasm due to asthma. The sound of wheezing is quite different from the snoring noise heard when your baby breathes in with a congested nose from a cold (see above). Both bronchiolitis and asthma are likely to cause breathing difficulties (rapid breathing, increased effort with each breath) over and above the cough and wheeze.

Bronchiolitis is very common, especially in winter. Many infants will have cold symptoms before the coughing and wheezing begin, and they may have been in contact with someone with a cold. For bronchiolitis treatments, see page 332 and the "Quick guide to common health conditions," page 415.

Asthma affects about 10% of children and is more common in babies whose families have a strong history of asthma, eczema, or hay fever. An asthma attack can be set off by a cold and can look almost identical to an episode of bronchiolitis. For asthma treatments, see the "Quick guide to common health conditions," page 414.

Once a child has had a couple of episodes of wheezing, especially if she responds well to puffers, she is usually considered to have asthma.

Urgent care: If you hear wheezing with a cough, especially if your baby shows signs of breathing difficulties, seek medical attention immediately.

Croup

Croup is a viral infection that primarily involves the voice box area, causing a seal-like, barky, hoarse cough. Croup is more common in the spring and fall, and usually follows a few days of cold symptoms. The cough tends to be most severe in the middle of the night. For croup treatments, see page 332 and the "Quick guide to common health conditions," page 418.

Urgent care: If this condition doesn't settle when you expose your baby to humidity (by running a hot water shower in a closed bathroom or taking her outside, for example), and particularly if you notice breathing difficulties or stridor (a high-pitched noise heard when breathing in), she needs immediate medical attention.

Whooping cough (pertussis)

If the coughing comes in fits, followed by a whoop, vomiting, or a blue spell, and an adult or teenager in your home has a chronic cough, your baby could have whooping cough. While incompletely immunized and unimmunized children are at much higher risk, even fully immunized babies may still get whooping cough on the odd occasion, although it is likely to be less severe. For whooping cough treatments, see page 279 and the "Quick guide to common health conditions," page 426, under Pertussis.

Urgent care: If you suspect that your baby may have whooping cough, consult your doctor immediately, especially if she is under 6 months of age.

Choking

It is not unusual for liquids to go down "the wrong way," causing a bit of a choke and a cough. Prevent choking episodes by keeping choking hazards away from your baby and cutting certain foods, such as hot dogs and grapes, into pieces small enough that they can't plug the airway. For choking treatments, see page 378.

Urgent care: If the cough settles quickly, there is usually nothing to worry about, but if it continues or your baby experiences any breathing difficulty, wheezing or stridor (a high-pitched noise heard when breathing in), immediate medical attention may be required.

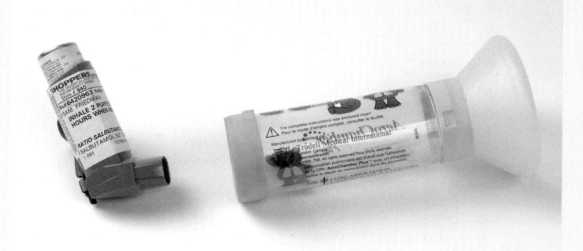

■ Puffer and spacer device.

Understanding developmental delay

An infant's first smile, initial tentative steps, and first words are some of the most eagerly anticipated and vividly remembered milestones we experience as parents. The process whereby an infant transforms from a completely dependent being into a mobile, independent child who becomes an increasingly fluent speaker is a remarkable and mysterious human experience.

While infant development is a "hard-wired" process that differs little from one corner of the world to another, this process can be delayed for various reasons that demand your immediate attention. There are many causes of delays in development — some are temporary, while others are permanent; some are serious, while others can be overcome. If you have concerns regarding delays in your baby's development, make sure to address them with your health-care provider.

Variability

Some skills acquired during infancy are extremely variable and are therefore not accurate indicators of development. For example, while some infants will walk independently at 9 months of age, other equally "normal" infants may begin walking at 15 months. Likewise, some infants are adept at rolling from their front to back and vice versa by 4 months of age, while some seem to hardly roll at all. (Now that infants are commonly placed on their back to sleep, many authorities have observed that infants seem to be less adept at rolling over from their tummy.) Some infants are very mobile, crawling with remarkable speed after 6 months of age, while others may never crawl but will instead proceed effortlessly from standing and cruising around furniture to walking independently at about 1 year of age.

All of these patterns of development, while quite different, are normal. There are, however, other developmental milestones that vary little between individuals. Variations in the development of gross and fine motor skills, vision, and hearing may be cause for concern and should be discussed with your health-care provider.

Developmental problem red flags

- **Gross motor skills:** See your health-care provider if your baby starts rolling over prior to 3 months or is not walking by 18 months.
- **Fine motor skills:** Behaviors of concern include holding hands tightly in fists for most of the time at 3 months and preferring the right or left hand before 18 months.

- **Vision:** By 2 months of age, an infant should demonstrate that she can fix her gaze and follow objects, especially faces, in her field of vision. In addition, your baby should be smiling. If you are concerned about your infant's vision, discuss it with your health-care provider. A parent's instinct should always be taken seriously.
- **Hearing:** Your baby's hearing should be fully developed at birth. Babies should respond to loud noises. By the age of 6 months, your baby should be showing some response to her name and should be starting to babble. If you have any concerns about your baby's ability to hear, or if other members of the family have hearing loss, discuss this with your child's health-care provider and take advantage of the newborn hearing screening programs offered in many areas.

Loss of skills

The loss of a previously acquired skill — for example, the ability to sit — is never normal and must be addressed by a health-care provider. However, as infants gain more sophisticated skills and behaviors, they may use some previously acquired skills less often. For example, a 9-month-old might be very keen on showing off her ability to "blow raspberries" or wave "bye-bye" on command, but these behaviors will generally become less frequent as she gets older and develops more sophisticated forms of communication.

Basic developmental milestones

Age	Motor skills	Communication
2 months		• Smiles responsively
4 months	• Reaches for objects • Can control head	• Coos • Laughs
6 months	• Can roll both ways • Sits when supported • Transfers an object from hand to hand	• Babbles ("bababa") • Turns when her name is called
9 months	• Sits unsupported • Puts objects in mouth	• Waves bye-bye
12–15 months	• Walks independently • Uses a spoon	• Understands "no" • Says a few single words

Recognizing failure to thrive

Parents almost always worry whether their baby is growing and gaining weight appropriately. In many cultures, a healthy infant is synonymous with a chubby infant, but there is a wide range of healthy weights in infancy. Some of the many factors that influence weight gain include maternal health during pregnancy and, most importantly, your baby's genetic makeup. The type of feeding also has a small influence on patterns of weight gain, with breast-fed infants gaining weight at a somewhat slower rate than formula-fed infants.

Genetic factors

As the expression goes, the apple does not fall far from the tree, and weight and growth patterns in children are strongly related to those of their parents and siblings. If you and your partner are small or slim, don't be surprised if your baby seems to be growing along one of the lower percentile lines on her growth chart (for example, the 3rd or 10th percentile).

Failure to thrive facts

The term "failure to thrive" (FTT) refers to infants whose pattern of weight gain is less than optimal. During well-baby visits, your health-care provider will monitor your baby's growth and will record and plot her measurements on a growth chart. There is, of course, no ideal weight for all infants. Much more important is the rate of weight gain over time. There is usually no cause for concern unless your baby has lost weight or her growth has "plateaued."

Failure to thrive red flags

If your baby shows the following signs and symptoms of failure to thrive, or if you have concerns about her general health, ask your health-care provider to help you determine the possible cause of the problem and recommend treatment to get your baby back on track.

- Your baby is losing or stops gaining weight.
- Your baby's weight gain is so small that she has fallen over two major percentiles (for example, from the 50th to the 10th) on the growth chart over the course of a few months.
- Your baby experiences persistent vomiting or diarrhea.

HOW TO
Manage failure to thrive

1. Establish that your baby is indeed failing to thrive, not just failing to meet your expectations of a chubby baby. You may not be able to establish this without the help of your health-care provider, using your baby's record of heights and weights since birth.

2. If your baby is truly failing to thrive, your health-care provider will set out to establish why. In many cases, there is no single cause; nevertheless, it is important to look at all the possibilities, many of which can be treated:

- **Inadequate calories:** The most common cause of FTT is inadequate intake of calories. In breast-fed babies, this may be caused by an insufficient supply of milk. Breast milk supply can be checked by pumping the breasts and measuring how many ounces come out or by weighing the baby before and after a feed to establish how much she is drinking (an accurate scale designed specifically for infants is required). A gain of 2 ounces (60 g), for example, would suggest that she has drunk 2 ounces (60 mL) of milk.

  More rarely, the powdered formula given to formula-fed babies may be overdiluted; it is important to review the dilution instructions on the container.

  Some babies simply are not able to take in the amount of calories required for weight gain. An example is babies with severe gastroesophageal reflux, who get heartburn when they feed and, as a result, develop an aversion to feeding because of the pain they associate with it. These babies often spit up and tend to be irritable and uncomfortable during feeds, sometimes pulling away from the breast or bottle. Babies with underlying diseases such as congenital heart disease can become very tired from the effort of feeding and do not have enough energy left to feed adequately.

- **Losing calories:** Another potential cause of FTT is calorie loss through vomiting or diarrhea. In diseases that result in chronic vomiting, the food does not stay in the stomach long enough to be digested and absorbed. In a number of conditions, inflammation of the intestinal wall can cause problems with digestion and absorption, resulting in ongoing diarrhea. Some examples include cystic fibrosis, celiac disease, and cow's milk protein allergy.

- **Increased metabolic rate:** Although rare, some chronic diseases (such as heart, lung, and kidney diseases and hyperthyroidism) result in an increased metabolic rate, which requires increased intake to ensure appropriate weight gain. With most of these diseases, you can expect the baby to have other difficulties in addition to poor weight gain.

Even if there is no specific cause or treatment for your baby's failure to thrive, there are a number of ways to increase the calories going into your baby, which usually results in improved weight gain. Any changes in diet should be discussed with your health-care provider.

Giving medicine to your baby

As many parents can attest, the decision to give medication, such as acetaminophen for fever or antibiotics for an ear infection, may be straightforward, but actually administering the medication to a baby can be far from easy. While some infants take medication without incident, others swallow it under protest and spit it up, to the utter frustration of their caregivers — and those who are doing the laundry. Fortunately, there is special equipment designed to help with this task, and you can benefit from techniques refined by experienced parents through trial and error.

Infant medications

Medications can be divided into those purchased over the counter (OTC) and those that are prescribed. OTC medications, such as cough and cold remedies, can be bought from any pharmacy, and these days from many supermarkets as well. To purchase prescribed medications, such as antibiotics, you'll need a prescription from your doctor, and the medicine must be dispensed by a licensed pharmacist. For a list of some of the over-the-counter and prescribed medications used in the first year of life, see the chart on pages 410–11.

Side effects

Almost all medications have the potential for unwanted side effects. While many of these are of minor importance, in rare circumstances more serious adverse effects, such as a severe allergic reaction, can result.

Side effects are certainly not limited to prescribed medications; they can also be caused by over-the-counter medications, as well as naturopathic and herbal remedies.

When you're deciding whether to give your infant a medication, it is always wise to weigh the risks and benefits. In the case of a urinary tract infection, for example, the benefit of antibiotic treatment far outweighs the risk of side effects. With the common cold, on the other hand, the risks of side effects from OTC cold remedies outweigh the benefits (which have not been proven in infants).

Equipment

Because most medications for babies come in liquid form, a dropper is the best way to give medication orally. Other tools include cylindrical dosing spoons (available in pharmacies and useful for babies who already eat by spoon), medication cups (better for older infants and children), and syringes.

Caution should be used when using syringes that come with caps on the end to prevent spillage — these small caps can be a choking hazard.

Infant medications

Name	Indication	Examples	Dose	Comments
Antipyretics and analgesics	• Fever • Discomfort	• Acetaminophen (Tylenol, Tempra) • Ibuprofen (Advil, Motrin)	• 10–15 mg per kg every 4–6 hours, or consult package • *Under 6 months:* 5 mg per kg every 8 hrs as necessary • *Over 6 months:* 5–10 mg per kg every 6–8 hours as necessary	• Do not use in babies under 3 months unless discussed with your doctor. • Do not use both acetaminophen and ibuprofen at the same time.
Antibiotics	• Bacterial infections: for example, ear infections, urinary tract infections, skin infections, pneumonia	• Amoxicillin	• 50 mg per kg daily (⅓ total dose given 3 times a day)	• 80–90 mg per kg daily may be required if child is attending daycare. • Different types of antibiotics are required depending on where the infection is, and to what the causative bacteria is sensitive. • Complete the full course of antibiotics as prescribed to avoid building up resistant bacteria.
Laxatives	• Constipation	• Glycerin suppository • Lactulose	• 1 infant suppository as necessary • 2.5–5 mL daily	• Mineral oil is generally contraindicated in babies because of the damage to the lungs if aspirated.

Name	Indication	Examples	Dose	Comments
Topical creams and ointments	• Eczema • Fungal infections	• 1% hydrocortisone cream • Nystatin ointment	• Apply 3 times daily to affected area	• Only mild steroid creams and ointments should be used on thin-skinned areas (face and diaper area). • Ointments are preferred in cooler or drier conditions.
Inhalers	• Asthma	• Salbutamol/ Albuterol (Ventolin)	• 2 puffs every 4 hours as needed by metered dose inhaler (MDI) with aerochamber • *For young infants:* 0.03 mL per kg per dose in 3 mL of normal saline via nebulizer	• Infants need to be able to breathe deeply enough to move the valve in the aerochamber. Otherwise, they require a nebulizer (compressor).

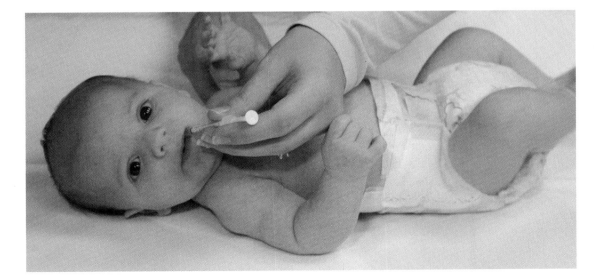

HOW TO
Give medications to your baby

Some medications are best given orally, by dropper or syringe. Others can be given by rectal suppository; this route is most helpful when your child is vomiting. Medicines can take 30 to 45 minutes to be absorbed or to pass through the stomach. If your child vomits within 15 to 30 minutes of being given an oral medication, the dose can be repeated.

Oral (by dropper or syringe)
- Check the storage directions. Some liquid medications, such as antibiotics, need to be stored in the refrigerator.
- Shake the bottle before use.
- Carefully check the dosage recommendations on the label. It is very easy to mix up mL and mg, and different formulations of antipyretics, for example, may have different strengths.

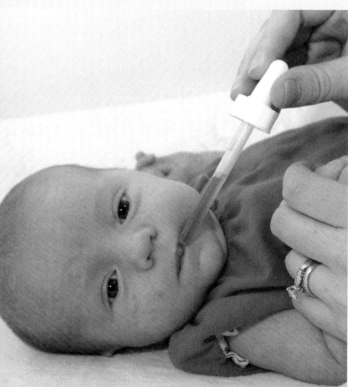

- Use a dropper or syringe to get the medicine into your baby's mouth. Place the tip of the dropper or syringe in her mouth so that the tip is pointing toward the cheek and slowly squeeze the dropper or press the syringe plunger.
- To help prevent gagging, avoid squirting liquid medication at the roof of the mouth or the back of the tongue. Small squirts into the space between the gum and cheek often work best. Use your finger to pull the cheek outward gently to find this helpful spot. It will also be harder for your infant to spit out the medicine this way.
- It is not uncommon for a child to spit out medication, or to vomit after taking it. If the medication is spat up or vomited within 15 to 30 minutes, it is usually appropriate to repeat the dose.

Rectal (by suppository)
- Place your baby's hips and knees in a flexed position to relax the anus and make administration easier.
- Insert the suppository gently into the anus using a small amount of petroleum jelly as a lubricant.

HOW TO
Give eye, nose, and ear drops

Infections involving the eyes, ears, and nose are not uncommon in infants. While it may be difficult to get the drops into these sensitive (and small) parts of the body, drops are often safer and more effective than other forms of administration because the medication goes directly to the site of the infection. In addition, because only a minimal amount is absorbed into the bloodstream, the risk of side effects is lower.

Eye drops

- Warm the bottle in your hands to avoid discomfort.
- Wrap your baby in a blanket.
- Lay your baby on her back and gently pull her lower eyelid down with your thumb, forming a pocket for the drops.
- If your baby resists opening her eyes, drop the liquid onto the inner corner of the eye and rub gently with your fingertip. As your baby opens her eyes, the medication will be absorbed.
- Never touch the eye with the dropper.

Nose drops

- Warm the bottle in your hands to avoid discomfort.
- Wrap your baby in a blanket.
- Lay your baby on her back so that her head falls back over your thigh, and support her head with your hand.
- Place the tip of the dropper just above the nostril and give the drops as prescribed.

Ear drops

- Warm the bottle in your hands to avoid discomfort.
- Wrap your baby in a blanket.
- Lay your baby on her side on your lap, with her infected ear facing up.
- Gently pull her earlobe down and back to straighten the ear canal.
- Drop, don't squirt, drops into ear.
- Keep your baby lying down for a minute to prevent the drops from running out.

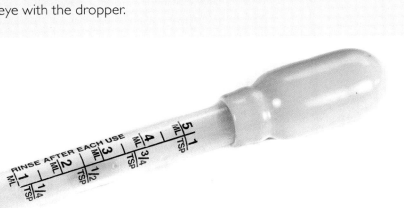

Quick guide to common health conditions

It is often a challenge to find the information you need to care for your sick baby when you need it. The following chart, with common health conditions listed in alphabetical order, condenses the information provided in this book and provides page numbers that will lead you to more detailed information.

Quick guide to common health conditions

Condition	Signs and symptoms	Treatments
Acrocyanosis (page 64)	Purplish blue discoloration of the newborn baby's hands and feet.	Normal — no treatment required.
Apnea of prematurity (page 113)	A pause in breathing that lasts for more than 15 seconds. The more premature the baby, the more frequently this occurs. If severe, apnea may cause a bluish color and/or slowing of the heart rate.	Usually resolves spontaneously, but may require gentle stimulation. If severe, the premature baby may require assistance with breathing. Stops occurring as the baby gets older.
Asthma (pages 332, 403)	Infants present with distressed breathing, which may include rapid respiration and increased effort with each breath. Asthma can result in audible wheezing, coughing, flaring of the nostrils, and sucking in of the skin between the ribs with each breath. It is more common in infants with a history of atopy (for example, eczema) or a family history of allergy (for example, asthma or hayfever). Episodes can be triggered by many things, including a viral cold or exposure to cigarette smoke or allergens from pets.	Keep the infant away from possible triggers — cigarette smoke, dusty environments, and other allergens. Babies are too young to go for allergy testing. Asthma medications can be divided into relievers and preventers. For relief of symptoms, most children will require a bronchodilator (Ventolin, Albuterol) given by a puffer and spacer device. An anti-inflammatory (corticosteroid) is usually given in syrup form for 5 days. For children with frequent attacks, a preventative medication is usually prescribed, commonly in the form of a steroid puffer and spacer, used every day.

Condition	Signs and symptoms	Treatments
Baby acne (page 97)	Looks similar to teenage acne, but occurs on the face of young babies.	No treatment required. Disappears over the first few months.
Birthmarks (page 219)	The most frequently seen is the salmon patch — a flat pink skin discoloration seen at birth, usually over the eyelid ("angel's kiss") or at the back of the neck ("stork bite"). Mongolian spots, bluish gray discolorations usually found over the lower back and buttocks, are common in babies with pigmented skin. Strawberry hemangiomas are raised reddish (or bluish) lumps; they tend to be very small or even absent at birth. They are actually small growths of blood vessels under the skin.	Salmon patches and Mongolian spots tend to disappear as the child gets older; treatment is never necessary. Strawberry hemangiomas grow quite rapidly in the first 6 months, then gradually shrink. By 9 years, 90% will have disappeared. Treatment is indicated only if the hemangioma is in a very sensitive area — for example, close to the eye, obscuring vision — or is causing bleeding from repeated trauma.
Bronchiolitis (pages 332, 403)	A viral infection affecting the small airways in the lungs. Occurs predominantly in winter. Presents with cough and cold symptoms, which may go on to increased work to breathe, with rapid respirations and increased effort with each breath. This can result in audible wheezing, flaring of the nostrils, and sucking in of the skin between the ribs with each breath. Infants with significant respiratory distress will often have difficulty feeding.	This is a self-resolving condition, similar to a cold, which will improve over the course of a week. Because it is a viral infection, antibiotics are not helpful. A minority of infants may benefit from inhaled medications, such as Ventolin (Salbutamol/Albuterol) to open up the small airways, which can be given through a puffer and spacer device or a compressor (similar to the treatment of asthma). If the baby has significant respiratory distress and is feeding poorly, she may require hospitalization so she can receive supplemental oxygen (by mask or prongs in the nose) and additional fluids (through an intravenous or nasogastric tube).

Condition	Signs and symptoms	Treatments
Bronchopulmonary dysplasia (BPD) (page 113)	A lung condition seen in premature babies. Occurs as a result of lung disease in preemies, combined with the extra oxygen required and the high pressures needed to ensure adequate breathing. Even after they have passed their due date, babies may have to work harder to breathe and may wheeze; in these cases supplemental oxygen is required.	Treatment depends on the severity of the condition, but many babies will go home on supplemental oxygen and other inhaled medications.
Candida yeast rash (pages 211, 212)	A bright red rash in the diaper area. Usually also involves the skin hidden between rolls of fat and may include small red blotches beyond the margins of the rash.	An antifungal topical cream, such as nystatin, is applied over the rash 3 times daily for about 5 days.
Caput (page 64)	Swelling of the newborn's scalp, caused by the tight squeeze through the birth canal. Can give the baby the appearance of a "conehead." Often accompanied by "molding" of the skull bones (a ridge may be felt under the scalp where one skull bone has overlapped another).	No treatment required. Will disappear over the first few days of life.
Cephalohematoma (page 64)	A large bruise under the scalp seen after delivery. May initially feel soft, but can harden over time. Can increase the risk of jaundice.	No treatment required. Will resolve over the course of weeks or months.
Chicken pox (page 272)	A very contagious viral infection. Usually causes fever, muscle aches, and an itchy rash. Complications are rare, but include secondary skin infections (for example, flesh-eating disease) and involvement of the brain (for example, encephalitis).	The varicella (chicken pox) vaccination will prevent most cases of chicken pox. Vaccinated children who get the disease tend to have a milder course. There is no specific treatment, although medications are often given to relieve the itch and treat the fever and achiness.

Condition	Signs and symptoms	Treatments
Club foot (page 220)	A baby is born with the heel and forefoot of one or both feet pointed inward. The foot is stiff and cannot be moved into the normal position.	An orthopedic surgeon may place a series of plaster casts over the foot to gradually correct the position, or it may require a surgical procedure.
Cold (page 274)	A viral infection. Babies usually present with nasal congestion and/or discharge, cough, decreased appetite, low-grade fever, and a bit less energy than usual.	Saline nasal drops may be helpful to loosen up the nasal congestion. Over-the- counter cough and cold remedies are not recommended in the first year because the risk of side effects outweighs the benefits. Acetaminophen or ibuprofen may be used to treat discomfort or fever (discuss with your doctor first if your baby is less than 3 months old).
Colic (page 209)	Inconsolable crying, often starting without warning, usually a few weeks after birth. The baby may go red in the face, clench her fists, and pull up her legs. Can last for hours, during which time she cannot be calmed down. Happens on most days, often at the same time, most often in the late afternoon or early evening.	No proven therapies that work in all cases, but colic resolves on its own by the age of 4 months. In a small percentage of cases, it may help if a breast-feeding mother avoids dairy products or if the formula given is changed to a hypoallergenic one. No safe, effective medications. Outside support for parents is valuable, as is ensuring that both parents take turns to get away from the crying.
Constipation (page 334)	Characterized by the passage of hard, painful stools, which often resemble small pellets. The frequency of stools does not indicate constipation; breast-fed babies, for example, may have 7 stools a day or 1 stool every 7th day. Both would be considered normal as long as the stool is soft.	Treatment may involve dietary changes, such as adding a few ounces of prune juice to the diet. Non-absorbable sugars, such as lactulose, may help to draw water into the bowel and soften the stool. Occasionally, a baby may require a suppository. Do not use mineral oil in the first year — it can cause a serious pneumonia if aspirated into the lungs.

Condition	Signs and symptoms	Treatments
Croup (page 332)	A viral infection affecting the voice box and windpipe. Most common in spring and fall. Usually starts with cold symptoms, followed by a loud, barking, seal-like cough, which is often worse in the middle of the night. In the most severe cases, the baby will have stridor (she will make a high-pitched noise when breathing in) and will have to work harder to breathe.	Many parents find that humidity helps — they either run a hot shower and allow the bathroom to become steamy or take the baby into the cool outside air. If croup causes your baby to work harder to breathe, an urgent visit to the doctor is required; treatment will likely involve epinephrine inhaled through a mask and anti-inflammatory corticosteroid medication.
Dehydration (page 275)	The most common cause of dehydration is loss of fluids through diarrhea and/or vomiting. Babies can become dehydrated quite quickly. Some of the more common signs include listlessness, decreased interest in feeding and playing, dry mouth and tongue, sunken eyes and decreased tears, and a decrease in the number of wet diapers.	Treatment involves getting more fluid into the baby. In general, she will have lost water and salts, so rehydration is best achieved with a commercially available solution such as Pedialyte, which can be purchased over the counter at most pharmacies. These solutions are often flavored to disguise the somewhat "yucky" salty taste. Water or juice may suffice in very mild cases, but they do not contain enough salt or sugar for the truly dehydrated baby. If your baby has signs of dehydration, have her assessed immediately by a health-care professional.
Developmental dysplasia of the hip (page 218)	A spectrum of conditions that occur when the top of the thigh bone is not properly covered by the pelvic bone. Not painful. Usually noticed by the doctor when she examines the baby's hips. Parents may notice decreased range of movement of the hip during diaper changes or a difference in the skin creases between the baby's thighs.	Treatment is supervised by an orthopedic surgeon. The baby may have to wear a special harness to keep the thigh bone in position until the hip joint develops properly, or surgery may be required.

Condition	Signs and symptoms	Treatments
Diaper rash (dermatitis) (pages 211, 212, 400)	Red, inflamed skin in the diaper area, often with raw areas. Unlike a yeast rash, diaper rash does not involve the skin between the creases that is not exposed to the irritants in the diaper.	Treatment involves frequent diaper changes, exposing the skin to fresh air, and the use of barrier creams. If these measures don't solve the problem, a mild corticosteroid cream, is usually prescribed and is applied topically 3 times a day for up to a week, or until the rash looks better.
Diarrhea and vomiting (page 275)	Diarrhea means more frequent, looser stools than normal. The most common cause of diarrhea and vomiting is viral gastroenteritis. This usually starts with vomiting for 24–48 hours, often accompanied by a low-grade fever, and followed by the onset of diarrhea, which can continue for several days to a week. Watch out for signs of dehydration.	If the symptoms are mild, babies are usually able to continue with their normal feeding schedule. Those with persistent symptoms and mild dehydration should be offered frequent small amounts of a commercial oral rehydration solution, such as Pedialyte. If the baby cannot keep anything down and is looking ill, see your doctor. Intravenous or nasogastric fluids are occasionally required. Medications to stop vomiting and diarrhea are not used for babies.
Diphtheria (page 270)	A potentially fatal bacterial infection that mainly affects the throat, obstructing the airway. Releases a toxin that affects the heart and nerves as well.	Prevented by vaccination, usually as part of the primary series at 2, 4, and 6 months, with two boosters later on.
Eczema (atopic dermatitis) (pages 278, 401)	Patches of dry skin that are often red, a bit raised, scaly, and itchy. The areas most commonly affected are the face, especially the cheeks, and the outer part of the knees and arms.	Eczema resolves spontaneously in up to 50% of children by school age, but there is no cure. To prevent flare-ups, avoid irritants (such as perfumed soaps, fabric softener, and woolen garments) and use hypoallergenic soaps and moisturizers to trap moisture in the skin. During flare-ups, a mild corticosteroid cream is often required for inflamed areas.

Condition	Signs and symptoms	Treatments
Erythema toxicum (page 97)	Very often seen in the first few days of life, this rash consists of tiny yellow or white pustules on a red background. They are usually found in groups and tend to come and go in a matter of hours.	Disappears spontaneously over the course of a few days. No treatment required.
Failure to thrive (FTT) (page 407)	Refers to babies with suboptimal weight gain. This includes any baby who stops gaining weight or loses weight over the course of weeks or months. It also includes babies whose growth slows so that they cross over two or more percentiles on their growth chart.	Requires a thorough assessment by your health-care provider. Treatment varies depending on the underlying cause of the problem, but will likely involve trying to get more calories into your baby. There are many strategies your health-care provider can recommend to achieve this.
Fetal alcohol spectrum disorder (FASD) (page 26)	Can occur if a pregnant mother ingests alcohol during pregnancy. Nobody knows what the safe level of alcohol in pregnancy is. Babies tend to be small, with small heads and a particular facial appearance. They tend to have failure to thrive and developmental delays.	Prevention is key — do not drink alcohol during pregnancy.
Food allergies (page 331)	Can present with hives, wheezing, or vomiting. Anaphylactic reactions are life-threatening and include swelling of the throat and a drop in blood pressure. Allergy to cow's milk protein can result in blood in the stool, diarrhea and vomiting, irritability, and poor weight gain.	Treatment consists of avoiding the offending foods. For severe allergies, a MedicAlert bracelet and EpiPen are necessities. Anaphylactic reactions are medical emergencies and require immediate attention and treatment with epinephrine, antihistamines, and corticosteroids.
Gastroenteritis	See Diarrhea and vomiting.	
Gastroesophageal reflux	See Spitting up.	

Condition	Signs and symptoms	Treatments
Hearing loss (page 222)	If the baby is not responding to her name or babbling by 6 months of age, she could have a hearing problem. A lack of response to loud noises is also worrisome. Hearing screening is now performed on all newborn babies in many jurisdictions.	Referrals should be made to an audiologist and an ear, nose, and throat specialist. Treatment will depend on the cause of the hearing loss, and may range from placement of tubes in the eardrum to placement of cochlear implants.
Heart murmurs (page 280)	A heart murmur is a noise heard by your health-care professional while listening with a stethoscope. It is caused by the blood flowing through the chambers and valves of the heart. At least 50% of children will have a heart murmur at some time in childhood, but very few will have a heart problem.	If a murmur is heard, the doctor will decide whether it is necessary to do any further investigation, such as an x-ray (to look at the size and shape of the heart), an electrocardiogram (to look at the electrical forces of the heart), or an echocardiogram (to take an ultrasound of the heart). Most murmurs do not indicate heart disease. If there are any abnormalities on the tests, medications or an operation may be recommended.
Heat rash (page 213)	When the sweat glands get blocked, a rash with tiny red bumps (prickly heat) usually results. Heat rash is most commonly seen where the skin is covered (for example, the upper back and chest).	Avoid overbundling the baby or exposing her to excessive heat and humidity. Cotton clothing tends to allow heat and moisture to escape more easily. Ointments, creams, and powders may further block the pores and make the rash worse.
Hemangiomas	See Birthmarks.	
Hemorrhagic disease of the newborn (page 68)	May occur in newborns and can result in serious bleeding problems in the first weeks of life.	Prevented by giving the newborn baby an injection of vitamin K.

Condition	Signs and symptoms	Treatments
Hepatitis B (pages 18, 272)	Inflammation of the liver caused by infection with the hepatitis B virus. Passed from person to person by the exchange of body fluids — for example, from a mother to her baby during birth. Many infected infants have no symptoms. Occasionally, children may get fever, lethargy, and jaundice and have a poor appetite. It can lead to long-term liver damage.	Mothers are checked for hepatitis B in pregnancy; if they are carriers, their newborns will be vaccinated as soon as they are born. Hepatitis B vaccination is provided to all children as part of their routine vaccination schedule, with the exact timing varying among jurisdictions.
Hernias (page 277)	Abdominal contents move through a weakened part of the abdominal wall, resulting in a "lump." This lump may come and go, or may be present all the time. The two areas most commonly affected are the belly button (umbilical hernia) and the groin (inguinal hernia).	Umbilical hernias almost always close by themselves before the child reaches school age, so no treatment is necessary. Inguinal hernias do not go away and therefore need to be surgically repaired by a general surgeon. This is usually an outpatient procedure.
Hypospadias and chordee (page 221)	The opening of the urethra in baby boys occurs somewhere along the shaft or at the base of the penis, instead of at the tip. This makes it very difficult for older boys to pee accurately when standing. It is often associated with chordee, in which the penis bends when erect.	Treatment is done by a urologist. Very minor degrees of hypospadias may not require treatment. Surgical repair is required for significant hypospadias. The foreskin may be used in the repair, so boys with hypospadias should not be circumcised.
Hypothyroidism (page 93)	Congenital hypothyroidism occurs when a baby has a decreased amount of thyroid hormone at the time of birth. Babies may present with prolonged jaundice, lethargy, constipation, feeding problems, low muscle tone, and developmental delays.	Will be diagnosed by the newborn thyroid blood screening test, performed in the first few days of life. Treatment involves supplementation with thyroid hormone.

Condition	Signs and symptoms	Treatments
Influenza (page 273)	Caused by the influenza A or B virus. Usually results in high fevers, with chills, headache, sore throat, muscle pains, weakness, and a dry cough. Young infants can look very sick. Influenza is sometimes mistaken for meningitis.	An annual influenza immunization, given in the fall, is recommended for all children between the ages of 6 months and 5 years (it cannot be given before 6 months) as a preventative measure. Treatment is usually with antipyretics, but infants are sometimes so sick that they may require hospitalization.
Intussusception (page 398)	A rare condition in which the wall of the intestine "telescopes" into the piece of intestine in front, causing a blockage of the bowel. Babies typically present with spasms of severe tummy pain separated by periods where they are quite comfortable. There may be blood in the stool, which is sometimes said to look like red current jelly.	Diagnosed by means of an ultrasound of the intestines. Can usually be fixed by pushing air in through the rectum, which forces the telescoped bowel back into its normal position, relieving the blockage. This "air enema" is done by a radiologist (x-ray specialist). Occasionally, a surgical procedure is required.
Irregular and noisy breathing (page 215)	Periodic breathing is normal in the first month of life. The baby breathes rapidly, then has an occasional deep breath and sigh, and may even pause between breaths for a few seconds. Because the newborn's nasal passages are so small, breathing may sound noisy and congested. The baby will sneeze from time to time to clear her nose; this does not mean that she has a cold.	No treatment required. If the baby appears to have to work harder to breathe on a regular basis, have her seen by your doctor. If she does have a blocked nose, you can try saline nose drops and an aspirator to see if this helps to clear some of the mucus out of her nose.

Condition	Signs and symptoms	Treatments
Jaundice (page 95)	A yellow pigment on the skin or in the whites of the eyes; seen in many newborn babies in the first few weeks of life.	Treatment varies depending on the cause of the jaundice. The most common treatments are help with the feeding process and the use of phototherapy lights, which allow the baby to break down bilirubin and excrete it.
Lip blister (page 96)	A blister or callus, usually in the middle of the newborn's upper lip, caused by vigorous sucking.	No treatment required; will heal on its own.
Measles (page 272)	A very contagious viral infection. The illness begins with fever, runny nose, red eyes, and cough, followed a few days later by a bright red rash. Complications include ear infections, pneumonia, and involvement of the brain.	Prevention is through immunization with the MMR vaccine. Two doses are required. Measles has no specific treatment, other than trying to make the child more comfortable with antipyretics and fluids.
Meningitis (pages 271, 279)	An infection of the lining of the brain. The classic presentation of bacterial meningitis, seen in older children, consists of neck stiffness, fever, and vomiting. In infants, the presentation can be much less specific and may include fever, lethargy, poor feeding, vomiting, and seizures.	The incidence of bacterial meningitis has dropped significantly since the introduction of the hemophilus B, pneumococcal, and meningococcal conjugate vaccines. Cases are treated with intravenous antibiotics and require close observation for complications.

Condition	Signs and symptoms	Treatments
Meningococcemia (page 271)	A rare but extremely dangerous and rapidly progressive infection in the bloodstream caused by a bacterium known as *Neisseria meningitides* (or meningococcus). Babies tend to have a fever and look very unwell, and may develop petechiae (pinpoint red spots on the skin) and purpura (pinkish-purple flat discolorations of the skin that look like bruises). These skin lesions do not disappear (blanch) if pressure is applied over the skin, suggesting that they are caused by bleeding just below the skin. The bacteria can spread to the brain, resulting in meningococcal meningitis.	With the introduction of the new meningococcal conjugate vaccine, the incidence of meningococcemia should decrease, but the vaccine does not cover all of the different types of meningococcus, so cases will continue to be seen. Meningococcemia is a medical emergency; treatment involves immediate intravenous antibiotics and intensive supportive care in the hospital.
Milia (page 97)	Tiny white bumps seen in newborns, particularly over the nose and cheeks. They are caused by a blockage of tiny glands in the skin, leading to a buildup of natural oils.	No treatment required; the bumps will disappear within a few weeks.
Mongolian spot (page 219)	Bluish gray pigmentation of the skin, most commonly found over the buttocks and lower back. It is most common in darker-skinned ethnic groups and is present from birth.	No treatment required; the spots will fade as the child grows older.
Mumps (page 272)	A viral infection that usually causes a headache, fever, aches, and pains, as well as a painful swelling around the angle of the jaw that makes the cheeks puff out.	Prevention is through immunization with the MMR vaccine. There is no specific treatment if your child gets the infection.

Condition	Signs and symptoms	Treatments
Necrotizing enterocolitis (NEC) (page 114)	A condition of the bowel, usually seen in premature babies, caused by decreased blood supply or oxygen to the bowel. Babies tend to present with intolerance to food, distended tummies, and some blood in the stool.	Treatment depends on the severity of the condition. Mild cases may be treated with resting of the bowel (by not feeding the baby) and intravenous antibiotics; severe cases require a surgical operation.
Otitis media (ear infection) (page 335)	Occurs as a result of an infection in the middle ear, behind the eardrum. It is uncommon before the age of 6 months and often occurs in the setting of a cold. Babies tend to be very irritable and often wake up crying in the middle of the night. They may pull on the ear, and occasionally the eardrum may burst, resulting in drainage of fluid from the ear and some pain relief.	It is important to treat the pain with acetaminophen or ibuprofen. Even though some ear infections resolve by themselves, antibiotics are generally prescribed in the first year or two of life. In fact, this is the most common indication for antibiotics at this age.
Pertussis (whooping cough) (pages 270, 279)	Babies usually present with coughing spasms that are often followed by a vomit, a whoop, or even a "blue" spell from lack of oxygen. Pertussis is usually preceded by a few days of cold symptoms and a cough.	Immunization has sharply decreased the number of cases, as well as the severity of the disease in those who are immunized but still get it. There is no effective treatment, but the baby and all close contacts are given antibiotics to reduce spread. Some young babies require hospitalization for supportive care, which includes oxygen and suctioning.
Phenylketonuria (PKU) (page 93)	A rare inherited metabolic disease that can lead to mental retardation and developmental delays. It is detected by the routine newborn PKU screen, performed in the first few days of life.	Treatment involves making significant adjustments to the baby's diet. This limits the intake of the protein she is unable to break down as a result of her disease. A buildup of this protein is what causes damage.

Condition	Signs and symptoms	Treatments
Pneumococcus (page 271)	A bacterium known more formally as *Streptococcus pneumoniae*. It can cause infection in many parts of the body, including the ears (otitis media), the lungs (pneumonia), the bloodstream (bacteremia), and, most seriously, the brain (meningitis).	Many cases can be prevented by the pneumococcal conjugate vaccine. Treatment consists of antibiotics, given either by mouth (for otitis media, for example) or intravenously (for meningitis, for example).
Pneumonia (page 271)	An infection of the lungs, often diagnosed when an abnormality of the lung is seen on a chest x-ray. Infants can have bacterial or viral pneumonia. In either case, they are likely to have a cough and some difficulty breathing, including flaring of the nostrils, an increased number of breaths per minute, and increased effort with each breath. They will also usually have decreased energy and will feed poorly. Babies with bacterial pneumonia often have a higher fever and look sicker than those with viral pneumonia.	Treatment involves supporting the baby while she fights off the infection. This means no treatment at all in mild cases of viral pneumonia. More severe cases may require hospitalization for supplemental oxygen (by mask or prongs in the nose) and additional fluids by intravenous or nasogastric tube. Bacterial pneumonia requires a course of antibiotics, which will be given either by mouth or intravenously, depending on how sick the baby is. Supportive care may also be required.
Polio (page 270)	A viral infection caused by the polio virus. Can result in minimal symptoms or in fevers, headaches, vomiting, pain, and weakness. Can also cause permanent paralysis.	With the introduction of polio immunization, this disease is now eradicated in North America, although outbreaks still occur in developing countries. The immunization is usually given at 2, 4, and 6 months, with boosters thereafter.

Condition	Signs and symptoms	Treatments
Pre-eclampsia (page 16)	Also known as toxemia, this condition may occur during the second half of pregnancy. The most common signs in the pregnant mother include high blood pressure; increased swelling over and above that normally seen in pregnancy, with sudden weight gain; and the spilling of protein into the urine (detected by placing a testing stick in a urine sample). Headaches and changes in vision may also occur.	Treatment depends on the severity of the condition. The only real cure is delivery of the baby. Mild cases may be treated with restriction of activity and close monitoring. More severe cases may require hospitalization, medications, and even premature delivery of the baby.
Pyloric stenosis (page 218)	An obstruction at the outlet of the stomach caused by a thickening of the pyloric muscle. Boys are more likely to be affected by pyloric stenosis than girls. Babies tend to present with projectile vomiting starting at 2–4 weeks of age.	Requires a surgical procedure and a brief stay of a couple of days in the hospital.
Respiratory distress syndrome (RDS) (page 113)	A problem affecting the lungs in very premature babies caused by the lack of a substance called surfactant. The premature newborn will have severe difficulty with breathing (respiratory distress).	Treatment usually involves attaching the newborn to a ventilation machine, giving supplemental oxygen and instilling surfactant into the lungs through a breathing tube that ends in the baby's windpipe. This occurs in the neonatal ICU.
Roseola (page 336)	Caused by human herpes virus 6 (HHV 6). The baby usually has a high fever and is quite irritable. Just as the fever settles, a flat or slightly raised pinkish rash may occur.	No treatment required; roseola is self-resolving. Acetaminophen or ibuprofen can be given for the fever and irritability.

Condition	Signs and symptoms	Treatments
Rubella (pages 18, 272)	Also known as German measles. Tends to be a mild illness in children. It can cause a rash, fever, and swollen glands. Most dangerous if a pregnant woman contracts rubella in the first 20 weeks of her pregnancy; this usually causes severe damage to the growing fetus.	Rubella is prevented by the MMR immunization. There is no specific treatment for the infection.
Seborrheic dermatitis (cradle cap) (pages 278, 401)	Looks like a scaly yellow eruption, with greasy reddened skin around and underneath the scales. Most commonly involves the scalp (cradle cap), but can involve the skin behind the ears, on the neck, over the eyebrows, and in the groin area. Usually seen in the first 3 months of life. It is generally not itchy.	If it is mild, it will resolve spontaneously and no treatment is necessary. In more severe cases, special shampoos or a corticosteroid lotion can be used.
Spitting up (gastroesophageal reflux) (pages 216, 397)	Regurgitation of feeds from the stomach through the mouth or nose; very common because the valve mechanism between the stomach and gullet doesn't work well in babies.	Spitting up is considered normal and gradually improves over the first 6–12 months. If it is associated with pain or poor weight gain, a number of treatments are recommended. Smaller, more frequent feeds, holding the baby upright for 30 minutes after the feed, or thickening the milk with some rice cereal may help. If not, medication to counter the acid in the stomach may be prescribed. Severe cases may require an operation.
Squint (strabismus) (page 333)	Misalignment of the eyes — the eye can be either turned in (esotropia) or turned out (exotropia). This can be normal in the first few months of life, but if it persists, it will need to be attended to.	Referral to an ophthalmologist. Treatment may involve glasses, patching of the eye, or surgical repair. If treatment does not occur promptly, the baby may develop a "lazy eye" (amblyopia), which can cause permanent loss of vision in that eye.

Condition	Signs and symptoms	Treatments
Subconjunctival hemorrhage (page 96)	A red streak seen in the white part of the eye. Commonly seen after delivery and also with coughing spells.	No treatment required; resolves within a week.
Sudden infant death syndrome (SIDS) (pages 241–43)	The sudden and unexpected death of an apparently healthy baby in the first year of life, with no cause found after an extensive investigation — 95% of cases happen in the first 6 months of life.	To reduce the risk, place the baby on her back to sleep in the first 6 months, breast-feed, do not expose her to cigarette smoke, do not overheat her, avoid bed-sharing, and place her on a firm sleeping surface, away from anything that may cause suffocation.
Tears and eye discharge (page 214)	Newborn babies may not have tears for the first few weeks, but will thereafter have tears with crying. Blocked tear ducts will result in the baby having teary eyes even when happy, sometimes with a milky discharge in the corner of the eye.	Use a clean piece of cotton wool to wipe away crusty material. Ask your doctor to show you how to massage the duct against the nose to help unblock it. If still blocked at 1 year, an ear, nose, and throat specialist can unblock it using a probe. If the eye discharge becomes very pussy and profuse and the eyelids are sticking together, ask your doctor whether your baby needs drops for bacterial conjunctivitis.
Tetanus (page 270)	Tetanus, or lockjaw, is a rare but serious disease caused by bacteria that live in the soil and enter the body through a break in the skin. Can cause paralyzing muscle spasms, as well as breathing problems and convulsions.	Prevention is through immunization in infancy, followed by periodic booster shots. Treatment involves cleaning the wound and giving the infected person antibodies from donated blood; even with treatment, tetanus is potentially fatal.
Thrush (page 213)	An overgrowth of yeast (fungus) in the mouth; very common in young infants. It looks like milk curds on the tongue, gums, or inside of the cheeks, but is difficult to remove.	The baby is given an oral antifungal liquid, such as nystatin. Breast-feeding mothers should treat their nipples with an antifungal cream. Place bottle nipples in boiling water for 5–10 minutes before use.

Condition	Signs and symptoms	Treatments
Undescended testicle (page 276)	The testis cannot be found in the scrotum; particularly common in premature boys (up to 30%).	Testis may descend spontaneously, but not likely to occur if it hasn't happened by 6 months of age. A simple outpatient operation can be performed at 9–15 months to bring the testis into the scrotum.
Urinary tract infection (UTI) (page 223)	UTIs include infections of the upper urinary tract (kidneys) and the lower urinary tract (bladder). In infants with UTIs, unlike in older children and adults, both the kidneys and the bladder tend to be infected. The signs and symptoms are non-specific; young babies may have only a fever and some irritability. Other helpful symptoms may include vomiting, poor feeding, decreased energy, and smelly urine.	If a UTI is diagnosed, the baby will require a 10–14 day course of antibiotics. The type of antibiotic and the method of delivery (by mouth or intravenous) will depend on her age, how sick she looks, and the type of bacterial germ grown in the urine sample (usually E. coli). Babies with UTIs generally require some standard investigations to rule out underlying abnormalities, including an ultrasound of the kidneys and a special x-ray called a voiding cystourethrogram (VCUG).
Volvulus (page 398)	Occurs when the intestines become twisted, causing a blockage; thankfully, it is very rare. The baby may have some tummy pain and distension and will usually have vomiting with dark green bile.	This is an emergency, requiring an immediate operation to untwist the intestines.
Wheezing (pages 332, 403)	A whistling or sighing noise when breathing out. Can be accompanied by increased work to breathe. Most commonly caused by bronchiolitis (a viral infection of the lungs) or an asthma attack.	Treatment depends on the cause of the wheezing. Inhaled bronchodilators, such as Ventolin (Salbutamol/Albuterol) will usually be used through a nebulizer or puffer and spacer device. This works well for asthma, but is often ineffective in bronchiolitis. Oxygen may also be required if the baby is having significant breathing difficulties.

Frequently asked questions

As family doctors and pediatricians, we answer many questions from parents. Here are some of the most frequently asked questions. Be sure to ask your health-care providers any other questions that arise. If they don't have the answers, they will refer you to a colleague who does.

Q: Should I get something at the drugstore for my baby's cold?

A: Dozens of over-the-counter medications marketed as treatments for cold symptoms — such as cough, runny nose, and congestion — are available at stores and pharmacies. Apart from medications that relieve discomfort and fever, such as acetaminophen and ibuprofen, these preparations have not been shown to benefit young infants and children, and in some situations, they can cause unwanted or harmful side effects. In general, these products should be avoided in children under school age.

Many products contain or are marketed as antihistamines or decongestants. Antihistamines can be useful in treating an older child with a runny nose or congestion caused by allergies, but they are of no benefit to infants with colds, which are caused by viruses. Decongestants usually contain compounds related to adrenaline, which are intended to restrict blood vessels in the nose. They generally provide minimal benefit (at best) in adults; in young children, they can lead to restlessness and poor sleep. Some antihistamine and decongestant preparations also contain ibuprofen or acetaminophen; if you're not aware of this, you may inadvertently give your baby too much of these medications.

If you're wondering whether to give your baby a cough suppressant, remember that coughing is a protective reflex in response to irritants in the breathing passages and lungs; it is the body's natural way of clearing mucus and irritants from the airway. Studies on cough suppressants have shown minimal benefit at best in adults. They are not recommended for young children.

Q: What should I do if my 6-month-old spits up her medication after I give it to her?

A: This is a common problem. In general, you can repeat the dose if it is spat up within 15 to 30 minutes of administration. If it looks as if only a portion is spat up, it is reasonable to repeat half the dose. Your infant will get the message after a few repeat doses and should stop spitting up.

Q: If my prescription says I need to give my son his antibiotic every 6 hours, should I wake him to take the dose?

A: Very few medications have to be given exactly every 6 or 8 hours. If he is sick, you both likely need your sleep. In the case of antibiotics and most other medications, it would be reasonable to give him a dose before he goes to sleep, and, if you are lucky enough that he sleeps for 7 or 8 hours, give him the next dose when he wakes up.

Q: My mother always told me to feed a cold and starve a fever. Is this true for babies?

A: Absolutely not — and it's not true for adults, either. Whenever a baby is unwell, whether with a cold or a fever, it is important that she remain well hydrated, so offer lots of liquids. Most babies lose their appetite when sick, but you should continue to offer them their regular foods — just don't be disappointed if they aren't eating as well as usual.

Q: What is a febrile convulsion? Is it dangerous? Will my baby always be prone to convulsions?

A: These are seizures that occur in normal children during the first 24 hours of an illness that is accompanied by fever. The baby is often absolutely fine when she is put down to sleep; then, the parents are awoken by the sounds of the baby having a seizure, at which point they notice the fever for the first time. Febrile convulsions are certainly not uncommon (they occur in 3% to 4% of normal babies), but they do not occur before 6 months of age.

Children with typical febrile convulsions will grow out of them by the age of 6 years; they are at minimally increased risk of convulsions after this, when compared to the general population.

The seizures are generally brief and do not cause any damage to the child, although the parent may be traumatized. Watching your baby have a seizure is an awful experience. Unfortunately, there isn't much you can do to prevent them; antipyretics, although often recommended, haven't been shown to decrease the chance of a febrile convulsion.

Q: My daughter is 6 months old. How should I be taking her temperature? I used to use a glass/mercury thermometer. Are the newer digital ones better?

A: A child has to be about 4 to 5 years old before you are likely to get an accurate result by taking her temperature orally. Ear thermometers are expensive and are not particularly accurate for children under 2 years of age. Rectal thermometers are the most accurate, but most children do not appreciate having their temperature taken rectally, so it is usually reserved for babies under 3 months of age, for whom an accurate temperature reading is more important. For a 6-month-old, we suggest taking her temperature under her arm.

We prefer digital thermometers because they read the temperature much more quickly, so you don't have to hold her down for long. With glass thermometers, there is always a risk, albeit very slight, that it will break — and the mercury inside is toxic.

Sam's Diary

January 23 (11½ months old)

Dad is amazed at how you seem to learn something new every day. You know where your hair, head, toes, eyes, teeth, ears, and nose are. You can identify many things — some of your favorites include car, train, milk, apple, and rice cake. You love to give high fives, and you blew on a whistle for the first time. You have three new teeth and don't seem at all bothered by them.

You are determined to feed yourself with your spoon and get

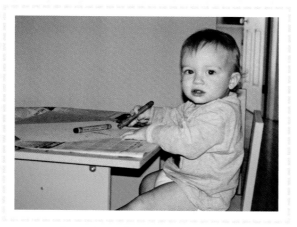

extremely frustrated and mad when we try to help you — you really want to be independent. When you are frustrated, you bang yourself on the head, which looks pretty painful. We feel so helpless watching you, as you will not accept help and we can see how desperate you are to achieve your goals. Dad says your determination will stand you in good stead when you are older. At times, you throw yourself flat on the floor and just cry — it's tough to watch.

It's amazing, but you are already helping us dress you. If you're holding a toy in one hand while we're putting on your top, you put the toy in the hand we aren't busy with and then swap it over. You are getting so much better at entertaining yourself — especially with books and anything with wheels on it. You have this cute habit of lying down and putting your little head on your favorite toys.

You are quite a little chatterbox, always engaging people, especially elderly folks, while we're waiting in the line-up at the grocery store. Perhaps they remind you of your grandparents?

February 9 (1 year old)
Happy birthday!

This year has passed so very quickly — it seems like just yesterday that you were born, though some of the days (and especially nights) seemed endless. It has been tiring, but exciting and wonderful. We count our blessings all the time. We are sitting in your bedroom, and you are listening to music and reading your books in between playing with your bears. When the music ends, you stand in front of your tape recorder, point your index finger, and say "Da!" which means "Put it on again without delay!" You enjoyed opening your birthday presents this morning, although you were far more interested in the paper and the boxes than the presents themselves. Your grandparents all phoned to wish you happy birthday; despite how talkative you usually are, you just said a few things and mostly listened quietly to the voices. You watched Dad make cupcakes for you last night, just as his mommy used to do for him, and we also got you a clown cake for later today.

A few days ago, you got your first pair of proper walking shoes (size 5), which make you look all grown up. You had fish (tuna lasagna) for the first time and seemed to enjoy it. You have gone to two birthday parties in the last week and, for the first time, you seemed interested in other little friends and enjoyed their company. You get around mostly by crawling or walking behind objects, and now you are walking on your knees, which must take a lot of effort. It seems much more difficult than walking on your feet would be, but we assume you know what you are doing. These days, if you want to attract someone's attention, you give them a smile — not just any smile, but a very funny, toothy grin. Your nose crinkles up, and your eyes and eyebrows frown. You especially like to try this while we're lining up at the supermarket, and it works every time. You love buses and call out "Sss" from the back of the car whenever we pass one. You always spot them before we do. You also love to wave and blow kisses.

Happy birthday, Sam, you precious little man.

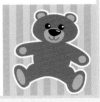

Baby Care Resources

A word about reliable resources…

The last decade has witnessed a dramatic transformation in the way people learn about things. The Internet and sophisticated search engines such as Google and Yahoo! have put vast amounts of information at the disposal of millions of people. Simply pick a topic, and hundreds, even thousands, of websites pertaining to a given subject become immediately available. We are now capable of informing just about everyone about pretty well everything.

There is one catch. People can get misinformation on the Internet just as easily. There is no requirement demanding that websites be screened for accuracy. Opinion can replace fact. What you read on any subject may or may not be either authoritative or true.

What, then, is a parent seeking advice to do when trying to filter all the available information? The solution is to seek answers from websites sponsored by well-respected professional organizations and official government agencies. The advice on these websites is carefully researched and written. Even so, trust your instincts: any advice you are given should make sense to you, regardless of the source.

We have provided here a short list of reliable and comprehensive North American resources. However, your child's health-care providers remain your best source of information.

Parenting Corner
American Academy of Pediatrics (AAP)
P.O. Box 927, Dept. C
Elk Grove Village, IL 60009-0927
Tel. 847-434-4000
www.aap.org/parents
Authoritative information in an American context, with links to other credible resources.

Caring for Kids
Canadian Paediatric Society (CPS)
2305 St. Laurent Boulevard
Ottawa, ON K1G 4J8
Tel. 613-526-9387
www.caringforkids.cps.ca
Authoritative information in a Canadian context, with links to other credible resources.

American College of Obstetricians and Gynecologists
P.O. Box 4500
Kearneysville, WV 25430
Toll-free tel. 800-762-2264
www.acog.com
Best source for information on pregnancy and childbirth in an American context.

Society of Obstetricians and Gynaecologists of Canada
780 Echo Drive
Ottawa, ON K1S 5R7
Tel. 613-730-4192
www.sogc.medical.org
Best source for information on pregnancy and childbirth in a Canadian context.

National Institute of Child Health and Human Development
Bldg. 31, Room 2A32, MSC 2425
31 Center Drive
Bethesda, MD 20892-2425
www.nichd.nih.gov
Official site of the U.S. government office on children's health.

Canadian Institute of Child Health
Suite 300, 384 Bank Street
Ottawa, ON K2P 1Y4
Tel. 613-230-8838
www.cich.ca
An advocate for children's health in a Canadian context.

About Kids Health
The Hospital for Sick Children
555 University Avenue
Toronto, ON M5G 1X8
www.aboutkidshealth.ca
Comprehensive source of practical guidelines for baby and child care.

Healthy Pregnancy
National Women's Health Information Center
U.S. Department of Health and Human Services
Suite 300, 8550 Arlington Boulevard
Fairfax, VA 22031
www.4women.org/pregnancy
Guide to resources for pregnant women in an American context.

Motherisk
The Hospital for Sick Children
555 University Avenue
Toronto, ON M5G 1X8
Tel. 416-813-6780 or 877-327-4636
www.motherisk.org
Evidence-based information regarding exposure to drugs and chemicals during pregnancy and while breast-feeding.

Child and Family Canada
www.cfc-efc.ca
A collective of more than 50 child health agencies.

La Leche League International
1400 North Meacham Road
Schaumburg, IL 60173-4840
Toll-free tel. 800-LA-LECHE
www.lalecheleague.org
Support for mothers who choose to breast-feed.

Acknowledgments

Many people have helped to create this book. Fortunately, too many cooks did not spoil the broth. The result of this team effort is our proud salute to parents and their babies across the world.

Special thanks and mention go to:

- Our contributing authors, Sherri Adams, Carolyn Beck, Catherine Birken, Sheila Jacobson, Michelle Shouldice, and Michael Weinstein: this book could not have been written without their outstanding contributions. Extra thanks to Sherri, Catherine, and Carolyn for taking time during their maternity leaves to write in "real time!"
- Bob Dees, Bob Hilderley, Marian Jarkovich, and the team at Robert Rose, whose enthusiasm, support, and talents have been much appreciated and far exceeded our expectations.
- Andrew Smith, Kevin Cockburn, and the team at PageWave Graphics, who have been very easy to work with and have done a superb job of presenting the information in a clear and easy-to-read format. And to Kveta for providing the illustrations.
- Heidi Falckh and her team from the Sick Kids Corporate Ventures office, for their support on the business side along the way; Denis Daneman, the pediatrician-in-chief, and Mary Jo Haddad, the CEO, at Sick Kids, for their visionary leadership and appreciation of the importance of disseminating the knowledge and experience that has accumulated inside this great institution; Tiziana Altobelli, for her administrative help and 110% effort every day; Lisa Lipkin and her team from Public Affairs, and Michael O'Mahoney and his team at the Sick Kids Foundation, who have been so helpful in promoting our books.
- Diogenes Baena and Robert Teteruck, the Sick Kids photographers, for their flexibility and creativity in doing the bulk of the photography for the book; Dr. Michael Sgro and Alex McDonald from St. Michael's Hospital, for the beautiful photographs from the newborn nursery; Tatiana Freire-Lizama, for the ultrasound pictures; and Beverley Daniels, for contributing some of the wonderful breast-feeding photographs.
- Daina Kalnins and Iola Panetta, for their review of earlier drafts of the feeding and breast-feeding sections; Shelly Weiss, for her help with the chapter on sleep; Howard Leibovich, for the piece on fathering; Dr. Trey Coffey, for her review of the manuscript.
- Our photographic models, who mainly included the members of our general pediatric team and their families — Sherri and Sam; Carolyn, Neil, and Simon; Catherine and Dahlia; Stacey and Katie; Eyal, Ali and Daphne; Emma and Bronwen — as well as Drs. Sheila Jacobson, Mike Peer, and Carolyn Taylor, and the patients from

Clairhurst Medical Clinic; Sharon and Ethan; Jennifer, Michael, and Elizabeth Gallop; Cara, Jamie and Michael Orsech; Kigeorgia and Jenae Morrison; Dr. Kirsten Smith and Elizabeth Beecroft; Natasha Flora, and Sydney and Bailey Flora-Kirsch; Rani and Noah Jamieson; Andrea Felsmann and Jack Felsmann Pires; Michelle Lee and Dr. Jonathan Maguire, who allowed us to take so many photographs to get the ones we needed to illustrate the point; and, of course, the many patients at Sick Kids who agreed to have their babies photographed for this book while they were in the hospital.

We are indebted to all of you for your efforts. Thanks for everything.

Dr. Jeremy Friedman
Dr. Norman Saunders

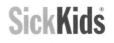

Photography Credits

All photos by Robert Teteruck and Diogenes Baena, © The Hospital for Sick Children, except: **5** © iStockphoto.com/Brian McEntire; **8** © Alex McDonald/St. Michael's Hospital; **12** © ImageShop/ Corbis; **15** © iStockphoto.com/Mark Thoburn; **17** © Stockbyte/Corbis; **21** © iStockphoto.com/ Eugeny Shevchenko; **27** © iStockphoto.com/Heiko Bennewitz; **35** © iStockphoto.com/Photo Inc.; **38** © Mike Gallop; **39** © Mike Gallop; **45** © iStockphoto.com/Foto Pfluegl; **47** © Masterfile; **48** © iStockphoto.com/Jan Michael Leung; **49** © image100/Corbis; **52–53** © Shelley and Jeremy Friedman; **54** © image100/Corbis; **57** © Thinkstock/Corbis; **58** © Alex McDonald/St. Michael's Hospital; **59** © iStockphoto.com/Crystal Kirk; **64** (left) © Alex McDonald/St. Michael's Hospital; **65** © Alex McDonald/St. Michael's Hospital; **67** © Alex McDonald/St. Michael's Hospital; **68** © Alex McDonald/St. Michael's Hospital; **70** © Beverley Daniels Photography; **81** © iStockphoto.com/ Felix Thiang; **83** © Alex McDonald/St. Michael's Hospital; **84** © Alex McDonald/St. Michael's Hospital; **85** © Alex McDonald/St. Michael's Hospital; **94** © Alex McDonald/St. Michael's Hospital; **95** © Shelley and Jeremy Friedman; **96** © Alex McDonald/St. Michael's Hospital; **97** (top left) © Alex McDonald/St. Michael's Hospital; **104** © iStockphoto.com/Nancy Catherine Walker; **109** © Alex McDonald/St. Michael's Hospital; **110** © Alex McDonald/St. Michael's Hospital; **111** © Alex McDonald/St. Michael's Hospital; **112** © Alex McDonald/St. Michael's Hospital; **117** © iStockphoto.com/Damir Cudic; **118–19** © Shelley and Jeremy Friedman; **123** © Beverley Daniels Photography; **126** © Beverley Daniels Photography; **127** © Beverley Daniels Photography; **157** © Beverley Daniels Photography; **199** © Alex McDonald/St. Michael's Hospital; **203** © iStockphoto.com/Paulus Rusyanto; **205** © iStockphoto.com/Trista Weibell; **207** © iStockphoto.com/ Galina Dreyzina; **208** © iStockphoto.com/Damir Cudic; **209** © iStockphoto.com/Dóri O'Connell; **210** © iStockphoto.com/Rosemarie Gearhart **220** © Alex McDonald/St. Michael's Hospital; **222** © iStockphoto.com/Kateryna Govorushchenko; **227** © iStockphoto.com/Heiko Bennewitz; **228–29** © Shelley and Jeremy Friedman; **251** © iStockphoto.com/Studio Zipper; **264** © Mike Gallop; **268** © iStockphoto.com/Dóri O'Connell; **274** © iStockphoto.com/Mr. Jamsey; **284–85** © Shelley and Jeremy Friedman; **301** © iStockphoto.com/Suzannah Skelton; **317** © iStockphoto.com/Brian McEntire; **318** © iStockphoto.com/Amanda Rohde; **323** © iStockphoto.com/Shawn Gearhart; **325** © iStockphoto.com/Zsolt Nyulaszi; **330** © iStockphoto.com/Photodora; **340–41** © Shelley and Jeremy Friedman; **346** © iStockphoto.com/Brian McEntire; **348** © iStockphoto.com/Kim Hall; **360–61** © Shelley and Jeremy Friedman; **366** © iStockphoto.com/Melissa King; **373** © iStockphoto.com/Jim Jurica; **387** © iStockphoto.com/Heiko Bennewitz; **388** © SW Productions/ Brand X/Corbis; **392** © iStockphoto.com/Fred Goldstein; **393** (left) © iStockphoto.com/Jaimie D. Travis; **413** © iStockphoto.com/Robert Brown; **434** © Shelley and Jeremy Friedman.

Every effort has been made to contact and obtain permission for the photographs in this book. If omissions and errors have occurred, we encourage you to contact the publisher.

Library and Archives Canada Cataloguing in Publication

Friedman, Jeremy
    The baby care book : a complete guide from birth to 12 months old / Jeremy Friedman, Norman Saunders.

Includes index.
ISBN 978-0-7788-0160-3

1. Pediatrics—Popular works. 2. Infants—Health and hygiene. 3. Infants—Care.
I. Saunders, Norman II. Title.

RJ61.F748 2007   618.92   C2007-900259-5

Friedman, Jeremy
    Canada's baby care book : a complete guide from birth to 12 months old / Jeremy Friedman, Norman Saunders.

Includes index.
ISBN 978-0-7788-0156-6

1. Pediatrics—Popular works. 2. Infants—Health and hygiene. 3. Infants—Care.
I. Saunders, Norman II. Title.

RJ61.F75 2007   618.92   C2006-905910-1

Index